Clinical Endocrinology and Diabetes

Clinical Endocrinology and Diabetes

EDITED BY

Michael C. Sheppard PhD FRCP

Professor, Department of Medicine,
University of Birmingham;
Honorary Consultant Physician, Queen Elizabeth Hospital,
Birmingham

Jayne A. Franklyn MD MRCP

Lecturer and Honorary Senior Registrar,
Department of Medicine,
University of Birmingham

With a foreword by

Sir Raymond Hoffenberg MD PhD
President of the Royal College of Physicians;
formerly William Withering Professor of Medicine,
University of Birmingham

CHURCHILL LIVINGSTONE
EDINBURGH LONDON MELBOURNE AND NEW YORK 1988

CHURCHILL LIVINGSTONE
Medical Division of Longman Group UK Limited

Distributed in the United States of America by Churchill
Livingstone Inc., 1560 Broadway, New York, N.Y. 10036, and
by associated companies, branches and representatives
throughout the world.

First published   1988

ISBN 0-443-03153-3

British Library Cataloguing in Publication Data

Sheppard, Michael C.
    Clinical endocrinology and diabetes.
    1. Endocrine glands — Diseases
    I. Title   II. Franklyn, Jayne A.
    616.4   RC648

Library of Congress Cataloging in Publication Data

Clinical endocrinology and diabetes / edited by Michael C. Sheppard,
    Jayne A. Franklyn; with a foreword by Sir Raymond Hoffenberg.
        p.   cm.
    Bibliography: p.
    Includes index.
    ISBN 0-443-03153-3
    1. Endocrinology.   2. Endocrine glands—Diseases.   3. Diabetes.
I. Sheppard, Michael C.   II. Franklyn, Jayne A.
RC648.C565 1988
616.4--dc19   87-33807
                                                              CIP

Printed and bound in Great Britain at The Bath Press, Avon

Foreword

During the thirteen years I spent as Professor of Medicine in Birmingham, I was fortunate enough to have in my department a series of bright and enthusiastic young lecturers who specialised in various branches of endocrinology and whose contributions form the major part of this volume. To them, and to the other authors who are in senior posts in Birmingham, I express my gratitude for their part in having made my stay so enjoyable. The regular endocrine meetings were always lively and challenging, and one was seldom able to get away with a loose or uncritical comment. Not surprisingly, they were all good teachers and this book gives tangible expression to their eagerness to impart their knowledge.

It is often argued that we already have enough books on enough topics. Why another? In this case, justification is to be found in the rapidly changing character of endocrinology. Not only has the basic science of endocrinology developed greatly over the past decade or so, but new clinical applications have emerged, as well as new clinical syndromes. A further justification exists in the kinship of the authors. In Birmingham the emphasis was always on clinical aspects of endocrinology, but understanding the scientific basis of the subject was regarded as essential. I believe this philosophy emerges from the book. I am delighted to see it in print.

Birmingham, 1988   Sir Raymond Hoffenberg

Preface

For a number of years the practice of clinical endocrinology and diabetes has thrived and expanded in Birmingham, with expertise being gained in many different aspects of both subjects. Colleagues with specialist experience in various branches of endocrinology and diabetes remain in Birmingham, or have moved on after a period of postgraduate training. It seemed logical therefore to bring together these colleagues, with their broad range of clinical skills and experience, to write a new textbook of endocrinology and diabetes, a textbook in which each chapter has been written by an author actively pursuing the specialist interest he describes.

It has been our aim to create a book which is up-to-date, easy to read and of practical use. It is a text which covers a broad range of topics, providing an insight into all aspects of the clinical practice of endocrinology and diabetes, and, we hope, is not to be used simply for reference purposes. We anticipate the book will be read by both under-graduate and postgraduate students, and may in general be of use to practising clinicians who do not have a specialist endocrine or diabetes interest.

We acknowledge gratefully the role of Sir Raymond Hoffenberg in providing the stimulus for the growth of endocrinology in Birmingham and we are indebted to him for his enthusiasm, guidance and support, and for bringing together the authors of this text. We also thank Professor David London for his lively and critical review of our clinical practice.

Birmingham, 1988

M. C. S.
J. A. F.

Contributors

P. H. Baylis MD FRCP
Senior Lecturer and Consultant Physician,
Department of Medicine, University of Newcastle
upon Tyne, UK

R. N. Clayton BSc MD FRCP
Head of Endocrine Research Group, Clinical
Research Centre, Harrow, Middlesex, UK

J. Dawson DM MRCP
Consultant Physician, Clatterbridge Hospital,
Wirral, UK

J. A. Franklyn MD MRCP
Lecturer and Honorary Senior Registrar,
Department of Medicine, University of
Birmingham, UK

S. Franks MD MRCP
Senior Lecturer in Reproductive Endocrinology,
St Mary's Medical School, London, UK

P. J. Hale DM MRCP
Senior Registrar, General Hospital, Birmingham,
UK

D. A. Heath MB FRCP
Reader in Medicine, University of Birmingham,
UK

P. M. Horrocks MD MRCP
Lecturer and Honorary Senior Registrar,
Department of Medicine, University of
Birmingham, UK

M. Nattrass PhD FRCP
Consultant Physician, General Hospital,
Birmingham, UK

P. H. W. Rayner BSc MB FRCP
Senior Lecturer in Paediatrics and Child Health and
Honorary Consultant Paediatrician, University of
Birmingham, UK

M. C. Sheppard PhD FRCP
Professor, Department of Medicine, University of
Birmingham, UK

A. D. Wright MB FRCP
Reader in Medicine, University of Birmingham,
UK

Contents

Hormone physiology and clinical presentation of endocrine disease

Endocrinology is the study of the actions of hormones and of the organs in which hormones are synthesised. A hormone is traditionally defined as a chemical messenger which is released into the circulation and which acts at a site distant from its site of production. The limit of the boundary of endocrinology has become blurred, however, by the recognition that such chemical messengers can be produced and released by endocrine and neural as well as other tissues, and may act as either circulating hormones, local regulators or neurotransmitters, or all of these. There is no sharp distinction between the endocrine and nervous systems and intimate links at the level of the hypothalamus serve to integrate the two systems which act together to maintain the function of the intact organism.

The majority of hormones are peptides or amino acid derivatives. These include the glycoprotein hormones, thyrotrophin and luteinising hormone, the small peptide, thyrotrophin releasing hormone, and the amino acid derivatives, thyroxine and dopamine. The remaining hormones are steroid molecules derived from the precursor cholesterol. These include gonadal and adrenal steroids, as well as vitamin D and its derivatives.

Hormone synthesis, processing and release

The major sites of hormone synthesis are the endocrine organs, although many peptide hormones are synthesised in the central nervous system and gastrointestinal tract. Transcription of the hormone gene is the first step in the synthetic pathway which is illustrated in Figure 1.1.

Messenger (m)RNA is processed within the cell nucleus and transported into the cytoplasm where translation of the mRNA occurs at the site of the ribosome. The first product of synthesis is often a large precursor molecule or prohormone which is progressively cleaved or processed to form the active molecule. An example of the importance of processing is pro-opiomelanocortin, which is efficiently converted to corticotrophin (ACTH) in the anterior pituitary gland. In the case of steroid hormones, the parent molecule cholesterol is modified by sequential cleavage and hydroxylation to form its varied products. After processing is complete, the hormone is packaged so that it is available for release into the circulation. In general there is a rapid turnover of synthesised hormone, stores being depleted within hours, or days if synthesis is inhibited. Exceptions to this rule are thyroglobulin which acts as a major reservoir for the hormones thyroxine and triiodothyronine, and vitamin D_3 or cholecalciferol which acts as a reservoir for the active hormone 1,25 dihydroxy vitamin D.

Hormone transport

Water soluble hormones are transported in the circulation in solution. Most hormones are insoluble in water and require specific transport proteins. Proteins such as albumin and prealbumin have a large number of low-affinity binding sites and act as transporters for a variety of hormones. Specific transport proteins are larger molecules with a smaller number of high-affinity binding sites. These include thyroxine-binding globulin, sex hormone-binding globulin and cortisol-binding

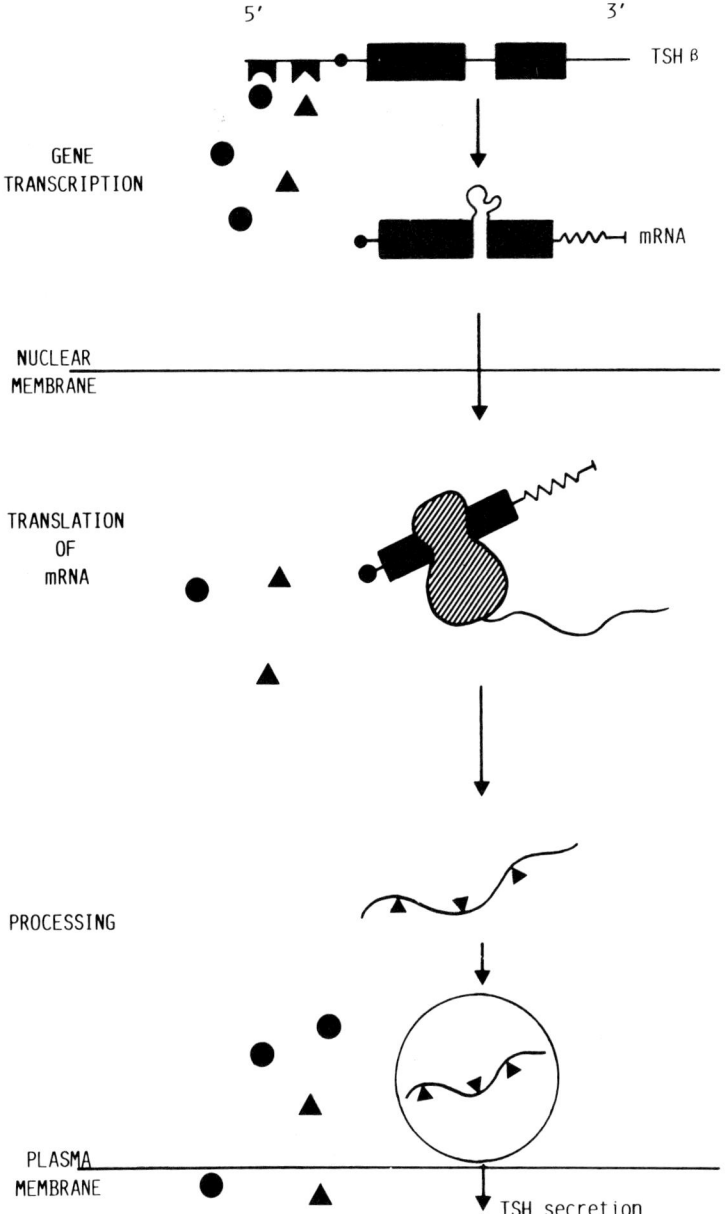

Fig. 1.1 Outline of thyrotrophin β subunit synthetic pathway.

globulin. In general, it is only the free or unbound hormone which enters the target cell and exerts its effect, so that protein bound hormone provides a large reservoir within the circulation. The small amount of free hormone in the plasma is in dynamic equilibrium with bound hormone. Increases or decreases in the amounts of specific transport protein have no effect on the function of the hormone but may cause diagnostic confusion by altering the total concentrations of hormone in the plasma.

Target organ effects

Hormones enter the target cell by a variety of processes. Many hormones are lipid soluble and

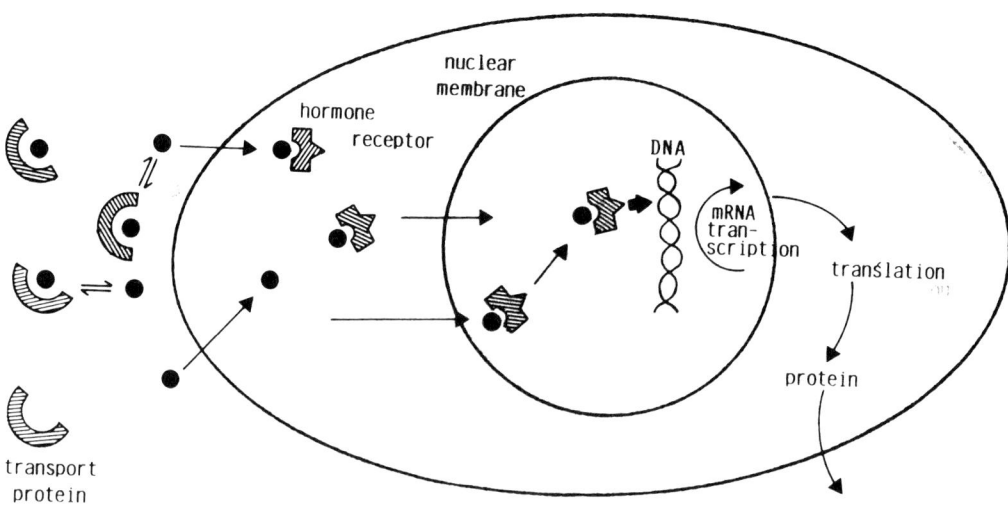

Fig. 1.2   Mechanism of action of steroid or thyroid hormones. 'Free' or unbound hormone enters the target cell and binds to specific receptors which may themselves bind to chromatin and hence modulate gene transcription.

enter by passive diffusion. Active uptake systems have also been described and in the case of peptide hormones that bind to cell surface receptors, the hormone-receptor complex may be internalised by endocytosis. This process of internalisation may be important in determining the rate of degradation of the hormone or the number of surface receptors available, but peptide hormone effects on the cell are mediated largely by activation of a complex system of intracellular second messengers including cyclic AMP and protein kinases. Steroid and thyroid hormones, on the other hand, have specific high-affinity intracellular binding sites — such sites or receptors being found in close association with nuclear chromatin (Fig. 1.2).

Another mechanism which targets the action of specific hormones is that of delivery into a defined circulation, such as the hypophyseal portal system or hepatic portal system. Because of dilution and rapid clearance, concentrations of hypothalamic and gastrointestinal hormones are much lower or even unmeasurable in the peripheral circulation. Local production of hormone from circulating precursors is another important mechanism which determines the site of hormone action, for example the production of dihydrotestosterone from testosterone in androgenic target tissues like the prostate.

The effects of hormones on the tissues are complex. A single hormone can exert different effects on a variety of tissues but a single tissue or metabolic process is often regulated by more than one hormone. Thyroid hormones, for example, exert diverse effects on the growth, development and function of most tissues of the body but the process of growth is regulated by complex interactions between thyroid, steroid and peptide hormones. The final common pathway through which hormones exert their cellular effects is not fully defined but interaction of hormone receptor complexes or intracellular messengers with specific regulatory sequences of DNA is known to promote or inhibit the transcription of genes and production of mRNA (Fig. 1.3).

Regulatory mechanisms

The most important regulatory mechanism is feedback control, a system in which the concentration of hormone determines the need for increased or

Transcription
rate

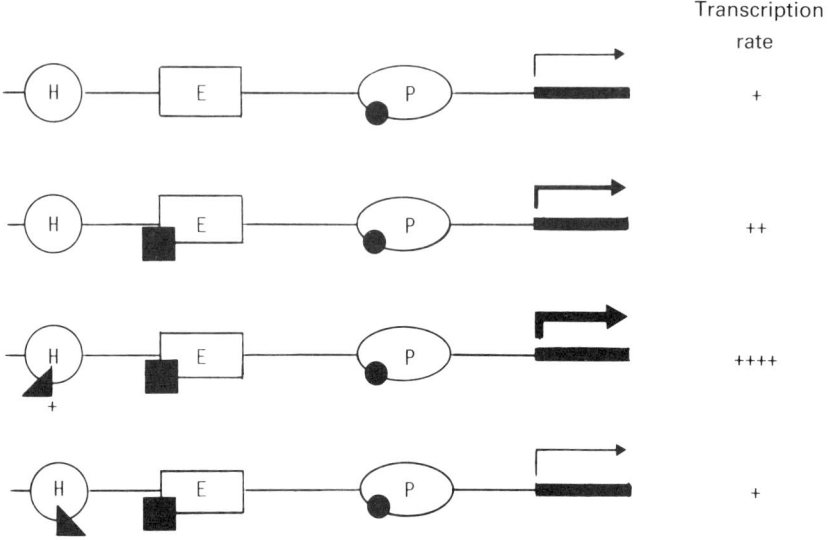

Fig. 1.3 Regulation of gene transcription. RNA polymerase links to the promoter (P) to initiate gene transcription. Binding of transacting factors to enhancer sequences (E) and hormone regulatory elements (H) further stimulates or inhibits the rate of transcription.

decreased synthesis and release. The best example of feedback regulation is the interaction of the anterior pituitary with the thyroid, adrenal and gonads.

Hormones produced from the target tissues feed back on the pituitary, and to a lesser extent the hypothalamus, and inhibit the production of the pituitary trophic hormones (Fig. 1.4).

Endocrine disorders can be divided into syndromes of hormone deficiency or excess.

HORMONE DEFICIENCY

Hormone deficiency may be due to diminished or absent secretion. The cause may be developmental as in thyroid or gonadal dysgenesis. Congenital enzyme deficiency may prevent hormone synthesis, such as 21-hydroxylase deficiency leading to congenital adrenal hyperplasia. More commonly, hormone deficiency results from damage or destruction of a normal endocrine gland. The destructive process may be one of infarction as in Sheehan's syndrome or pituitary necrosis, or may result from direct trauma due to surgery or radiotherapy. Infiltrative processes, such as

granulomatous infiltration of the pituitary in sarcoidosis or malignant infiltration of the adrenals, form another category. Infections such as tuberculosis also lead to destruction of endocrine tissues. A common category is that of autoimmune destruction which may involve a variety of organs including the thyroid, gonads, adrenals and rarely the pituitary.

The syndrome of hormone deficiency may result not only from a reduction in hormone production, but also from production of abnormal hormone or resistance to hormone action. For example, diabetes results rarely from a single gene mutation leading to production of an abnormal insulin molecule which binds ineffectively to the insulin receptor. In general, hormone resistance results from abnormality of the hormone receptor, from blocking of the hormone receptor by an abnormal ligand or reflects abnormality of postreceptor events. For example, pseudohypoparathyroidism results from an herditary abnormality of the guanosine triphosphate binding protein in cell membranes which normally activates adenylate cyclase after binding of parathyroid hormone to its

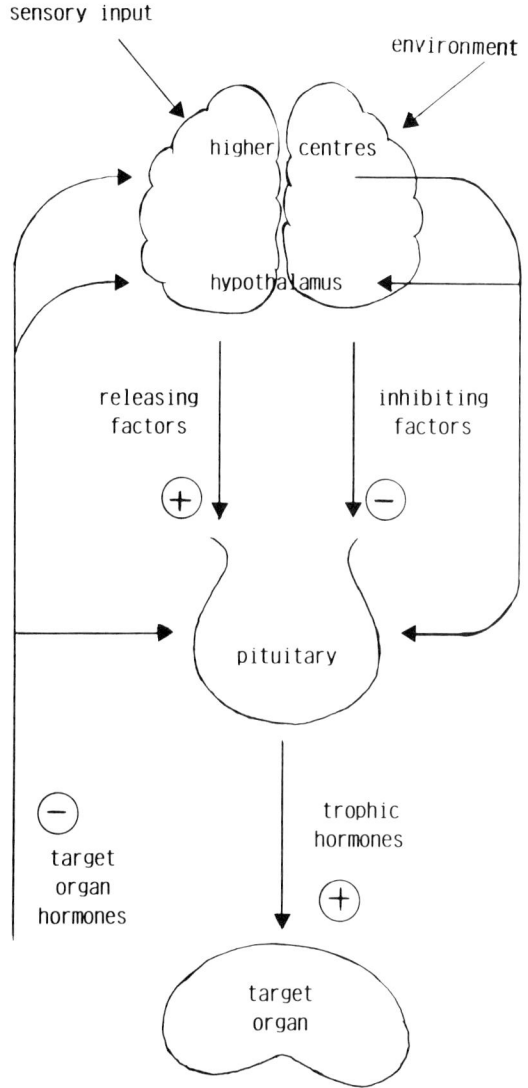

Fig. 1.4 Feedback regulation of the hypothalamic—pituitary—target organ axes.

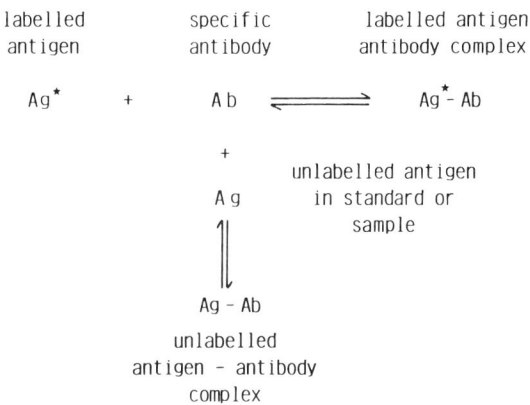

Fig. 1.5 The principle of radioimmunoassay.

cortex. Hyperplasia of endocrine cells may also lead to excess hormone production, for example in the parathyroids or adrenals, and may in turn result from excess secretion of the trophic hormone, such as adrenocorticotrophic hormone (ACTH) from the anterior pituitary. Tumours of non-endocrine tissues may assume an endocrine function and secrete hormones 'ectopically', such as production of ACTH and arginine vasopressin from bronchial carcinomas. Occasionally immunoglobulins function as hormones, for example thyroid-stimulating immunoglobulins which interact with the thyrotrophin receptor on the thyroid follicular cell, leading to stimulation of thyroid hormone synthesis and release.

Investigation of endocrine disorders

The principles of investigation of endocrine disorders are, firstly, definition of hormone deficiency or excess by measurement of circulating concentrations of specific hormones and, secondly, localisation of the abnormality. Measurement of circulating hormone concentrations in serum or plasma has been revolutionised by the progression from cumbersome and non-specific bioassays to the development of specific and sensitive radioimmunoassays. The basis of radioimmunoassay (Fig. 1.5) is the competitive inhibition of binding of radioactively-labelled hormone to antibody by unlabelled hormone contained in standards or in unknown samples. Circulating concentrations of

cell surface receptor. Hormone resistance may be hereditary, as in testicular feminisation syndrome, or acquired, as in the insulin resistance of obesity.

HORMONE EXCESS

Syndromes of hormone excess similarly have a variety of causes. Tumours, either benign or malignant, can affect endocrine glands, for example adenoma or carcinoma of the adrenal hormones may be measured in the basal state or, more usefully, in the dynamic situation where hormone suppression or stimulation is sought. The feedback control of hormone secretion is the basis for most dynamic tests of endocrine function and disturbances in this feedback relationship are often found in pathological states of hormone deficiency or excess.

Localisation of endocrine pathology may be aided by biochemical assessment of the condition, such as by measurement of plasma ACTH in the patient with Cushing's syndrome, or by seeking a 'step-up' in hormone concentration in samples taken from multiple sites. Usually, however, localisation and assessment of the extent of pathology requires radiological investigation with either plain X-ray or often by computerised tomography.

CLINICAL PRESENTATION OF ENDOCRINE DISORDERS

The modes of presentation of endocrine diseases are many and varied. Symptoms and signs may be non-specific, such as changes in weight, anorexia, lethargy, weakness, sweating, muscle aches and so on. Features of the history may point to an organic cause for the symptoms described. For example, loss of weight occurring over a short period may be the presenting symptom of diabetes mellitus or hyperthyroidism. Associated features such as thirst and polyuria, or palpitations and enlargement of the neck may lead to the diagnosis. Obesity on the other hand is a common problem and rarely has a specific endocrine cause. Hypothyroidism may lead to weight gain, but by the time it is pronounced, more characteristic features of myxoedema are present. Cushing's syndrome is another uncommon cause of obesity, but rarely presents without other more obvious features. The occurrence of 'funny turns' is another non-specific complaint, but one which may again result from endocrine disorders such as hypoglycaemia due to an insulinoma or from arrhythmias and hypertension due to a phaeochromocytoma.

In addition to some of the non-specific symptoms mentioned above, endocrine disease may present with symptoms and signs which more readily prompt investigation of the endocrine system. These include local symptoms and signs related to enlargement of endocrine organs, such as the development of a goitre or headache and visual disturbance due to enlargement of a pituitary tumour. Other symptoms and signs pointing to an endocrine diagnosis include abnormalities of stature (tall or short), abnormalities of puberty (precocious or delayed), hirsutism, gynaecomastia, polyuria and polydipsia. Nonetheless, although growth and puberty are primarily under endocrine control, disorders of other systems can result in abnormalities. Examples of this include chronic illnesses of childhood such as coeliac disease or renal failure, which result in growth retardation and delayed puberty.

The family history of a patient with suspected endocrine disease often proves very valuable. An autosomal recessive pattern of inheritance is seen with some single gene disorders such as in some cases of growth hormone deficiency or congenital adrenal hyperplasia. Rarely, sex-linked inheritance is seen such as in vitamin D-resistant rickets, or autosomal dominant inheritance as in multiple endocrine adenomatosis syndromes. More commonly a positive family history for endocrine diseases emerges, with no clear pattern of inheritance. This is often the case for diseases which are autoimmune in origin, for example first-degree relatives may have a positive history for a spectrum of related disorders including myxoedema, Graves' disease, Addison's disease and diabetes mellitus. The family history may also point to the absence of significant endocrine disease such as in cases of tall or short stature or delayed puberty where the height or age of puberty of parents show that constitutional factors, and not specific pathological processes, are responsible.

The past medical history is often of importance too in establishing an endocrine diagnosis. Previous infertility, surgery or radiotherapy, for example to the central nervous system in childhood leukaemia, may all suggest a later diagnosis of endocrine dysfunction.

It must be remembered that with few exceptions endocrine disorders present with a wide spectrum of symptoms and signs and delay in diagnosis may result from failure to suspect the underlying cause. Diagnosis is, however, usually worthwhile since most of the conditions to be described are readily amenable to treatment.

Hypothalamus and anterior pituitary

In order to understand clinical disorders of the anterior pituitary gland it is essential to appreciate the normal regulatory mechanisms for anterior pituitary hormone secretion. This chapter therefore begins with a brief review of the physiology of the hypothalamic-pituitary-target organ axes.

HYPOTHALAMIC CONTROL OF ANTERIOR PITUITARY HORMONE RELEASE

The idea of hypothalamic regulation of anterior pituitary hormone secretion arose following the demonstration of a vascular connection between the base of the brain and the adenohypophysis, the hypothalamo-hypophyseal portal system. The hypothalamus is a highly specialised area of the brain containing groups of neuroendocrine cells which synthesise small peptide molecules (releasing and inhibiting hormones) which are released into the hypothalamo-hypophyseal portal venous system thereby reaching their target cells in the anterior pituitary. The hypothalamus receives neural inputs, largely from catecholaminergic and serotoninergic neurones, from many brain areas which act as signals for the release (and synthesis) of releasing and inhibiting hormones. Accordingly, the hypothalamus is a final integrator, for both neural and hormonal feedback messages and provides the essential basic regulation (through releasing and inhibiting hormones) of the adenohypophysis. A schematic representation of the neural control of anterior pituitary hormone secretion is shown in Figure 2.1.

In recent years, major releasing and inhibiting hormones for all the anterior pituitary hormones have been isolated from the hypothalamus, their structure determined, and the peptides chemically synthesised in pure form suitable for clinical use. The structure and actions of the releasing and inhibiting hormones are depicted in Table 2.1.

Table 2.1 Structure and function of hypothalamic releasing hormones

Hypothalamic hormone	Peptide length (no. of amino acids)	Releases/Inhibits
TRH (thyrotrophin releasing hormone	3	TSH (thyrotrophin) PRL (prolactin)
GnRH(gonadotrophin releasing hormone)	10	LH (luteinising hormone FSH (follicle stimulating hormone)
CRF (corticotrophin releasing factor)	41	ACTH (adreno-corticotrophic hormone + related peptides
GRF (growth hormone releasing factor)	40–44	GH (growth hormone)
GRIH (somatostatin) (growth hormone release inhibiting hormone)	41	GH TSH
PIF (dopamine) (prolactin inhibiting factor)	—	PRL

These structures have been highly conserved during evolution, with only very minor changes between fishes, birds, reptiles and mammals. It should be noted that releasing hormones not only stimulate anterior pituitary hormone

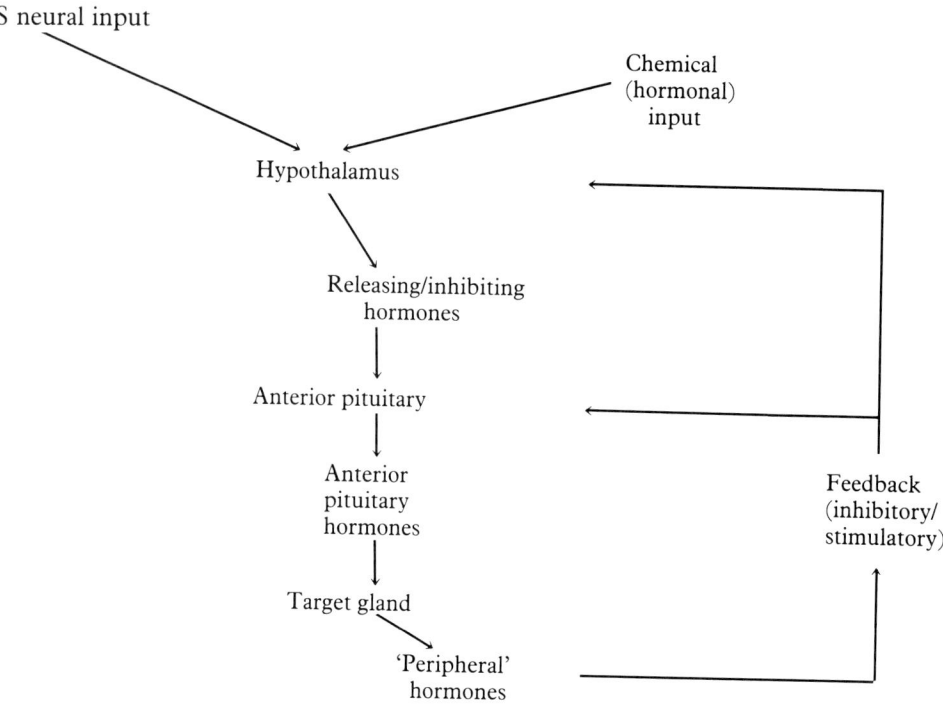

Fig. 2.1 Schematic representation of anterior pituitary hormone regulation.

release, but also their synthesis, and as such are trophic hormones. All the anterior pituitary hormones are under stimulatory control by releasing peptides with the exception of prolactin (PRL) which is under tonic inhibition by dopamine. Although exogenous thyrotrophin-releasing hormone (TRH) will release PRL, the role of TRH as a physiological prolactin-releasing factor has not been established.

Somatostatin, named because of its ability to specifically suppress growth hormone (GH) secretion, was first isolated from the hypothalamus but has subsequently been found in a variety of extrahypothalamic tissues (see Ch. 8). In addition to its suppressive effect on GH secretion, somatostatin inhibits the release of a number of other hormones, including insulin and glucagon from the pancreas. The demonstration of somatostatin in axon terminals within the central nervous system suggests a neurotransmitter function. Many other small peptide hormones, originally isolated from the gastrointestinal tract have been found in the hypothalamus and extrahypothalamic brain tissue, e.g. cholecystokinin, vasoactive intestinal polypeptide (VIP), gastric inhibitory polypeptide.

This has led to the concept of peptidergic, in addition to classical cholinergic and catecholaminergic, neurotransmission. VIP is also a potent stimulator of GH and PRL release, though its physiological role in this regard is not known.

In general, endogenous hypothalamic releasing hormones are not detectable in the peripheral circulation because of their very low concentration and rapid degradation. Thus, there is no readily available direct test of hypothalamic function. When measured at very frequent intervals (10 min or less), however, the serum levels of many anterior pituitary hormones (LH, FSH, GH, ACTH and PRL) show distinct peaks (pulses) and troughs. This has been best described for the gonadotrophins (LH and FSH) where periodicity or frequency of pulses is approximately 1 per 2 h. Since each LH pulse presumably occurs in response to a preceding pulse of gonadotrophin releasing hormone (GnRH), hypothalamic activity can be inferred indirectly from measurement of the peripheral gonadotrophin hormone levels, therefore GnRH is released from the hypothalamus in a pulsatile manner. The hypothalamus acts as a pulse generator, with an intrinsic frequency which can be modulated by neural input. This same principle may also hold for corticotrophin-releasing factor (CRF), growth hormone releasing factor (GRF) and dopamine. The pulsatile nature of releasing hormone secretion has important therapeutic implications (see below).

Clinical application of hypothalamic hormones

Synthetic hypothalamic releasing hormones are used in the biochemical assessment of anterior pituitary hormone secretion (see below).

Gonadotrophin releasing hormone, in addition to its role in the assessment of gonadotroph function, may be used clinically for induction of ovulation, and sometimes spermatogenesis, in hypogonadotrophic hypogonadism (see Ch. 6). In contrast to its use in the treatment of infertility, long-acting agonist analogues of GnRH may be used to induce a medical gonadectomy. This therapeutic approach depends upon the phenomenon of 'desensitisation' of LH secretion, which occurs when large doses of GnRH or its synthetic analogues are administered. This form of treatment has the advantage that it is fully reversible when stopped.

GnRH is the first hypothalamic hormone for which a therapeutic role has been defined (Table 2.2). It is likely that a similar therapeutic role for GRF may emerge in the treatment of children with isolated GH deficiency (see below). The role of the hypothalamic hormone somatostatin is also being explored. Its greatest clinical impact has been in the control of gastrointestinal bleeding. Theoretically somatostatin is ideal to use in this situation because of its effects of reducing gastric acid secretion, splanchnic blood flow and portal vein pressure, but the results of clinical trials of its efficacy in the management of haematemesis and variceal bleeding have been conflicting. Other reported benefits of somatostatin include inhibition of symptoms of the dumping syndrome, and inhibition of abnormal hormone secretion in patients with acromegaly, insulinoma, glucagonoma, VIPoma and carcinoid syndrome.

Feedback regulation of pituitary hormone secretion by peripheral hormones

The preceding section described the primary regulation of anterior pituitary hormone secretion by hypothalamic hormones (Fig. 2.1). This section deals briefly with some aspects of end-organ hormone modulation of pituitary responsiveness to releasing hormones. In general, end organ hormones exert inhibitory feedback on secretion and synthesis of anterior pituitary hormones, feedback operating largely at the pituitary level. Though there is probably also an inhibitory effect on secretion of hypothalamic-releasing hormones, this is minor. The one important exception to the general principle of negative feedback occurs in the hypothalamic-pituitary-ovarian axis. While this is described in detail in Chapter 6, it is worth emphasising that rising serum oestradiol concentrations exert stimulatory feedback effects on gonadotrophin secretion at the mid-point of the menstrual cycle, and are responsible for the preovulatory LH surge essential for normal female reproductive function. Thus, oestradiol is both inhibitory and stimulatory to pituitary gonadotrophin release, a unique feature of this hormone in females, with no male counterpart.

HYPOPITUITARISM

Hypopituitarism may be classified as partial when the deficiency is limited to one or two of the anterior pituitary hormones or complete, when

Table 2.2 Therapeutic uses of gonadotrophin releasing hormone and agonist analogues

Stimulation of fertility	Inhibition of gonadal function
Pulsatile low-doses of GnRH 1. females with hypothalamic amenorrhoea and hypogonadotrophic hypogonadism 2. males with isolated gonadotrophin deficiency	1. Hormone dependent cancer — prostate/breast 2. True precocious puberty 3. Endometriosis 4. ? Contraceptive for males 5. ? Premenstrual tension

all anterior pituitary hormone secretion is absent. Thus, the clinical picture will depend upon which hormone is absent or deficient. Additionally, the age of onset of hormone deficiency will determine the clinical presentation. Thus, GH deficiency is of little consequence in adults, but a major cause of delayed growth when occurring during infancy and childhood. In general the hypothalamo-pituitary axis is more susceptible to damage in infancy and childhood and the consequences are correspondingly more severe. This has become particularly apparent with the widespread use of combination chemotherapy and craniospinal irradiation for treatment of childhood leukaemia, lymphomas and intracranial tumours.

Causes of hypopituitarism

These may be classified as primary when the cause is within the pituitary, or secondary when hypothalamic releasing hormone secretion is impaired. Occasionally, secondary partial hypopituitarism may be reversible. This applies specifically to the reduction in gonadotrophin secretion (secondary to decreased GnRH output) accompanying severe loss of weight (with or without anorexia nervosa). Upon gaining weight gonadotrophin secretion is restored. Some of the less common causes of primary hypopituitarism, e.g. granulomatous conditions, may also involve the hypothalamus and vice versa. The causes of hypopituitarism are listed in Table 2.3 with the commonest listed first. With progressively enlarging pituitary tumours, normal pituitary tissue is gradually destroyed. This may give sequential hormone deficiencies of gonadotrophins, GH, TSH and ACTH. This sequence of hormone loss is not invariably followed. When the pituitary stalk is involved, the interruption of dopamine supply to the anterior pituitary results in modest hyperprolactinaemia (see section on prolactinoma). Hypoprolactinaemia has no clinical sequelae in the non-pregnant individual, its only consequence being failure to lactate postpartum.

Clinical features of hypopituitarism

These are discussed with respect to each pituitary hormone deficiency; complete hypopituitarism will

Table 2.3 Causes of hypopituitarism

Primary	Secondary

Post-treatment of pituitary tumours
  Hypophysectomy
  Radiotherapy
	Tumours
	  Craniopharygiomas
	  meningiomas/gliomas
	  Pinealomas
	  Metastases

Pituitary tumours
  Non-functional adenomas (non-hormone secreting)
  Functional adenomas (hormone secreting)
  Metastatic deposits (v. rare)
	Irradiation/chemotherapy
	  Craniospinal
	  Combination chemotherapy

Pituitary infarction
  With pituitary tumours
   (either functional or non-functional)
  Post-partum necrosis
  (Sheehan's syndrome)
	Developmental
	Hypothalamic GRF deficiency
	Hypothalamic GnRH deficiency
	  (Kallman's syndrome when anosmia and
	  colour blindness)
	With cerebellar ataxia and retinitis pigmentosa
	Congenital rubella

Chemotherapy	Trauma Head injury with pituitary stalk transection

Granulomas
  sarcoidosis
  Tuberculosis
  Syphilis
  Histiocytosis
	Granulomas
	As primary

Autoimmune	

Table 2.4 Clinical features of gonadotrophin deficiency

Prepuberty	Postpuberty
Tall	Fine wrinkled skin
Span>height	Loss of 2° sex hair
Obesity	Reduced libido
Prepubertal genitalia	Impotence
Small soft testes (< 3ml volume)	Testicular atrophy and oligo/azoospermia
Absent facial, pubic and axillary hair	Dyspareunia/vaginal dryness
Primary amenorrhoea	2° amenorrhoea and infertility

present with the appropriate combination of symptoms and signs.

Gonadotrophin deficiency

The clinical features are dependent upon the age of onset of deficiency and range from delayed puberty → arrested puberty → secondary hypogonadism, if occurring before, during and after puberty respectively. The clinical features are summarised in Table 2.4. In gonadotrophin deficient patients the rate of linear growth is normal before puberty but the failure of pubertal epiphyseal closure, consequent upon lack of oestrogen and testosterone secretion from the gonads, results ultimately in eunuchoid skeletal proportions (Fig. 2.2). Such individuals must be tested for sense of smell and questioned about colour blindness (Kallman's syndrome).

Growth hormone deficiency

This often occurs in association with gonadotrophin deficiency. In childhood and adolescence GH deficiency typically causes retarded skeletal growth (see section on short stature); in adults it is of little consequence, rarely causing fasting hypoglycaemia due to increased insulin sensitivity.

Thyrotrophin deficiency

This causes the usual symptoms of hypothyroidism (see Ch. 4) in the absence of a goitre. Symptoms of TSH deficiency appear 4–8 weeks after complete hypophysectomy. If TSH deficiency is present in childhood, growth and epiphyseal closure are delayed. Tests of growth hormone secretion may be impaired but return to normal with thyroid hormone replacement (see section on tests of pituitary function). Thus, GH deficiency cannot be diagnosed in a hypothyroid patient until reassessed in the euthyroid state.

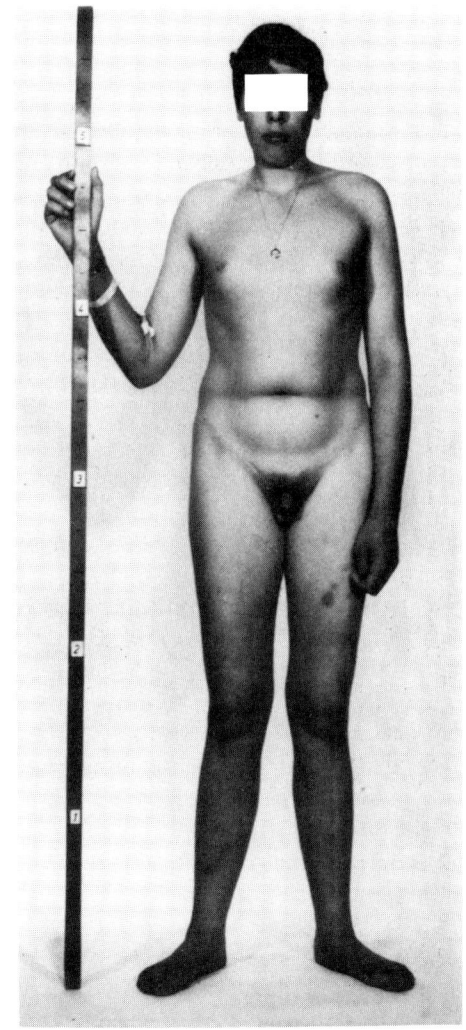

Fig. 2.2 Eunuchoid features in a patient with Kallman's syndrome.

Adrenocorticotrophic hormone deficiency

This is often partial and by itself causes few symptoms, usually being found in combination with other trophic hormone deficiencies after hypophysectomy or pituitary irradiation. Complete ACTH deficiency is associated with symptoms of cortisol lack i.e. weight loss, weakness, vomiting and abdominal pain (see Ch. 5). Since adrenal mineralocorticoid secretion is largely under control of the renin-angiotensin system, electrolyte disturbances are rare in pituitary hypoadrenalism. ACTH deficiency is associated with pale skin and impaired ability to tan on exposure to sunlight. Although insulin sensitivity is increased, spontaneous hypoglycaemia is rare. Cortisol deficiency results in increased renal tubular water reabsorption and decreases urinary output in patients with cranial diabetes insipidus. Occasionally, diabetes insipidus may be 'unmasked' by hydrocortisone replacement therapy.

Investigation of hypopituitarism

The aims of investigation of hypopituitarism are firstly to establish the extent and degree of anterior pituitary hormone insufficiency, and secondly to identify the pathology responsible. The first of these aims centres exclusively on dynamic hormonal tests and is a biochemical definition. Identification of the cause of documented hypopituitarism usually requires additional radiology (discussed in section on pituitary tumours) and visual field charting.

Simple screening tests should be performed first in patients with symptoms or signs suggestive of pituitary hormone deficiency. Measurements of pituitary hormones in random serum samples are uninterpretable unless target gland hormones are measured simultaneously. Impaired pituitary function is suspected when the target gland hormone level is low and the pituitary trophic hormone level is also low, i.e. failure of the normal negative feedback response, e.g. serum free T4 — low, TSH — low; serum testosterone — low, LH and FSH — low.

A low random serum cortisol or GH level is unhelpful in making the diagnosis of ACTH or GH deficiency; ACTH and GH secretion can be examined only with provocative testing. The most important provocative test is the combined pituitary stimulation test, which includes insulin hypoglycaemia for assessment of ACTH/ cortisol and GH reserve, and administration of TRH for TSH, and GnRH for gonadotrophin reserves. The details of this and the interpretation of results are given in Tables 2.5 and 2.6 Insulin hypoglycaemia is hazardous in patients with a history of ischaemic heart disease and should be avoided. The 'stress' of hypoglycaemia tests the integrity of the hypothalamus as well as the pituitary. The recent introduction of synthetic CRF and GRF allows selective testing of pituitary ACTH and GH reserves, respectively. These tests do not depend upon a stress reaction and are therefore safer than insulin hypoglycaemia; they do not, however, test the integrity of the hypothalamus. Parts of the combined pituitary stimulation test described in Table 2.5 can be performed in isolation, e.g. TRH test, GnRH test, insulin hypoglycaemia alone. Radiological investigation is considered in the section on pituitary tumours. Formal assessment of visual fields should be performed when X-rays are abnormal. General investigations aimed at elucidating the cause of hypopituitarism should include full blood count and ESR, biochemical profile, and chest X-ray. Specific additional tests are performed in the light of radiological and hormonal results.

Treatment of hypopituitarism

The primary treatment depends upon the cause of pituitary failure. When hypopituitarism is due to a pituitary tumour or previous hypophysectomy or radiotherapy, hormone deficiency is rarely reversible and long-term hormone replacement is indicated. A standard regimen for hormone replacement is shown in Table 2.7.

Short stature

After birth the velocity of linear growth declines rapidly for the first 2 years; it then decelerates more slowly until puberty when an adolescent growth spurt, secondary to adrenal and gonadal steroid production, is seen. In developed countries, the adolescent growth spurt peaks at age 12 in girls (range 9.5–14.5 years) and precedes the menarche. In boys, peak growth velocity is later, average age 14 (range 10.5–16 years).

Table 2.5 Details of combined pituitaru stimulation test

Patient preparation

fast patient from midnight, weigh patient and record weight

Insert intravenous cannula at 8:00 (30–60 min before commencing test)

Draw up 20 ml of 50% dextrose ⎫ by bedside for immediate i.v.
Hydrocortisone 100 mg   ⎭ administration

Clotted blood sample (40 ml time 0, 20 ml all other times) except for glucose in fluoride bottle

Test procedure and samples to be analysed

Time (min)	Glucose	GH	Cortisol	TSH	LH	FSH	PRL	Testosterone or E^2	T_4/fT_4
0	\	\	\	\	\	\	\	\	\
30	\	\	\	\.	\	\			
60	\	\	\	\	\	\			
90	\	\	\						
120	\	\	\						

After time 0 blood sample inject i.v.: TRH (200 μg), GnRH (100 μg)
Insulin (normal dose 0.15 u/kg; obesity, acromegaly, Cushing's 0.3 u/kg; suspected hypopituitarism 0.1 u/kg)

Notes

1. Symptoms of hypoglycaemia (sweating, drowsiness, pallor) — record time in notes
2. Blood glucose *must* fall below 2.2 mmol/l. Send samples to lab. at +30 and +60 min for urgent glucose
   If 60 min result >2.2 mmol/l repeat i.v. insulin and start again for glucose, cortisol and GH
3. If patient markedly drowsy, take blood for urgent glucose (noting time), give either i.v. dextrose or glucose drink *without* waiting for result, and *continue* sampling. Administration of glucose (after clinical hypoglycaemia) *does not* invalidate test since stimulus has already been achieved
4. To check cortisol (ACTH response) in patient on dexamthasone or prednisolone change to equivalent dose of hydrocortisone 10 days before test and stop hydrocortisone 48 h before test.
5. To check TSH response to TRH patient must have been off thyroxine replacement for 6 weeks
6. For adequate assessment of GH response patient must be euthyroid and eugonadal (normal testosterone or oestradiol)

Table 2.6 Interpretation of results of combined pituitary stimulation test

Pituitary function normal if:
1. Cortisol response — at least one value >550 nmol/l (<400 nmol/l — probably abnormal)
2. ★Growth hormone response — at least one value >15mu/l
3. TSH response — consult laboratory
4. LH response — females: varies with stage of mentrual cycle
   peak 2–4 × basal value
   — males: peak 2–4 × basal value
5. basal prolactin should be <500 mu/l

★ Patient must be euthyroid and have normal testosterone or oestradiol. If hypogonadal the test should be repeated for GH measurements after 3 days treatment with testosterone (testosterone undecanoate 80 mg b.d.) or oestrogen (50 μg/day).

Table 2.7 Hormone replacement therapy in hypopituitarism

TSH deficiency	— L-thyroxine 100–200 μg/day
ACTH deficiency	— hydrocortisone 20 mg mane, 10 mg nocte
GH deficiency	— only consider treatment prior to fusion of epiphyses (see section on short stature)
Gonadotrophin deficiency	—
males:	testosterone enanthate 250 mg i.m. every 2–3 weeks or testosterone undecanoate 80 mg b.d. orally
females:	cyclical oestrogen (PILL)

Simulation of ovulation and spermatogenesis with human FSH and human chorionic gonadotrophin or pulsatile GnRH is considered in Chapter 6.

In the assessment of stature, the height of an individual should be compared with that of a population of children on a centile chart, the 50th centile representing the average height for children of a given age. Since height is governed by many genetic and environmental factors, a child's centile position should be related to the mean centile position of the parents. A single abnormal height measurement does not necessarily demand investigation; management is directed instead by

Table 2.8 Causes of short stature

Primary	Secondary

Skeletal dysplasia:
  Achondroplasia
  Hypochindroplasia
  Dyschondrosteosis
  Multiple epiphyseal dysplasia
  Fibrous dysplasia
	Intrauterine growth retardation:
	  Infections
	  Maternal illness
	  Placental insufficiency

	Malnutrition

Chromosomal abnormalities:
  Down's syndrome
  Turner's syndrome
	Gastrointestinal disease:
	  Coeliac disease
	  Cystic fibrosis
	  Inflammatory bowel disease

Inborn errors of metabolism:
  Mucopolysachharidoses
  Glycogen storage diseases
	Renal disease:
	  Chronic parenchymal disease
	  Renal tubular acidosis

Genetic short stature, e.g. Pygmies	Cardiorespiratory disease:
	  Congenital heart disease
	  Asthma

	Endocrine disease — se Table 2.9 Psychosocial deprivation Constitutional (idiopathic) growth delay

documentation of growth velocity, i.e. rate of growth over a period of 6–12 months. A useful classification of the aetiology of short stature depends upon whether the defect is intrinsic to the skeletal system (primary) or secondary to factors outside the skeletal system. In primary defects the potential for bone growth is severely impaired and skeletal age is not retarded; when short stature is secondary to factors outside the skeletal system, a potential for catch-up growth exists and bone age is retarded. Common causes of primary and secondary growth deficiency are listed in Table 2.8. The endocrine causes of short stature are shown in Table 2.9. The clinical problem of short stature can be subdivided into two categories based upon age at presentation: 1. infants and children prior to their adolescent growth spurt often presenting to the paediatrician, 2. delayed adolescent growth spurt (normally with delayed puberty) presenting to the endocrinologist.

Table 2.9 Endocrine causes of short stature

Hypopituitarism
Isolated growth hormone/growth hormone releasing factor
  deficiency
  Laron dwarfism — failure of peripheral tissue response to GH
Hypogonadism and delayed puberty
Cushing's syndrome
Pseudohypoparathyroidism
Androgen/oestrogen excess (precocious puberty)

The subject of delayed puberty is considered in detail in Chapter 6.

A practical approach to the diagnosis is outlined in Figure 2.3.

Investigation of short stature

After initial clinical examination, general and other more specific investigations may be warranted (Table 2.10). Radiology should include bone age

Table 2.10 Laboratory investigation of short stature

General
Biochemical profile

Full blood count, red cell folate,
serume iron binding capacity

Radiological: bone age (hands)
              knees for growth potential

Specific

According to suspected cause

Endocrine

Thyroid function tests

Basal gonadal steroids and gonadotrophins

Combined pituitary stimulation test primarily
for growth hormone response

X-ray pituitary fossa (looking for suprasellar calcification)

? Proceed to CT scan

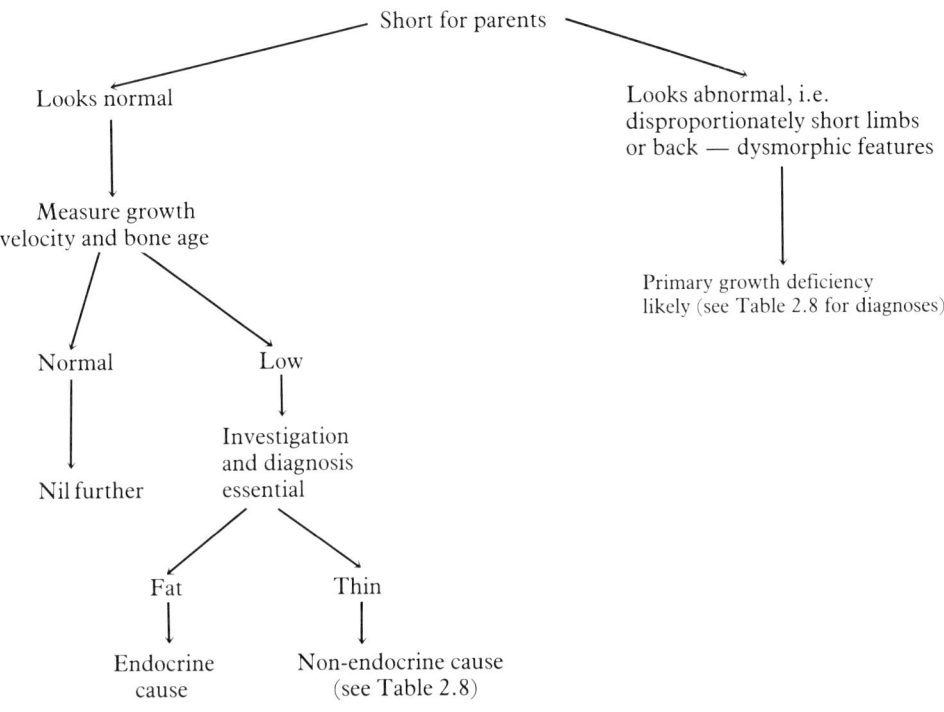

Fig. 2.3 Scheme for diagnosis of small stature.

(consult Greulich and Pyle *Atlas*), which is generally retarded from chronological age by more than 3 years in secondary causes of short stature. X-ray of the knees indicates the state of epiphyseal fusion and the potential for catch-up growth.

It has recently been realised that children with partial villous atrophy, without any haematological or biochemical evidence of malabsorption, may present with delayed growth; growth velocity resumes after removal of gluten from the diet. If endocrine and other causes have been excluded a jejunal biopsy is a safe and simple procedure which may provide the diagnosis.

Growth hormone deficiency

A random GH sample is unhelpful since resting GH may be undetectable in normal subjects. Exercise may be used as a simple provocative screening test. A value of >15 mu/l after 20 min of vigorous exercise excludes GH deficiency. If a screening test gives GH values <10 mu/l then a definitive test

should be performed. The insulin hypoglycaemia test is useful in that cortisol (ACTH) reserve may be evaluated in addition to GH reserve. This test is usually performed as part of a combined pituitary stimulation test (Table 2.5). If serum GH is <5 mu/l after adequate hypoglycaemia (<2.2 mmol/l), a single test is sufficient to diagnose GH deficiency. Where values between 5 and 10 mu/l are recorded, a second provocative test, such as arginine infusion, is required to confirm hormone deficiency. It is essential that the patient is tested when euthyroid and in cases where the result is low or borderline (peak GH 10–15 mu/l) the test should be repeated after oestrogen or testosterone administration for 3 days.

Treatment of GH deficiency This should be confined to regional referral centres and treatment undertaken only if criteria for GH deficiency are strictly fulfilled. Only human GH is effective, that from other species being useless (in contrast to insulin). Human GH extracted from cadaver pituitaries has been administered until recent years, but has now been withdrawn following the development of Jakob-Creutzfeldt disease in several young adults treated with cadaver-extracted GH. Synthetic human GH produced by recombinant DNA technology is now widely used. Successful treatment is accompanied by increased growth velocity and advancing skeletal maturation. Failure may occur if the patient develops hypothyroidism or hypoadrenalism during treatment and this should be monitored. Ultimate height attained should be close to that predicted from the mean parental height.

It is now clear that GH deficiency on provocative testing rarely reflects inability to synthesise the hormone, but more often reflects abnormality of hypothalamic secretion of GRF. Administration of GRF in GH deficient subjects has been shown to increase growth velocity and is another treatment option.

Constitutional growth delay

This is seen in infancy, childhood and in adolescence, the latter usually associated with delayed puberty. In the syndrome of constitutional growth delay, which is of unknown aetiology, growth velocity during infancy and childhood declines rapidly and height measurements fall below the 5th centile. Bone age is delayed compared to chronological age, but by not more than 2–3 years. Subsequently, growth rate increases and the final height achieved is normal or low-normal, though growth continues into the late teens in females and early twenties in males. The onset of puberty, which seems to be linked to bone age, is also delayed, but eventual fertility is unaffected.

A family history of growth delay or delay in pubertal development in parents is often obtained. Psychological stress is a common accompaniment, especially in adolescence. Management should be by reassurance which is best achieved by demonstration of a return of growth velocity to normal.

Tall stature

The causes of tall stature are shown in Table 2.11, the most common being constitutional tallness and early puberty.

Constitutional or genetically determined tallness produces most anxiety in girls. Physical

Table 2.11 Causes of tall stature

Constitutional/genetic
Premature prepubertal growth spurt
Klinefelter's syndrome
Marfan's syndrome
Homocystinuria
Growth hormone excess (gigantism)
Hyperthyroidism
Cerebral gigantism (Soto's syndrome)

examination is normal and no tests are required. Attempts to limit ultimate height with oestrogen therapy to induce epiphyseal fusion are generally unsuccessful, since most individuals present with a bone age of 12–13 years, when little potential for further growth remains. The disadvantages of oestrogens (in big doses) thus outweigh potential benefits and should be used only in exceptional circumstances. Early puberty may be evident on physical examination and does not prejudice final height although true precocious puberty causes short stature if untreated). Marfan's syndrome is characterised by tall stature, arachnodactyly and a variety of other skeletal abnormalities. Similar features are seen in homocystinuria, normally in association with mental retardation. Cerebral gigantism is characterised by prominent forehead, high-arched palate, hyperteleorism, pointed chin and mental retardation. Pituitary gigantism is caused by a GH-secreting pituitary tumour (see section on pituitary tumours).

PITUITARY TUMOURS

Clinically these present with either local effects due to expansion and compression of surrounding structures or excess hormone secretion (functional tumours). A classification of intrasellar and suprasellar tumours is shown in Table 2.12. Approximately 50% of intrasellar tumours are hormone secreting, of which the majority (about 60%) are prolactinomas. GH secreting tumours account for about 25% and ACTH secreting tumours 15% of functional adenomas. An anatomical classification, based on size and degree of extension (Table 2.13) is useful for defining pituitary adenomas (especially prolactinomas) since this determines the form and results of treatment.

Table 2.12 Classification of intrasellar and suprasellar space occupying lesions

Functional (hormone secreting) pituitary adenomas	ACTH secreting → Cushing's syndrome GH secreting → acromegaly/gigantism PRL secreting → amenorrhoea/infertility (very rarely TSH → hyperthyroidism)
Non-functional (non-hormone secreting) pituitary adenomas	Pressure effects Hypopituitarism No symptoms
Crangiopharyngiomas	Pressure effects Hypopituitarism
Dermoid cysts, meningiomas, chordomas, metastatic tumours	Pressure effects Hypopituitarism

Table 2.13 Classification of pituitary tumours according to size and extension

Confined to sella turcica:
1. Microadenoma < 1 cm diameter
2. Macroadenoma > 1 cm diameter

Suprasellar extension — non-invasive

Invasive extension
1. Localised destruction of sella anteriorly with extension into sphenoid sinus, or laterally into cavernous sinus
2. Diffuse — widespread invasion and suprasellar extension

Investigation of pituitary tumours

The aims of investigation are to define pituitary function (see section on investigation of hypopituitarism) and to define excess hormone seretion (PRL, GH, ACTH) (see below). The size of a pituitary tumour is defined by pituitary radiology.

Plain lateral skull X-ray is the first investigation. This may show a clearly expanded sella turcica, with or without destruction of the floor (Fig. 2.4). A localised bulge in the fossa floor is common with microprolactinomas, a double contour suggesting a larger macroadenoma. Antero-posterior views may show a sloping floor on one side. Lateral tomography of the pituitary fossa provides clearer definition when there is doubt about interpretation

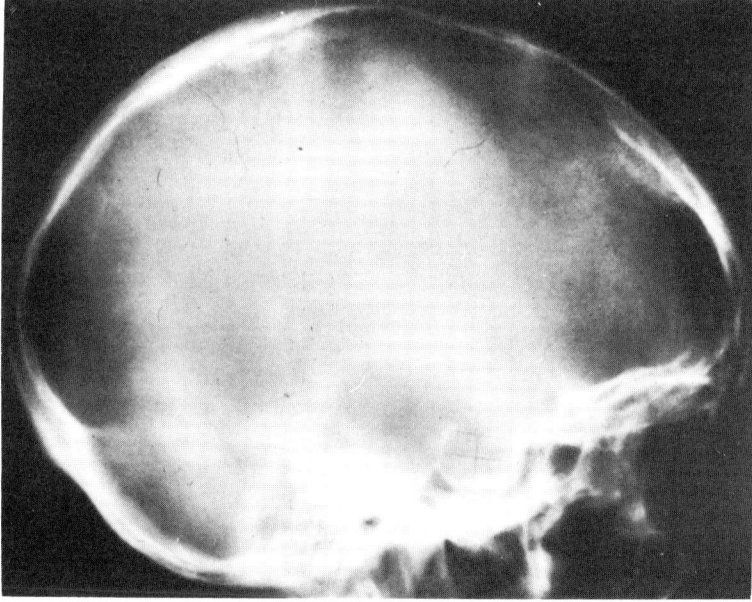

Fig. 2.4 Skull X-ray showing enlarged pituitary fossa due to pituitary tumour.

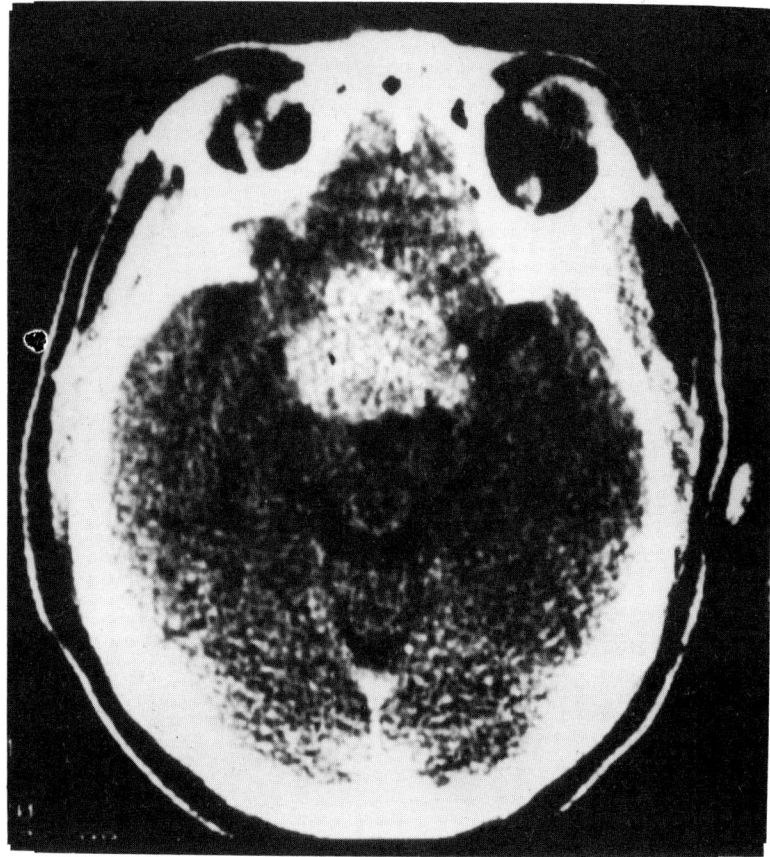

Fig. 2.5 CT scan of skull showing massive pituitary tumour.

of the plain X-ray. Supra or intrasellar calcification suggests a craniopharyngioma.

Computerised tomography, with contrast enhancement, should be performed if the skull X-ray is abnormal to define the presence and extent of any suprasellar extension. This is important to determine the operative approach for hypophysectomy. To delineate the optic nerves, pituitary stalk, and the presence of an empty sella, metrizamide cisternography with computerised tomographic (CT) scanning has replaced the air encephalogram.

Empty sella syndrome This is a radiological diagnosis and is usually made on CT scan by demonstration of a dark hole, (filled with cerebrospinal fluid) in the sella turcica. The most common cause is previous hypophysectomy or radiotherapy for pituitary tumours. Occasionally

this syndrome occurs spontaneously; a past history of sudden violent headache may raise the possibility of pituitary infarction as the cause. In spontaneous cases hormone deficiency is unusual. Visual field defects may arise from prolapse of the optic nerves or chiasm into the pituitary fossa and stretching over the diaphragma sellae. This condition must be excluded (by CT scanning) before pituitary surgery or radiotherapy is contemplated. After hypophysectomy, metrizamide cisternography with CT scanning is the best method for defining the position of the optic nerves and chiasm.

Clinical features of non-functional tumours

The clinical picture depends upon whether there is significant extrasellar extension. Headache is common, is typically intermittent and can be supraorbital, frontal, or temporal in location. Visual field defects result from compression of the optic chiasm or nerves. Classically, suprasellar extension of an intrasellar tumour produces first an upper quadrantic bitemporal field loss, which then proceeds to a full bitemporal hemianopia; visual deficit may, however, be variable, especially with suprasellar or parasellar tumours (craniopharyngiomas and meningiomas). An atypical and asymmetrical quadrantanopia does not preclude the presence of a pituitary space occupying lesion. Likewise, in the early stages of optic nerve compression, impaired visual acuity may be the first sign of a suprasellar lesion. Occasionally, lateral parasellar extension into the cavernous sinus produces unilateral III, IV, and VI nerve palsies. Suprasellar extension into the hypothalamus may rarely produce disturbance of appetite, sleep, mood, and temperature regulation. Hypopituitarism occurs when more than 75% of the normal pituitary is destroyed; this may be partial, or complete with larger lesions. Isolated gonado-trophin or GH deficiency are most commonly associated with primary suprasellar lesions (e.g. craniopharyngiomas, dermoid cysts). Moderate hyperprolactinaemia may result from compression of the pituitary stalk. Diabetes insipidus may also occur.

Craniopharyngioma

This is a suprasellar/intrasellar benign tumour arising from the remnants of Rathke's pouch. About 60% of such tumours are encapsulated cysts containing yellow oily fluid, 15% are solid and the remainder are mixed. Craniopharyngioma is primarily a childhood tumour with a peak incidence in the second decade, though asymptomatic cases presenting with suprasellar calcification on skull X-ray are found at all ages. Presentation is usually with signs and symptoms of a space occupying lesion: headache, nausea and vomiting and visual disturbance. About 40% of craniopharyngiomas present with pituitary hormone deficiency, often GH or LH, probably secondary to destruction of the hypothalamic centres producing GRF or GnRH.

Supra- or intrasellar calcification on skull X-ray is a feature of craniopharyngioma in children (80%

of cases), being less common in adults (40% of cases). A CT scan should be performed to delineate the extent of the lesion.

Treatment by neurosurgical excision of the tumour is the best therapeutic option. Total removal is often impossible, and recurrence is common, especially in cystic lesions. These tumours are radiosensitive and radiotherapy has been shown to reduce the recurrence rate.

Treatment of pituitary tumours

The management of pituitary tumours is dependent upon two factors: 1. their size and degree of extension, and 2. hormone secretion.

The most important definitive therapy for pituitary tumours is hypophysectomy. This is usually performed by the transphenoidal route for microadenomas and non-invasive macroadenomas. With this approach it is often possible to remove a localised adenoma, leaving normal pituitary tissue intact, thus reducing the likelihood of hypo-pituitarism. Large and invasive pituitary tumours may require a transcranial approach for removal. Large tumours presenting with progressive visual impairment represent a neurosurgical emergency and urgent craniotomy is required for relief of compression on optic nerves or chiasm.

Hypophysectomy should be covered with par-enteral hydrocortisone during and after surgery, hydrocortisone dosage being reduced to 30 mg/day within 2 weeks of operation. A combined pituitary stimulation test should be performed about 2 months after surgery to assess the need for long-term hydrocortisone and thyroxine replace-ment. Complications of hypophysectomy include transient diabetes insipidus, cerebrospinal fluid rhinorrhoea and basal meningitis (<1–2% of cases).

External radiotherapy is used if hypophysectomy fails to normalise excessive hormone secretion, or if significant tumour bulk remains and further treatment is required. Occasionally, external radiotherapy may be used as first line treatment, though suppression of hormone levels is slow and it may take years to be effective. Provided the total radiation dose does not exceed 4500 rad, and is given in divided doses, radiation optic neuritis and cerebral necrosis occur only rarely.

Table 2.14 Causes of hyperprolactaemia

Physiological

Pregnancy and lactation
Stress

Drugs

Phenothiazines
Tricyclic antidepressants
α-Methyl dopa
Rauwolfia alkaloids

Pituitary tumours

Prolactinomas — microadenoma (serum PRL 1000–5000 mu/l)
　　　　　　　macroadenomas (serum PRL > 5000 mu/l)

Hypothalamic and stalk lesions (serum PRL usually <2000 mu/l)

Non-secreting adenoma with suprasellar extension
Suprasellar tumours — craniopharyngiomas
Trauma with stalk transection
Hypothalamic granulomas — sarcoidosis
　　　　　　　　　　　　histiocytosis
　　　　　　　　　　　　basal meningitis

Chest wall (mediated by neural reflex)

Chronic nipple stimulation
Herpes zoster

Renal failure

Delayed metabolic clearance of prolactin

Severe hypothyroidism

Because of the continued risk of hypopituitarism following radiotherapy, long term annual follow-up is required. Other forms of pituitary irradiation include yttrium-90 implantation and proton beam irradiation but these are available only in specialised centres.

Prolactinomas

Pituitary prolactin secretion is normally under tonic inhibitory control by dopamine. Hyper-prolactinaemia accounts for about 30% of cases of amenorrhoea and is an important cause of infertility.

There are a number of causes of hyper-prolactinaemia (serum PRL >500 mu/l) of which prolactinomas form a major group (Table 2.14). A careful history and examination often elicit the cause of hyperprolactinaemia and drug therapy must be excluded.

The presentation of prolactinomas in females is with disorders of menstruation, ranging from amenorrhoea to more subtle abnormalities such as anovulatory menstrual cycles and defective luteal phases. Spontaneous galactorrhoea occurs in only about 35% of hyperprolactinaemic women. All infertile women should have a serum PRL level measured as a screening test. In males, prolactinomas normally present late when very large, often with pressure symptoms. Endocrine sequelae in males consist of impotence and loss of libido, due to the hypogonadism that accompanies sustained elevation of PRL.

Initial investigations for hyperprolactinaemia include biochemical profile, thyroid function tests and lateral skull X-ray. Generally the serum PRL level correlates well with the size of prolactinoma. Microadenomas are less than 1 cm in diameter and often no abnormality is seen on plain skull X-ray. Macroadenomas are greater than 1 cm in diameter and plain skull X-ray usually shows an abnormal sella, often a double floor. Provocative tests for PRL release (TRH, metoclopramide) are generally unhelpful in distinguishing between the various causes of hyperprolactinaemia.

Management of prolactinomas depends upon whether restoration of fertility is required and upon the size of the adenoma. The therapeutic options are outlined in Figure 2.6. If fertility is not required and symptoms are absent, observation of the patient may be sufficient. If infertility is a problem, dopamine agonists, such as bromocriptine or pergolide, provide a good chance of restoring PRL concentrations and fertility. Generally a dose of 5–15 mg/day of bromocriptine is sufficient and is well tolerated provided the dose is increased gradually (2.5 mg increments per week) and is taken with meals. The dose of dopamine agonist administered should be adjusted to the minimum which will maintain serum PRL within the normal range. Using this approach serum PRL is returned to normal in 95% of patients (even with large tumours); this may occur within 1 week of starting bromocriptine, menses resuming in 6–8 weeks. Permanent suppression of serum PRL is found in about 10% of microadenomas after stopping bromocriptine, though levels normally rebound within 1 month; medical treatment is thus rarely curative.

Pregnancy following bromocriptine is safe; there is no increase in spontaneous abortion or congenital

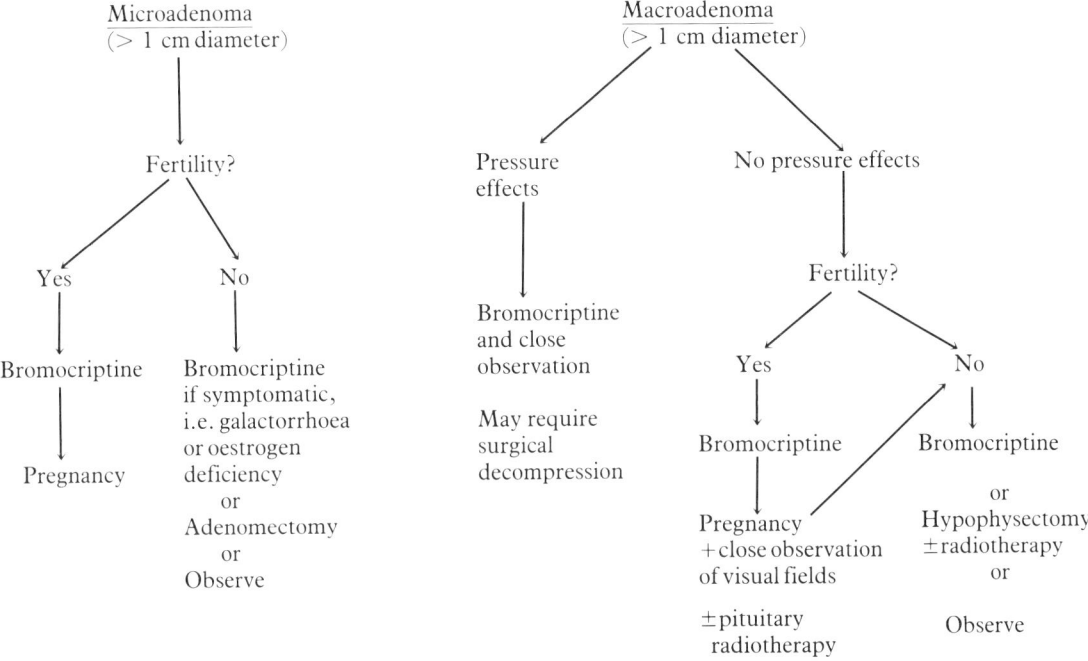

Fig. 2.6 Management of prolactinomas.

abnormalities. Since the pituitary gland of normal women enlarges during pregnancy, vision should be monitored regularly during pregnancy in women with prolactinomas; this applies particularly to patients with macroadenomas. Some centres have advocated prophylactic pituitary irradiation during early pregnancy in women with macroadenomas, although this may prejudice subsequent chances of fertility.

Hypophysectomy represents a definitive therapeutic option in the management of micro- and macroadenomas. Selective adenomectomy by the transphenoidal route provides a cure-rate for microadenomas of 70–90% in specialist hands, although recent reports indicate a significant (up to 50%) recurrence rate 4–6 years after surgery. For macroadenomas, initial cure rates are less than 50% with recurrence rates as high as 80–90% at 5 years.

Prolactinomas presenting with pressure symptoms, especially visual impairment, require urgent treatment. Such tumours are generally treated by transcranial hypophysectomy. In recent years, however, medical treatment with bromocriptine has emerged as a useful alternative. Bromocriptine has been shown to restore full vision rapidly (within a few days) and tumour shrinkage, documented by

CT scanning, occurs in 40–50% of patients with large prolactinomas. Close observation of the patient and regular monitoring of visual fields to detect deterioration is essential. Shrinkage of a large prolactinoma prior to hypophysectomy may make a subsequent neurosurgical approach easier.

Males with hyperprolactinaemia usually present with pressure symptoms from large tumours and require neurosurgery, but bromocriptine may be tried as first-line treatment, with careful monitoring.

Growth hormone secreting adenomas

These tumours present with acromegaly in adults or pituitary gigantism in preadolescents. As well as being a disfiguring disease, acromegaly decreases life-expectancy, especially in men, due predominantly to its cardiovascular complications. Early diagnosis and treatment, before excessive disfigurement and other complications have occurred, are therefore essential. Many patients present late because of the slow, insidious progression of the disease and lack of symptoms. Acromegaly is often diagnosed in this group at presentation of unrelated complaints and may not require aggressive therapy.

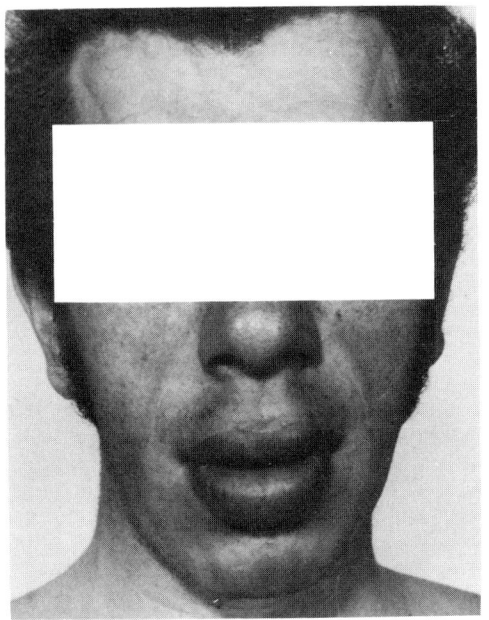

Fig. 2.7 Agromegalic facies.

Active acromegaly in a young individual (<40 years) requires treatment.

Early clinical features of GH hypersecretion are coarsening of facial features and soft tissue swelling of fingers, hands and feet (Figs. 2.7 and 2.8). Other manifestations of GH hypersecretion are shown in Table 2.15. Basal GH levels may

Table 2.15 Clinical manifestations of GH hypersecretion

	Approx % patients
Coarse facial features and soft tissue overgrowth	100
Organomegaly — liver, spleen, salivary gland	common
Excessive sweating	60–70
Degenerative joint disease	60
Weight gain	40
Abnormal glucose tolerance test	50
Clinical diabetes mellitus	10
Carpal tunnel syndrome	20
Hypertension	20–30
Goitre	25
Decreased libido (males)	20
Headache	90
Enlarged sella turcica	80–90
Visual impairment	variable

Rarer complications

Galactorrhoea (high serum PRL in 30%)
Cardiomyopathy
Hypercalcaemia and hypercalcuria

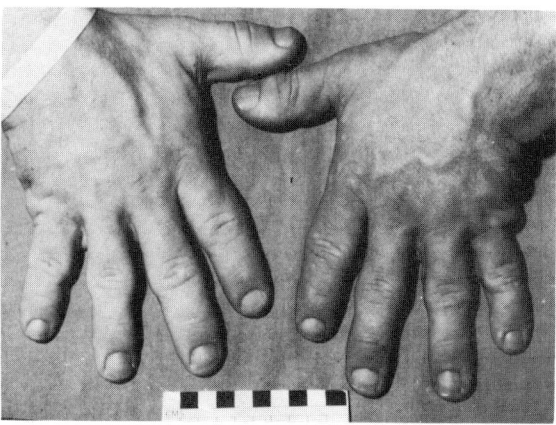

Fig. 2.8 Agromegalic hands.

be grossly elevated (>50 mu/l) or only slightly raised; a single abnormal value does not establish the diagnosis. Definitive diagnosis of acromegaly is based upon GH measurements during a 75 g standard oral glucose tolerance test. Normally at least one GH value should be <5 mu/l; failure to suppress below that value is strongly suggestive of acromegaly and often a paradoxical rise in serum GH is seen. Pituitary reserve should be tested and radiological assessment of pituitary tumour size is required.

Hypophysectomy represents the best chance of cure; selective adenomectomy via a transphenoidal approach is often possible with preservation of normal pituitary tissue. The clinical improvement in soft tissue swelling after successful reversal of GH hypersecretion is often dramatic and rapid, patients noticing loosening of rings within a few days. Assessment of treatment with repeat glucose tolerance test and measurement of GH should be performed 2 months after hypophysectomy and if GH secretion is still elevated, external pituitary irradiation is indicated. Alternative first-line therapies for acromegaly include yttrium-90 implantation (at selected centres), or radiotherapy. The latter is reserved for older patients who have relatively minor symptoms. No treatment is warranted in the elderly, asymptomatic patient who has long-standing disease.

Bromocriptine may normalise GH secretion in about 20% of cases of acromegaly and is accompanied by good symptomatic improvement. There are no predictive tests of likely response to bromocriptine and doses of up to 30 mg/day may be required.

GH suppression, if present, occurs rapidly so that biochemical response can be determined within 2–3 months. Long-acting somatostatin analogues have been shown to be effective in controlling GH secretion in a number of cases.

Rarely, acromegaly may be due to ectopic secretion of GRF. Pancreatic tumours synthesising GRF have been described, and a similar tumour producing GH has been reported.

ACTH secreting adenomas

The investigation and management of Cushing's disease are described in Chapter 5.

Posterior pituitary

PHYSIOLOGY

Two principal hormones are secreted by the posterior pituitary gland, or neurohypophysis, into the systemic circulation in man. These are arginine vasopressin (AVP) and oxytocin (OXT). Both are basic nonapeptides composed of a six amino-acid ring containing a disulphide bridge with a tripeptide tail. Substitution of two amino-acids, isoleucine for phenylalanine at position 3 and leucine for arginine at position 8, changes AVP to OXT. Both AVP and OXT are synthesised principally in two groups of magnocellular neurones called the supraoptic and paraventricular nuclei located in the hypothalamus. Large precursor molecules composed of the carrier protein (neurophysin) and the active hormone are synthesised and packaged together to form neurosecretory granules. These granules pass along the neuronal axons and processed AVP and OXT are stored in neuronal terminals before secretion. The neuronal pathways which transport the neurohypophyseal hormones from the supraoptic and paraventricular nuclei to the various points of discharge are shown in Figure 3.1. A major tract (I) passes from the hypothalamus into the pituitary stalk and terminates in the posterior pituitary, from which both hormones are secreted into the systemic circulation. A second tract (II) travels to the median eminence where AVP and OXT are released into the hypothalamo-hypophyseal portal vessels which supply blood to the anterior pituitary gland. Tract III goes to the floor of the third ventricle and it appears that AVP and probably OXT are actively secreted into the cerebrospinal fluid. The fourth tract (IV) passes posteriorly out of the hypothalamus to the brain stem and continues down the spinal cord. Fibres also pass to the forebrain.

Control of AVP secretion

Both AVP and OXT have short plasma half lives of approximately 3–5 minutes. The factors that control AVP secretion are given in Table 3.1. In

Table 3.1 Factors controlling the secretion of arginine vasopressin into the systemic circulation.

Major	Minor
Plasma osmolality (sodium)	Nausea, emesis
Blood pressure	Plasma angiotensin
Blood volume	Hypoglycaemia
	? Stress ? Pain ? Emotion

normal healthy adults, plasma osmolality is the major determinant of AVP release from minute to minute (see below). Large falls in blood pressure and/or volume can stimulate the release of enormous quantities of AVP, but the minor fluctuations which occur during normal daily activities probably have little effect. Whether hypertension influences AVP secretion remains controversial. Numerous minor factors influencing AVP release have been described, but their physiological and pathophysiological significance needs to be established.

Osmoregulation of AVP secretion

One of the essential homeostatic mechanisms for life is the maintenance of constant solute concentrations within tissues. In complex organisms,

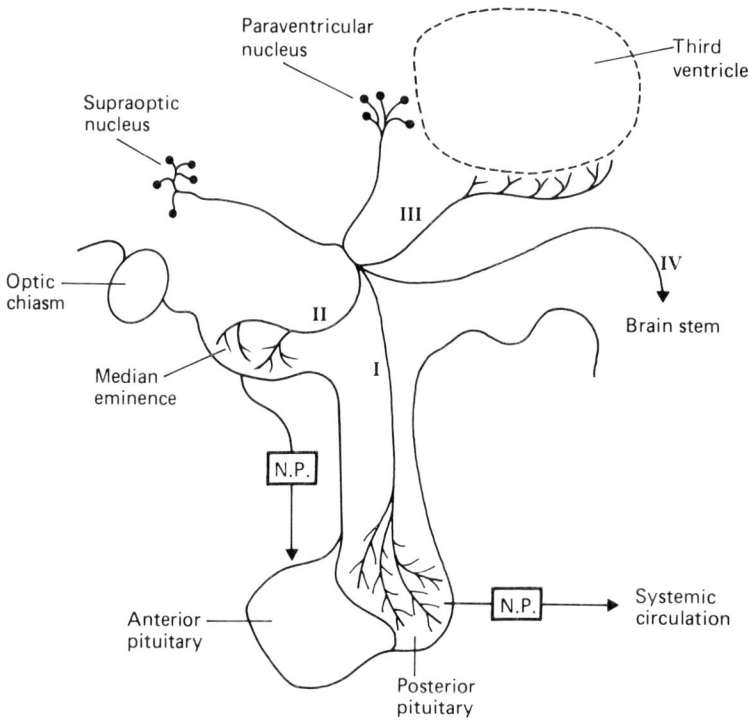

Fig. 3.1 Diagrammatic representation of the hypothalamus and the pituitary gland. Neuronal pathways from the supraoptic and paraventricular nuclei to the median eminence, posterior pituitary, floor of the third ventricle, brain stem and spinal cord. N.P. = neurophysin peptide complex.

the control of water intake and excretion is a major factor in maintaining solute concentrations. Water intake and excretion are in turn determined by thirst and by the action of AVP.

As the body loses water, so plasma osmolality rises. This stimulates the release of AVP into the systemic circulation, so that it may act on the renal tubules to conserve water and, in consequence, lower plasma osmolality again. The relationship between plasma osmolality and plasma AVP concentration, in healthy adults, is given in Figure 3.2. At plasma osmolalities of less than about 280 mOsmol/kg, AVP secretion is minimal and plasma AVP concentration becomes undetectable. This allows large quantities of dilute urine (approximately 15–20 litres per 24 hours) to be excreted. As plasma osmolality increases, so plasma AVP concentration increases, but at plasma AVP values of about 5 pmol/l, urine is maximally concentrated, and further rises in plasma AVP fail to conserve

more renal water. Plasma osmolalities slightly greater than those required to stimulate sufficient AVP release to produce maximally concentrated urine are necessary to stimulate severe thirst, increase water intake, and in turn lower plasma osmolality. As a consequence of the sensitive relationship between plasma osmolality and AVP secretion, and the ability of the kidney to respond to small changes in plasma AVP concentration, plasma osmolality in healthy adults is maintained within very narrow limits, 280–296 mOsmol/kg.

The cells that are sensitive to changes in plasma osmolality are located in the anterior hypothalamus, and are probably situated in the circumventricular organs. It is not known whether the osmosensitive cells that regulate AVP secretion also stimulate thirst sensation. Solutes vary in their capacity to stimulate AVP secretion. Sodium, the major cation in extracellular fluid, is one of the most potent solutes known to stimulate the release of AVP. Urea has a

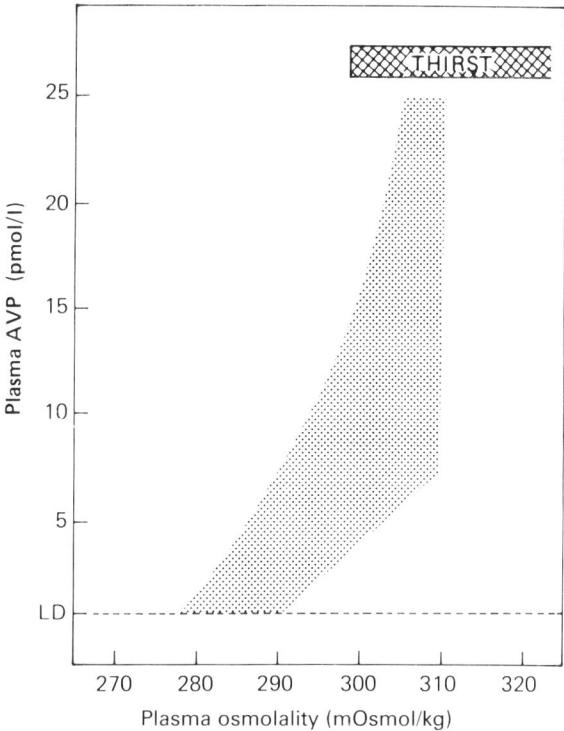

Fig. 3.2 Relationship between plasma AVP and plasma osmolality during hypertonic saline infusion into healthy adults (stippled area). Onset of severe thirst occurs, on average, at plasma osmolality of 298 mOsmol/kg. LD is the limit of assay detection.

smaller stimulatory effect and glucose fails to release AVP.

Baroregulation of AVP secretion

It is well recognised that large falls in blood pressure and/or volume result in the release of large quantities of AVP. The sensory input for the baroregulatory control of AVP secretion arises from high and low pressure receptors which are situated in the arch of the aorta, carotid vessels, the atria of the heart and the great veins within the thorax. Afferent fibres are carried in the vagus and glossopharyngeal nerves to the vasomotor nuclei of the brain stem. Sensory information then passes through the brain stem to both supraoptic and paraventricular hypothalamic nuclei. A fall in blood pressure of 10–20% is required to increase plasma AVP sufficiently to induce maximal antidiuresis but there is considerable individual variation in the degree of AVP response to hypotension.

Other factors controlling AVP secretion

Many factors have been implicated in the control of AVP secretion (Table 3.1). Early animal experiments suggested that pain and emotion trigger AVP release, so that many regard AVP as a 'stress hormone'. Convincing evidence that this is so in man is lacking. Nausea and vomiting are extremely potent stimulators of AVP release. It is believed that the emetic stimulus is mediated via the vagus nerve to the brain stem nuclei and sensory information then passes forward to the hypothalamus. It is possible that emesis associated with surgery may result in the postoperative antidiuresis so often observed in surgical patients. In addition, hypoglycaemia releases AVP in man. There is also a close association between the renin-angiotensin system and AVP secretion, infusion of angiotensin stimulating the release of modest amounts of AVP. Only a few agents are known to inhibit AVP secretion. Acute administration of alcohol or phenytoin reduces plasma AVP concentration and increases free water clearance. Recent evidence suiggests that atrial natriuretic factor may inhibit AVP release.

Thirst

Factors that stimulate thirst are similar to those controlling AVP secretion. As plasma osmolality rises to above 298 mOsmol/kg, thirst is perceived by means of osmotically-sensitive cells in the hypothalamus. The intensity of thirst does not increase with further rises in plasma osmolality. Salt is a greater dipsogenic agent than glucose. Isotonic hypovolaemia and large falls in blood pressure also stimulate thirst. The importance of the thirst mechanism in water balance is recognised when patients become adipsic. These patients, who also often have abnormalities of AVP secretion, are at risk of life-threatening hypernatraemia (see below).

Actions of AVP

Over the past few years many effects of AVP have been described in man and animals (Table 3.2). Its major systemic action is on the renal tubule.

Table 3.2 Actions of arginine vasopressin

Renal

Increase in cellular membrane permeability of collecting tubules to water, thus causing diuresis

Stimulation of sodium, potassium adenosine triphosphatase activity in the thick ascending limb of Henle's loop

Vascular

Constriction of smooth muscle in arterioles

Metabolic

Stimulation of liver glycogen phosphorylase activity
Increase in lipolysis

Anterior pituitary

Augmentation of release of andrenocorticotrophin

Cerebral

? Enhance memory and learning

Kidney

The principal site of action of circulating AVP is the collecting tubule, where it increases water permeability across the tubular cell. The antidiuretic action of AVP depends upon the generation of a solute gradient across the tubular cell. This is achieved by a counter-current system which creates a hyperosmolar interstitial renal medulla and permits hypotonic urine to enter the collecting tubule which itself passes through the medulla. Under the influence of AVP, the water permeability of these tubules increases, thus allowing solute-free water to move across the gradient from the lumen of the nephron into the renal medulla, and, in consequence, the urine becomes concentrated. This action of AVP is mediated by a membrane-bound adenylate cyclase system which, in turn, activates intracellular protein kinases and modifies intracellular microtubules and microfilaments. Renal prostaglandins reduce the antidiuretic action of AVP.

AVP also stimulates adenylate cyclase and sodium, potassium adenosine triphosphatase activities in the thick ascending limb of Henle's loop, with the result that sodium chloride is pumped into the renal medulla thus increasing its osmolality, raising the osmolar gradient and augmenting the antidiuretic action of AVP.

DIABETES INSIPIDUS

Diabetes insipidus has been recognised for many centuries, and in the past was differentiated from diabetes mellitus by physicians appreciating that the patient's urine was not sweet. This uncommon disorder, which may present at any age, usually presents with polyuria, thirst (polydipsia) and nocturia. Diabetes insipidus may result from lack of AVP (cranial, central or neurogenic diabetes insipidus) or from resistance to the antidiuretic action of AVP (nephrogenic diabetes insipidus).

Cranial diabetes insipidus

Lack of AVP results in the production of large quantities of dilute urine throughout the day and night. Plasma osmolality rises but fails to stimulate AVP secretion. Thirst is, however, stimulated and the constant intake of water maintains water homeostasis. Should thirst not be appreciated by the patient, or the thirsty patient be denied water, then progressive hypernatraemia may threaten life. The majority of patients with cranial diabetes insipidus do not have a complete lack of AVP, but more commonly they have inadequate quantities of AVP released in response to rises in plasma osmolality. If no AVP is secreted into the systemic circulation, patients may pass up to 20 litres of urine per 24 hours. Occasionally, patients have normal AVP responses to non-osmotic stimuli (e.g. hypotension or hypoglycaemia), but their osmoregulated AVP secretion is deficient.

Cranial diabetes is a rare disorder. Its causes can be divided into two major groups, familial and acquired (Table 3.3). The familial variety may be inherited as either a dominant or recessive trait, and becomes manifest in infancy. Another familial form of diabetes insipidus, which develops later in childhood, is associated with a number of abnormalities: diabetes mellitus, optic atrophy, nerve deafness and atonia of the ureters and bladder, and has been given the mnemonic DIDMOAD, although a more appropriate term is the Wolfram syndrome, after the original reporter's name. Atonia and dilatation of the renal tract is not unique to this syndrome however, but has been observed in many patients who have polyuria of any cause for prolonged periods.

In the older reviews of the causes of cranial diabetes insipidus, up to 50% of cases were idiopathic, although the more recent surveys suggest a figure of 30% for the idiopathic

form. Histological examination of the supraoptic and paraventricular nuclei shows atrophy of the magnocellular neurones. Within the idiopathic group, a subgroup of patients has been identified with circulating antibodies which bind to the cell membrane of AVP-synthesising neurones. Trauma to the pituitary stalk or hypothalamus accounts for about 30% of patients with cranial diabetes insipidus. Transient diabetes, which resolves after approximately 24–48 hours, is observed in many patients after hypophysectomy. Pituitary tumours rarely cause diabetes insipidus, but metastatic deposits or granulomatous diseases of the hypothalamus are well recognised causes of the disorder accounting for 30% of cases.

Nephrogenic diabetes insipidus

In nephrogenic diabetes insipidus the renal tubule fails to respond to AVP in either a complete or partial manner despite normal AVP secretion in response to osmotic stimulation. Dilute urine is therefore passed leading to loss of body water and an increase in plasma osmolality. Thirst is in turn stimulated to maintain water homeostasis. Nephrogenic diabetes insipidus may be due rarely to an inherited defect (sex-linked recessive) but more commonly is due to an acquired abnormality (Table 3.4). Metabolic disorders (hypercalcaemia or hypokalaemia) cause polyuria by a variety of mechanisms which include (i) inhibition of AVP-stimulated adenylate cyclase, (ii) inhibition of cyclic AMP-dependent protein kinases, (iii) reduction of sodium (and therefore solute content) in renal interstitial medulla, (iv) inhibition of sodium, potassium adenosine triphosphatase in the renal membranes and (v) deposition of calcium within

Table 3.3 Causes of cranial diabetes insipidus

Familial	Acquired
Dominant inheritance Recessive inheritance Cranial diabetes insipidus associated with diabetes mellitus, optic atrophy, nerve deafness, bladder atonia (DIDMOAD or Wolfram syndrome)	Idiopathic Antibodies to vasopressin-producing neurones Trauma (neurosurgery, head injury) Tumours (large pituitary tumours, metastases to hypothalamus, craniopharyngioma, pinealoma) Granulomas (sarcoidosis, histiocytosis X, eosinophilic granuloma) Infections (meningitis, encephalitis) Vascular (Sheehan's syndrome, aneurysms, sickle cell anaemia)

Table 3.4   Causes of nephrogenic diabetes insipidus.

Hereditary	Acquired
Sex-linked recessive inheritance	Metabolic (hypercalcaemia, hypokalaemia) Solute diuresis (glycosuria) Post obstruction to renal tract outflow Poisons (lithium, analgesics) Amyloid disease Medullary cystic disease Sickle cell anaemia Interstitial and tubular nephritis Prolonged water diuresis

the nephron. The presence of large quantities of glucose in the luminal fluid reduces the osmotic gradient across the tubule, thus reducing the effect of AVP and leads to polyuria. A similar mechanism operates after prolonged water diuresis, since solute is then flushed out of the renal interstitium, thereby lowering the osmotic gradient across the tubule. Amyloid deposition in the kidney, medullary cystic disease and sickle cell anaemia interfere with the action of AVP by causing structural damage to the nephron.

Cranial and nephrogenic diabetes insipidus must be differentiated from primary polydipsia or increased water drinking. In this condition increased drinking leads to a decrease in plasma osmolality, reduction in AVP secretion and, in consequence, production of dilute and copious urine. In this situation there is a tendency for the polyuria to be most noticeable during the day, unless the patient continues to drink throughout the night. It may be due to habitual drinking, persistent dry mouth which is occasionally caused by drugs such as anticholinergic agents or antidepressants, or a structural lesion affecting the hypothalamic thirst centre. Primary polydipsia is often observed in association with neurotic or psychotic illness.

Differential diagnosis of polyuria

Polyuria is defined as a urine output $\geq$ 3 litres per 24 hours. The conventional way to investigate the polyuric patient is by means of a water deprivation test. Although this test is satisfactory for patients with gross abnormalities, it is less good in establishing the diagnosis in mild diabetes insipidus. Other methods of investigation have therefore been devised (see below).

Table 3.5   Protocol for water deprivation test.

Preparation of patient

1. Water intake encouraged overnight
2. Light breakfast: no tea, coffe or alcohol and no smoking

Dehydration

1. No fluids for up to 8 hours. Small amount of dry food if necessary
2. Supervision essential
3. Weigh patient at hourly intervals; stop dehydration if weight loss greater than 5% of initial weight
4. Urine passed hourly, record volume and osmolality

Response to Desmopressin

After dehydration administer desmopressin (DDAVP) 2µg intramuscularly
2. Patient allowed to eat normally and drink, but no more than the volume of urine passed during dehydration period, over the next 12 hours
3. Urine passed at 1, 3, 5 and 12 hours after desmopressin, record volume and osmolality

Water deprivation test. The basis of this procedure is simple, but in practice it is often difficult to perform sufficiently well to establish an unequivocal diagnosis. The test is divided into two stages; during the first, urine and plasma osmolalities are measured at regular intervals while the patient is deprived of all fluids. Exogenous vasopressin (desmopressin) is then administered and urine and plasma osmolalities are recorded over the following 12 hours. Details of the procedure and its interpretation are given in Tables 3.5 and 3.6. It is essential that during the first stage of the test plasma osmolality rises adequately to stimulate AVP to produce maximal antidiuresis. On average plasma osmolality should reach 290–295 mOsmol/kg at the end of 8 hours of fluid restriction. Healthy adults and some patients with primary polydipsia will attain urine osmolalities in

Table 3.6   Interpretation of results from water deprivation test.

Urine osmolality (mOsmol/kg)		Diagnosis
After dehydration	*After desmopressin*	
> 750	> 750	Normal, primary polydipsia
< 300	> 750	Cranial diabetes insipidus
< 300	< 300	Nephrogenic diabetes insipidus
300–750	< 750	Partial diabetes insipidus or primary polydipsia

excess of 750 mOsmol/kg after dehydration and urine osmolality may or may not rise further after desmopressin. Patients who have marked disorders of cranial or nephrogenic diabetes insipidus will have unequivocal results, but those with partial disorders will be difficult to differentiate from primary polydipsia. This may be because prolonged polyuria itself washes out the solute in the renal interstitium, thus reducing the osmotic gradient across tubular cells and leading to partial AVP resistance (nephrogenic diabetes insipidus). If the clinician is unable to establish a firm diagnosis he may either suggest a therapeutic trial of desmopressin or, if plasma AVP measurements are available, wish to measure directly plasma AVP in response to osmotic stimulation.

Hypertonic saline infusion test. Because of wide individual variations, random measurements of plasma AVP are difficult to interpret; some form of dynamic test is therefore required. Infusion of 5% (850 mmol/l) hypertonic saline for 2 hours with measurements of plasma AVP and plasma osmolality provides a quick and reliable test that readily differentiates cranial diabetes insipidus, even the most minor forms, from other causes of polyuria. The protocol for the test is given in Table 3.7. Figure 3.3 shows the pattern of results that may be obtained. All patients with cranial diabetes insipidus will have subnormal concentrations of plasma AVP in relation to plasma osmolality, although under basal conditions there may be overlap with normal subjects. Some patients will have undetectable plasma AVP despite marked rises in plasma osmolality and could be termed complete cranial diabetes insipidus. By far the majority of patients perceive thirst normally but a few remain adipsic. Patients with nephrogenic diabetes insipidus and primary polydipsia have entirely normal plasma AVP responses to osmotic stimulation.

It is not appropriate to apply non-osmotic stimuli of AVP release to diagnose cranial diabetes insipidus, for many patients with this disorder have normal AVP responses to hypotension or hypoglycaemia.

Plasma AVP and urine osmolality. Patients with nephrogenic diabetes insipidus may be most readily distinguished from other polyuric patients by relating plasma AVP concentration

Table 3.7   Protocol for infusion of hypertonic saline

Preparation of patient
1. Water intake encouraged overnight
2. Fast from midnight
3. No tea, coffee or alcohol. No smoking

Procedure
1. Patient empties bladder
2. Weigh patient
3. Insert 2 cannulae, one into each antecubital vein
4. After patient has rested 30 minutes, take 2 basal venous blood samples, separated by 10 minutes
5. Infuse 5% (850 mmol/l) saline at the rate of 0.06 ml/kg/min for 2 hours
6. Blood samples taken at 30 minute intervals from non-infused arm after start of infusion
7. Note time of onset of severe thirst
8. Final blood sample taken 15 minutes after infusion stopped
9. Check blood pressure at 15-minute intervals during study
10. Avoid ingestion of large quantities of fluid at the end of study

Processing of blood
1. Take blood into cooled syringe and transfer immediately to lithium heparized tube on ice
2. Centrifuge tubes at 4°C within 10 minutes
3. Plasma aliquot for osmolality measurement should be kept at 4°C and aliquot for AVP should be immediately deep frozen at −30°C

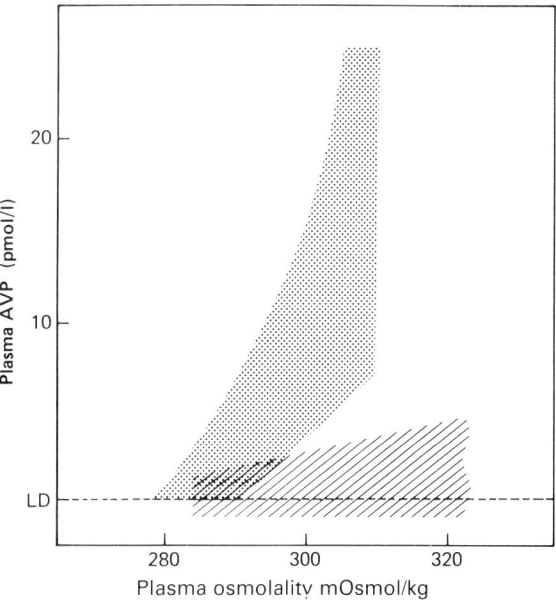

Fig. 3.3   Plasma osmolality and plasma AVP responses to hypertonic saline infusion. Patients with cranial diabetes insipidus (cross-hatched area) are differentiated from normal subjects (stippled area) by inappropriately low plasma AVP concentrations with respect to plasma osmolality. LD is limit of assay detection.

to urine osmolality after a period of dehydration. These patients have inappropriately high concentrations of plasma AVP with respect to their urine osmolalities, while patients with cranial diabetes insipidus have results in the normal range.

Therapeutic trial of desmopressin. Reliable AVP assays are not widely available at present so many clinicians need to rely on indirect methods to establish the diagnosis of diabetes insipidus. A carefully controlled therapeutic trial of desmopressin may be useful in this situation. Administration of desmopressin (10μg) intranasally once daily for two weeks will improve thirst and polyuria in patients with cranial diabetes insipidus. Those with the nephrogenic disorder will experience little or no improvement. Primary polydipsic patients will develop progressive dilutional hyponatraemia with weight gain and increase in urine osmolality. Since severe hyponatraemia may develop quickly in polydipsic patients who continue to drink in the presence of sustained antidiuresis, all patients undergoing such therapeutic trials should be monitored closely in hospital.

Treatment of cranial diabetes insipidus

Patients who suffer from mild degrees of polyuria (urine volume < 4 litres/24 hours) may require no treatment providing they are able to drink as much fluid as they desire. An intact thirst mechanism will protect them from extreme dehydration and hypernatraemia. More severe untreated polyuria may lead to distension and atonia of the bladder, hydroureter and hydronephrosis, as well as considerable social inconvenience. Such patients do require drug treatment. The following are the types of preparations that are available:

1. Desmoressin (DDAVP)
2. Lysine vasopressin
3. Oral agents (chlorpropamide, clofibrate, carbamazepine, thiazide diuretics)
4. Pitressin.

The synthetic analogue of AVP, desmopressin (DDAVP), is the treatment of choice. The antidiuretic action of DDAVP persists for about 12 hours; its antidiuretic potency is twofold greater than natural AVP and its pressor activity is minimal.

Desmopressin is administered either intranasally or parenterally. There is considerable individual variation in the dose required to control thirst and polyuria (5–40 μg per 24 hours, intranasally). Dilutional hyponatraemia may occur as a result of overtreatment, but this complication may be avoided by advising patients to become polyuric for a few hours each week.

If desmopressin is unavailable, an alternative preparation, lysine vasopressin, can be given. It acts for only about 4 hours and possesses pressor activity. Like desmopressin it must be given intranasally. Pitressin tannate in oil, an extract from animal posterior pituitary gland has been used extensively in the past, but is no longer available in many countries. It is administered intramuscularly, but it is most important that the vial contents be warmed and well mixed prior to injection. Its action may last for 24–72 hours, and it, too, possesses pressor activity.

Although desmopressin is the drug of choice for cranial diabetes insipidus irrespective of the degree of severity, a few clinicians still prefer to use oral agents for the treatment of partial cranial diabetes. These agents act mainly by potentiating the antidiuretic action of the low circulating concentrations of AVP present in partial forms of the disorder. Chlorpropamide is capable of reducing urine volume by 50%, but its maximum effect may take several weeks to achieve. Hypoglycaemia is often a troublesome side-effect. Carbamazepine and clofibrate are less effective than chlorpropamide at reducing urine volume in cranial diabetes insipidus.

ADIPSIC HYPERNATRAEMIA

Hypernatraemia (plasma sodium > 150 mmol/l) in adults is usually the result of water deficiency, either due to large losses from the gastrointestinal tract, skin, lungs or kidneys, or from decreased intake of fluid. Adipsic or hypodipsic hypernatraemia is a rare disorder in which little fluid is taken because of thirst deficiency. The thirst osmoreceptors are presumed to be damaged, and there is often an associated abnormality of osmoregulated AVP release, commonly manifest as cranial diabetes insipidus. Vascular abnormalities, neoplastic disease, granulomas or trauma are associated with adipsic hypernatraemia.

Treatment of such patients is very difficult because they no longer have a thirst mechanism to stimulate drinking when dehydration and hypernatraemia develop secondary to polyuria. The administration of a fixed daily intake of water does not maintain a steady plasma osmolality even in addition to administration of desmopressin. The variation in daily insensible fluid losses from changes in temperature, physical activity and diet still lead to wide fluctuations in plasma sodium and osmolality. One method to control plasma osmolality is to devise a sliding scale of water intake related to changes in daily body weight. A fixed dose of desmopressin should be given if there is insufficient endogenous AVP secretion. Regular checks of plasma sodium and/or osmolality ensure that there are no extreme fluctuations in electrolytes.

SYNDROME OF AVP EXCESS

Persistent excessive secretion of AVP together with continued drinking of fluid results in hyponatraemia. Retained water is distributed throughout the total body water space so that a clinically detectable increase in extracellular volume is absent (Table 3.8). Hypovolaemic conditions causing hyponatraemia can usually be readily identified by the clinical features of postural hypotension, tachycardia, decreased skin turgor and thirst, while the hypervolaemic group generally have dependent pitting oedema and signs of the underlying disease. The following are the characteristics of the syndrome of inappropriate antidiuretic hormone secretion, more correctly named the syndrome of inappropriate antidiuresis:

1. Dilutional hyponatraemia
2. Urine osmolality greater than plasma osmolality (usually)
3. Excessive renal sodium excretion
4. Normal renal and adrenal function
5. Absence of hypotension, hypovolaemia and oedema-forming states

Causes of the syndrome of inappropriate antidiuresis

Some of the conditions in which there is evidence of persistent excessive AVP secretion are given in Table 3.9. Three major groups of disorders have been identified: malignant, neurological and respiritory. Probably the commonest cause of the syndrome is oat cell carcinoma of the bronchus. It is presumed that most of these patients synthesise and release AVP-like peptides from neoplastic tissue although there is evidence that some carcinomatous patients have abnormal secretion of AVP from the neurohypophysis. Whether such patients secrete a tumourous factor which stimulates AVP release from the posterior pituitary or whether the tumour interferes with the normal non-osmotic AVP regulatory system (e.g. disruption of baroregulatory sensory input) is not known. Neurological disorders probably influence the neurohypophysis directly or interfere with the mechanisms which control AVP secretion.

From the few studies in which plasma AVP concentration has been measured in patients with the syndrome of inappropriate antidiuresis it is evident that the absolute concentration of circulating AVP may not be elevated but that it is inappropriately high for the plasma osmolality.

Table 3.8 Disorders associated with hyponatraemia.

Hypervolaemic	Normovolaemic	Hypovolaemic
Heart failure	SIAD[+]	Adrenal insufficiency
Nephrotic syndrome	SCS[*]	Diuretic therapy
Cirrhosis	Inappropriate	Renal salt wasting disease
Hypothyroidism	intravenous therapy	Burns
Inappropriate		Gastrointestinal loss
intravenous therapy		

+ Syndrome of inappropriate antidiuresis
* Sick cell syndrome

Table 3.9 Some cuases of the syndrome of inappropriate antidiuresis.

Malignancy	Chest disorders
Carcinoma (bronchitis, pancreas, ureter, duodenum, prostate)	Pneumonia
	Tuberculosis
Thymoma	Empyema
Mesothelioma	Cystic fibrosis
Lymphoma, leukemia	Asthma
Ewing's sarcoma	Pneumothorax
Nervous system disorders	*Miscellaneous*
Meningitis, encephalitis	Drugs (vincristine, vinblastine,
Brain tumour, abscess	vasopressin, oxytocin, cis-platinum,
Head injury	chlorpropamide, thiazide, phenothiazines)
Hydrocephalus	Endocrine (hypothgyroidism)
Cerebellar & cerebral atrophy	Acute psychosis
Shy-Drager syndrome	Delirium tremens
Porphyria	Idiopathic
Guillain-Barré syndrome	

Treatment

The clinical features of hyponatraemia (Table 3.10) depend not only on the absolute value of plasma

Table 3.10 Clinical features of hyponataemia.

Anorexia	Cramps	Headache
Nausea	Myoclonus	Confusion
Vomiting	Abdominal ileus	Convulsions
Fatigue	Ataxia	Coma

sodium, but also on the rate of development of hyponatraemia. In general, patients who have persistent plasma sodium concentrations greater than 125 mOsmol/kg rarely have significant symptoms or features of hyponatraemia, and specific therapy should not be required. Patients with lower plasma sodium values might need treatment, and it is worth remembering that therapy directed at the underlying cause of the persistent AVP excretion is the most rational approach. If this is not possible, or direct treatment of the hyponatraemia is required, then conventional therapy is fluid restriction. It is necessary to reduce fluid intake to about 500 ml per 24 hours with the aim of raising plasma sodium to approximately 130 mmol/l and then allowing a slightly greater fluid intake. Fluid restriction for prolonged periods can be very distressing

for patients. For this reason drug therapy to reduce endogenous AVP secretion or to inhibit the antidiuretic action of AVP has been advocated as follows:

1. Demeclocycline hydrochloride
2. Lithium carbonate
3. Phenytoin
4. Frusemide with sodium chloride supplementation
5. Infusion of hypertonic saline (dangerous procedure)

Demeclocycline and lithium carbonate cause partial nephrogenic diabetes insipidus and allow excretion of excess water. Demeclocycline (600–1200 mg in divided doses per 24 hours) is more reliable and less toxic than lithium, but its maximum effect may not occur for 3 weeks. Drugs which suppress AVP secretion (phenytoin and ethanol) are considerably less useful than demeclocycline. An alternative therapy involves administration of oral frusemide (40–80 mg daily) together with salt supplementation, up to 3 g daily.

Rapid increase in plasma sodium induced by infusion of hypertonic saline is not recommended unless the patient's life is threatened by hyponatraemia. Cautious infusion with 5% hypertonic saline at a rate of approximately 1–2 ml/min for

4–6 hours to increase plasma sodium concentration by no more than 10–15 mmol/l, can be considered, but it must be appreciated that the effects of the infusion are short-lived and this sudden rise in plasma sodium may induce convulsions or death and has been implicated in the development of central pontine myelinolysis.

OXYTOCIN

Although there is considerable knowledge about the physiology of OXT, no significant clinical disorders have been attributed to hyper- or hypo-secretion of the hormone.

Control of secretion

In contrast to AVP, the release of OXT from the posterior pituitary gland is episodic; each spurt of OXT increases plasma OXT concentrations about 10-fold above basal values. There are two major reflexes that control secretion of OXT in females. The first is the neuroendocrine reflex involving tactile stimulation of the nipple (suckling) causing release of OXT and, in turn, leading to contraction of the myoepithelial cells around the breast ducts, and milk ejection. The second reflex concerns stimulation of the stretch receptors of the lower genital tract, which is most evident at the time of parturition, and leads to the release of large quantities of OXT at delivery. Vaginal distension of non-pregnant female animals also appears to cause OXT secretion, and coitus in humans leads to OXT release in females but not males.

Little is known about the control of OXT secretion in males, but there is evidence that osmotic and haemodynamic stimulation increases the release of OXT in a similar fashion to AVP. From a pharmacological aspect, prostaglandins, dopamine and oestrogens all stimulate OXT release, while endogenous opiates appear to inhibit release.

Actions of OXT

The major target organs for OXT secreted into the systemic circulation are the uterus and breast (Table 3.11). Both possess high affinity receptors for OXT. Early in pregnancy plasma OXT con-

Table 3.11 Actions of oxytocin.

Uterine
Stimulation of uterine contraction

Breast
Contraction of mammary myoepithelium

Vascular
Constriction of arteriolar smooth muscle

Renal
Increase water permeability of collecting tubules

Metabolic
Increase in glucose uptake
? Stimulation of insulin and glucagon release

Anterior pituitary
Inhibition of adrenocorticotrophin secretion
? Modulation of gonadotrophin release

Cerebral
? Increase maternal behaviour
? Impairment of memory

centrations are low, but they tend to rise in later pregnancy and are high at parturition. The role of OXT in milk ejection is well established. The hormone causes contraction of mammary myoepithelial cells. Whether OXT also has effects on the composition and secretion of milk remains controversial.

Disorders of OXT function

No significant syndromes associated with OXT deficiency or excess have been described. OXT has been recovered from some tumours, and it is probable that ectopic production of OXT from neoplastic tissue does occur. No specific clinical features have been attributed to OXT-producing tumours, although one might anticipate a mild syndrome of inappropriate antidiuresis from the slight antidiuretic properties of OXT, if the hormone were released in large quantities.

Patients who have severe cranial diabetes insipidus do not have any difficulties with spontaneous vaginal deliveries. Administration of oxytocin (as Syntocinon) to induce uterine contractions at parturition, rarely causes dilutional hyponatraemia if given in excess together with large quantities of fluid.

Thyroid

PHYSIOLOGY

Synthesis and secretion of thyroid hormones

The thyroid gland is composed of follicular structures in which epithelial cells (follicular cells) surround a central lumen containing colloid. Colloid consists of a concentrated solution of a glycosylated iodine-containing protein, thyroglobulin which is the major synthetic product of the follicular cell and is the precursor and storage form of the thyroid hormones, thyroxine (T4) and triiodothyronine (T3). The thyroid follicular cell traps iodine at the base of the cell by an active transport mechanism. Following trapping, iodine is oxidised or organisied and this oxidised form of iodine is incorporated into the tyrosyl groups of thyroglobulin with the formation of monoiodotyrosine and diiodotyrosine residues in the glycoprotein. In the thyroglobulin molecule the iodotyrosines undergo oxidative coupling to form T4 and T3 and small amounts of reverse triiodothyronine (rT3).

Transport of thyroid hormones and their entry into tissues

T4 and T3 are poorly soluble in water and circulate in the plasma bound to three transport proteins, thyroxine binding globulin (TBG), thyroxine binding prealbumin (TBPA) and albumin. Of the three proteins TBG binds the most T4 and T3 in normal subjects. Normally some 70% of circulating T4 and T3 is bound to TBG, 20% to TBPA, and 10 per cent to albumin. A dynamic equilibrium exists between the binding proteins and the hormones, wherein free (unbound) hormone and proteins with unoc-cupied binding sites co-exist with hormone-protein complexes. The major part of both hormones circulates in the protein-bound form, with only a very small percentage in the free state (0.03% of circulating T4, 0.3% of circulating T3). Nevertheless, this small fraction has considerable significance, since hormones enter the target cell unattached to binding proteins. Thus in vitro measurements of free hormones are used as indices of thyroid function in vivo.

Thyroid hormone action at the cellular level

T3 is the biologically active thyroid hormone, possessing five times the metabolic activity of T4. T4 has assumed the role of a prohormone and whether T4 has any intrinsic activity or whether it first needs to be converted to T3 to achieve an effect remains a matter of controversy. In man, 80% of T3 is produced by 5′-monodeiodination of T4 outside the thyroid gland, T4 to T3 conversion occurring mostly in the liver and kidney. Reverse T3 (rT3) is the other product of monodeiodination of T4, and is the biologically inactive isomer of T3. The conversion of T4 to T3 and the deiodination of rT3 by the enzyme 5′-monodeiodinase may be inhibited in a number of situations, such as chronic illness or surgical stress, when a fall in T3 concentration is usually accompanied by a rise in rT3 – the 'low T3 syndrome'.

The most important cellular effects of thyroid hormones are on protein synthesis, mitochondrial respiration and ATP production. T3 probably produces most, if not all, of its cellular effects by binding to a specific receptor located in the cell nucleus. The binding of T3 to nuclear receptors has been correlated with many thyroid hormone dependent tissue responses, including induction of specific messenger RNAs and synthesis of thyroid hormone dependent proteins.

Regulation of the hypothalamic-pituitary-thyroid axis

The glycoprotein hormone TSH, released from thyrotrophs of the anterior pituitary into the peripheral circulation, stimulates the secretion of T4 and T3 from the thyroid gland. TSH is composed of two subunits, α and β. The β subunit confers immunological and biological specificity but requires combination with an α subunit for receptor binding and biological activity. TSH interacts with a specific receptor on the plasma membrane of the thyroid cell and transmits information to the cell via activation of adenylate cyclase and accumulation of cAMP. The essential control of this system is via negative feedback in which thyroid hormone acts on the anterior pituitary to suppress the release of TSH. Both T4 and T3 are active in this respect although studies have indicated that most of the T4 action involves its intrapituitary deiodination to T3. Superimposed on this system is the tonic stimulatory effect of thyrotrophin releasing hormone (TRH). TRH is a tripeptide which is transported from the hypothalamus through the portal vessel circulation to the anterior pituitary where it acts on the thyrotroph via specific plasma membrane receptors. The complexity of the system is increased by the interaction of a number of other hormones, peptides and neurotransmitters, e.g. somatostatin, dopamine and steroid hormones.

LABORATORY DIAGNOSIS OF THYROID DISEASE

Thyroid disease is common, often not diagnosed and usually easy to treat. Thyroid function tests are carried out for several reasons:
1.   To confirm a clinical diagnosis.
2.   To exclude the diagnosis in patients with unexplained abnormalities (e.g. weight loss, atrial fibrillation) that might be attributed to thyroid dysfunction.
3.   To monitor response to therapy in patients with confirmed thyroid disease.
4.   To screen for neonatal hypothyroidism.

Following the development of specific and reliable radioimmunoassay techniques there has been a marked change in the pattern of thyroid function testing with emphasis now directed towards the direct measurement of circulating thyroid hormone and TSH levels.

Serum thyroxine

Measurement of total serum T4 was until recently the standard test for assessing thyroid function, radioimmunoassay having replaced the imprecise competitive protein binding assays. Many factors, however, are known to influence the circulating concentration of the principal binding protein, TBG (Table 4.1) and thus it is essential to make allowance for the concentration of serum

Table 4.1   Causes of alteration of TBG

Increased TBG	Decreased TBG
Oestrogens, oral contraceptive pill, pregnancy	Androgens, corticosteroids
Phenothiazines, clofibrate	Asparaginase
Hypothyroidism	Acromegaly
Congenital increase	Nephrotic syndrome, protein losing enteropathy
Viral hepatitis	Starvation, severe illness
Acute intermittent porphyria	Thyrotoxicosis
	Congenital decrease or absence

TBG when interpreting the result of a total T4 measurement. This problem of marked variation in total T4 consequent on changes in TBG has been overcome by calculation of a free thyroxine index (FTI) or a T4:TBG ratio. The FTI is an estimate of free or unbound T4 concentration derived from measures of total T4 concentration and the number of unoccupied protein binding sites, the latter being defined by adding radiolabelled T3 to serum ('T3 uptake test'). The T4:TBG ratio provides another estimate of free or unbound thyroxine concentrations and relies upon direct measurement of circulating TBG by radioimmunoassay or immunoelectrophoresis. Both of these calculations of free T4 concentration correct for variations in TBG, although at extremes of TBG concentration inaccurate results may be obtained.

The advent of simple direct radioimmunoassays for measurement of free T4 now means that derived indices such as FTI and T4:TBG ratio are proving increasingly unnecessary. Measurement of free T4 concentration is unaffected by changes in TBG concentration due to inherited defects or the pill. Measurement of free T4 concentration is similarly unaffected by circulating concentrations of TBPA or albumin. Spurious elevation of free T4, as well as total T4 level, may occur in patients with circulating antibodies to iodothyronines and in patients with hereditary abnormalities of albumin or TBPA with increased affinity for T4 (see below).

Serum triiodothyronine

Serum T3 concentrations are measured by radioimmunoassay and like T4 values can be altered by changes in thyroid hormone binding proteins. A free T3 index, derived from total serum T3 concentration and T3-uptake, or a T3:TBG ratio both provide an indirect measure of free T3 concentration but neither method has been widely used. Commercial methods for the direct radioimmunoassay of free T3 have been developed and make these indirect measurements largely obsolete. The most important indication for the measurement of serum T3 is in the diagnosis of 'T3 toxicosis' where hyperthyroidism results from an excess of circulating T3 without an increase in total or free T4. The high T3 reflects preferential thyroidal secretion and may be an early feature of many cases of classical thyrotoxicosis (see below).

The term 'T4 toxicosis' has been applied to the syndrome of hyperthyroidism, in which serum T4 is elevated but serum T3 is normal. In almost all cases intercurrent non-thyroidal illness is present causing inhibition of 5'-monodeiodinase activity with reduction of T4 to T3 conversion. The marked fall in serum T3 in non-thyroidal disease demonstrates that T3 is inappropriate as a single test of thyroid function.

TSH and TRH stimulation test

TSH secretion is very sensitive to alterations in serum thyroid hormone concentrations, small decreases augmenting TSH secretion and small increases inhibiting it. In hyperthyroidism, high levels of circulating T4 and T3 suppress TSH secretion and in hypothyroidism, TSH secretion is increased. The value of basal or unstimulated serum TSH measurements has been limited to the diagnosis of hypothyroidism, since conventional radioimmunoassays are not sufficiently sensitive to distinguish serum TSH concentrations in euthyroid and thyrotoxic subjects; more sensitive assays have been developed and a difference between normal and suppressed levels can now be determined.

The TSH response to intravenous injection of TRH has had an important place in the diagnosis of thyroid dysfunction. Little or no response of TSH 20 or 30 minutes after administration of TRH (200 µg) is seen in hyperthyroidism, with an exaggerated response in hypothyroidism. Lack of response of TSH to TRH is not, however, diagnostic of hyperthyroidism since the TSH response may be absent or impaired in some euthyroid patients with autonomously functioning thyroid adenomas or multinodular goitres, in treated Graves' disease in remission, in ophthalmic Graves' disease, in normal subjects receiving thyroxine and in hypopituitarism. A normal TSH response to TRH may be used to exclude the diagnosis of thyrotoxicosis in a patient with suggestive symptoms but non-confirmatory tests of circulating thyroid hormones. Assessment of the

TSH response to TRH plays little part in the assessment of hypothyroidism, but may identify an exaggerated response in patients with borderline or minimal elevations of basal TSH.

There is a close correlation between basal serum TSH concentration, measured in a sensitive assay, and the TSH response to TRH and it is likely that sensitive TSH measurements will replace the need for TRH testing in assessing thyroid disease. A detectable TSH value will exclude hyperthyroidism; suppressed values are found not only in hyperthyroidism but also in euthyroid subjects with goitre, in those who have previously received antithyroid therapy as well as in the elderly and in patients with non-thyroidal illness.

Radioisotope uptake tests

Thyroidal radioisotope uptake measurements as tests of thyroid function have been largely replaced by laboratory assays of circulating thyroid hormones and are seldom used today for this purpose. Measurement of the uptake of ^{131}I or $^{99}Tc^m$ may, however, be of value in the differential diagnosis of thyrotoxicosis (see below).

Tests of peripheral tissue function and associated laboratory abnormalities

A number of laboratory procedures have been developed in an attempt to quantitate the effects of thyroid hormones on various tissues. The most widely used have been basal metabolic rate, Achilles tendon reflex contraction and relaxation time, and cardiac systolic time interval. These tests are not, however, sufficiently sensitive or specific to be useful in the diagnosis of thyroid dysfunction.

A number of non-specific biochemical abnormalities are found in patients with thyroid disease. In hyperthyroidism they include hypercalcaemia, hypocholesterolaemia, increased serum sex-hormone binding globulin, decreased serum creatine phosphokinase, increased red blood cell glucose-6-phosphate dehydrogenase and carbonic anhydrase, and increased red cell sodium and zinc concentrations. Biochemical abnormalities which have been recorded in hypothyroidism include the widely recognised hyperlipidaemia as well as dilutional hyponatraemia and increases in serum aspartate transaminase, lactate dehydrogenase, creatine phosphokinase and serum magnesium; suppression of adrenal steroid production and the cortisol and growth hormone responses to hypoglycaemia may also occur. None of these changes specifically reflects an excess or deficiency of thyroid hormone and are of no diagnostic value; it is important, however, that the potential cause of these is recognised and the patient not subjected to unnecessary investigation prior to management of the thyroid problem.

Autoantibodies

Microsomal and thyroglobulin antibodies

Circulating antibodies to various thyroid components are found in patients with thyroid disease as well as in up to 15% of the normal female population and 5% of males. Specific antibodies against thyroid microsomal and thyroglobulin antigens are found in many patients with Graves' disease and Graves' ophthalmopathy, in their relatives and in patients who have histological Hashimoto's thyroiditis. Contrary to earlier reports there is probably little difference in the incidence of antibody to microsomal antigen when comparing Graves' and Hashimoto's diseases, and in both conditions antibody to thyroglobulin, though not uncommon, is found less frequently. Measurement of these antibodies is of no value in the biochemical diagnosis of thyroid dysfunction but gives an indication of the aetiology. Antibody tests are not useful in monitoring response to drug therapy or predicting relapse, although it has been suggested that subjects with negative tests for antibody are less likely to become hypothyroid after treatment for thyrotoxicosis.

Microsomal antibodies are directed against a lipoprotein in the membrane of vesicles containing newly synthesised thyroglobulin, and are usually IgG. They are cytotoxic in nature and are routinely detected by immunofluorescence or by a complement fixation technique. Thyroglobulin antibodies, which are usually IgG and are directed against normal thyroglobulin, may be detected by a number of techniques; these include precipitin tests, the more sensitive tanned erythrocyte agglutination test, immunofluorescence of fixed thyroid sections and an extremely sensitive competitive binding radioassay.

TSH receptor antibodies

The presence and titre of circulating antibodies to the TSH receptor can be detected by a number of different techniques, but these assays are not as yet generally available for the routine investigation of thyroid disease. Their presence may indicate the cause of the hyperthyroidism but is of no value in the biochemical assessment of the thyrotoxic state. Measurement of TSH receptor antibodies may be clinically useful in the following situations: the diagnosis of Graves' disease in the absence of eye signs; the diagnosis of ophthalmic Graves' disease; assessment of the risk of neonatal hyperthyroidism and possibly in the prediction of relapse of hyperthyroidism after a course of antithyroid drugs.

HYPERTHYROIDISM

Aetiology

Hyperthyroidism or thyrotoxicosis is the clinical syndrome that results from an excess of circulating thyroid hormones. The prevalence of overt hyperthyroidism in females is around 20/1000 and in males approximately 2/1000. The great majority of cases (>90%) are due to Graves' disease with diffuse hyperplasia and hypertrophy of the thyroid, or from toxic multinodular goitre (Plummer's disease) and toxic adenoma. Other causes have been described (Table 4.2) and are important to recognise as their clinical presentation, laboratory diagnosis, and treatment may differ substantially.

Graves' disease

Graves' disease is an autoimmune disorder of the thyroid producing a syndrome of hyperthyroidism, diffuse goitre, eye signs and occasionally localised myxoedema. It is a common disorder affecting females 5–10 times more frequently than males. Graves' disease occurs at all ages but peaks at 20–40 years of age (compared with toxic nodular

Table 4.2 Causes of hyperthyroidism

Graves' disease
Toxic nodular goitre:
   multinodular
   single toxic adenoma
Neonatal thyrotoxicosis
Jod-Basedow (exogenous iodide)
Thyroiditis
Inappropriate secretion of TSH by pituitary:
   tumour
   non-tumour
Choriocarcinoma and hydatidiform mole
Thyrotoxicosis factitia
Thyroid carcinoma
Struma ovarii
Embryonal testicular carcinoma

goitre which has a peak incidence between 40 and 70 years).

There is considerable evidence that Graves' disease is related to the presence of autoantibodies to the TSH receptor of the thyroid follicular cell. This was first demonstrated in studies of mice injected with serum from patients with Graves' disease. The prolonged time-course of the release of iodine from the thyroid led to the serum component being called a long-acting thyroid stimulator (LATS). Immunoglobulin IgG, prepared from the serum of patients with Graves' disease, activates adenylate cyclase and increases thyroid hormone production in the thyroid cell; it also inhibits binding of labelled TSH to the thyroid cell membrane. These characteristics have resulted in a number of descriptive terms being applied to such immunoglobulins including LATS, LATS-protector (defined as a serum component from LATS-negative patients with Graves' disease that inhibits the binding of LATS to human thyroid tissue), thyroid stimulating immunoglobulin (TSI) and TSH binding inhibitory immunoglobulin (TBII).

Clinical and immunological family studies have demonstrated a convincing familial predisposition to thyroid disease and thyrogastric autoimmunity (i.e. presence of thyroid and gastric autoantibodies) in patients with Graves' disease. The HLA associations (B8 and DW3) and the greater rate of concordance for Graves' disease among monozygotic twins (50% compared with 5% for dizygotic twins) indicates the importance of hereditary determinants.

Patients with certain genotypes may be predisposed to a defect in the response of suppressor T lymphocytes to thyroid antigen.

Toxic nodular goitre

Multinodular goitre (Plummer's disease)

A nodular goitre is often present in older patients with hyperthyroidism and eye signs are usually absent. Radioisotope imaging of the thyroid gland reveals one or more active nodules. Some subjects with a nodular goitre may have co-existing Graves' disease indicated by circulating thyroid or TSH receptor antibodies.

Single toxic nodule

Single autonomously functioning thyroid nodules are an uncommon cause of thyrotoxicosis (approximately 5%), again found in older patients (40–50 years). The diagnosis is suspected in hyperthyroid patients with a solitary or dominant nodule in an otherwise palpably normal thyroid gland. Radionuclide imaging confirms the presence of a single functioning nodule.

The aetiology of toxic nodular goitre is not known, but the disorder may form part of the spectrum of endemic or sporadic goitre.

Clinical features of hyperthyroidism

The onset of the disease is usually gradual over a period of months to years but occasionally is dramatic and florid. The diverse and numerous clinical features of hyperthyroidism are listed in Table 4.3, but the symptoms and signs which are present most commonly are palpitations, tiredness, heat intolerance, excessive sweating, nervousness, loss of weight, thyroid enlargement and tachycardia or atrial fibrillation.

The thyroid gland is usually, but not invariably, enlarged. It is characteristically diffusely enlarged in Graves' disease but may be asymmetrical and nodular in cases of toxic nodular goitre. Increased vascularity is an important sign of thyroid overactivity and is best demonstrated as a systolic bruit. Cardiac rate and cardiac output rise and, in addition to palpitations and exercise intolerance, the patient may develop tachyarrhythmias. Ten to 15% of

Table 4.3 Clinical features of hyperthyroidism

General	Weight loss
	Fatigue, irritability
	Sweating, heat intolerance
Cardiovascular	Palpitations, dyspnoea, angina
	Sinus tachycardia, atrial fibrillation
	Collapsing pulse
	Cardiac failure
Neuromuscular	Nervousness, agitation, psychosis
	Tremor
	Muscle weakness, proximal myopathy
	Periodic paralysis
	Myasthenia gravis
Gastrointestinal	Vomiting
	Diarrhoea, steatorrhoea
Reproductive	Oligomenorrhoea
	Infertility
Skin	Itching
	Palmar erythema
	Pretibial myoedema
Goitre	Diffuse ±bruit
	Nodular
Ocular	Lid retraction, lid lag
	Periorbital puffiness
	Chemosis
	Proptosis, corneal ulceration
	Ophthalmoplegia, diplopia
	Papilloedema, loss of visual acuity

patients have atrial fibrillation; 60% of these revert to sinus rhythm when euthyroidism is restored. Cardiac failure is uncommon except in the elderly, when it may be a presenting feature.

Most patients with thyrotoxicosis show mild ocular involvement, usually lid lag and lid retraction, with little or no proptosis (Fig. 4.1). Occasionally,

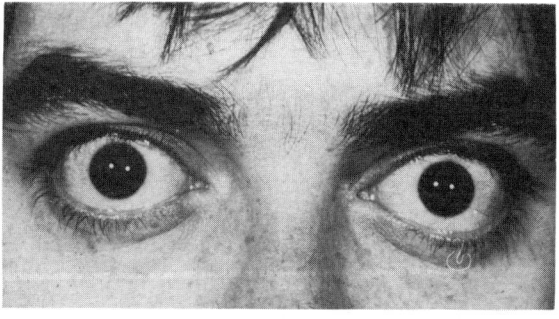

Fig. 4.1 Eye involvement in thyrotoxicosis. Lid retraction is seen.

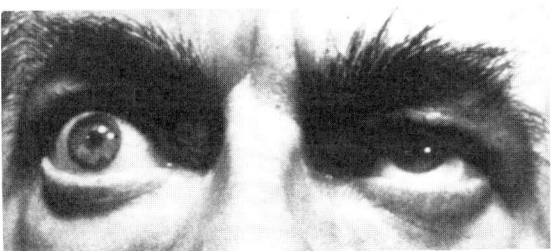

Fig. 4.2 Unilateral restriction of upward gaze in Graves' disease.

however, in Graves' disease the involvement is more severe with swelling of the retrobulbar tissues, lymphocytic infiltration and later fibrosis and contractures that restrict the mobility of the extraocular muscles (ophthalmoplegia) (Fig. 4.2). The swollen retrobulbar tissues tend to push the eye forwards causing proptosis and if the pressure in the retrobulbar space increases markedly, impairment of orbital venous drainage and optic nerve function with papilloedema may result. Oedema accumulates in periorbital tissues, eyelids and conjunctivae. As proptosis progresses the eye is pushed forward from the protective coverage of the lids; the patient acquires a staring expression and a gritty sensation in the eye due to corneal drying. Exposure keratitis and even corneal ulceration may result. Severe exophthalmos is usually, but not invariably, bilateral.

The term 'ophthalmic' Graves' disease is used to describe patients with the ocular manifestations of the disease in the absence of hyperthyroidism or a past history of hyperthyroidism. Eye signs are more often asymmetrical, ophthalmoplegia is commoner, the patients tend to be older and a goitre is present in one-third of patients. A sensitive TSH measurement or TSH response to TRH is abnormal in about 75% of patients and in a similar number thyroglobulin or microsomal autoantibodies can be detected. Antibodies directed against the TSH receptor are present in about one half of these subjects.

Localised myxoedema occurs in about 5% of patients with Graves' disease and the swelling is characteristically pretibial in site. The face, feet and toes are sometimes affected. The skin is coarse, purplish-red in colour and often tender due to infiltration of superficial layers with the

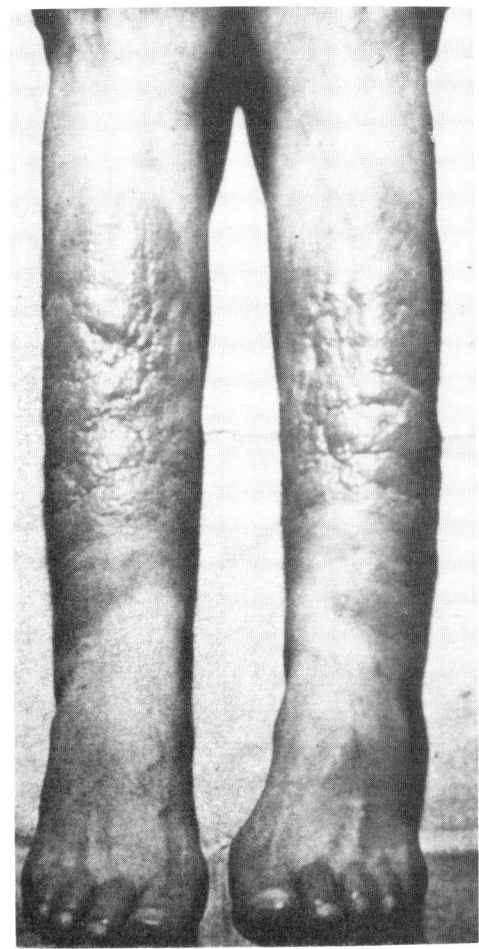

Fig. 4.3 Pretibial myxoedema

mucopolysaccharide hyaluronic acid (Fig. 4.3). Pretibial myxoedema is usually associated with high titres of TSH receptor antibodies and is said to develop particularly after radioiodine or surgical treatment for hyperthyroidism. Thyroid acropachy is clubbing associated with Graves' disease and resembles hypertrophic pulmonary osteoarthropathy.

T3-toxicosis results from an excess of circulating T3 without an increase in T4. The frequency of T3-toxicosis varies in different areas and in some parts of the world (particularly iodine-deficient areas) the syndrome is thought to account for 10–15% of cases of hyperthyroidism. In the UK the figure is probably less than 5%. Any variety of hyperthyroidism may be associated with T3-toxicosis, but it seems to be more common in patients with autonomous thyroid nodules, as an early finding in Graves' disease and in recurrences following surgical or radioiodine therapy.

Thyroid storm or crisis is a sudden life-threatening acceleration of the disease, fortunately uncommon, with accentuation of the symptoms and signs of hyperthyroidism accompanied by fever and tachycardia. In most cases hyperthyroidism is known to exist and a precipitating cause can be identified such as thyroidectomy in an inadequately prepared patient, rarely ^{131}I administration, or concurrent severe illness. The condition has a significant mortality and the patient may lapse rapidly into cardiac failure, delirium, stupor or coma.

Neonatal thyrotoxicosis is a rare condition which occurs only in infants born to mothers who are, or who have been, thyrotoxic. The condition is believed to arise from transplacental passage from the maternal circulation of thyroid stimulating antibodies which stimulate the fetal thyroid gland. The onset of hyperthyroidism may be dramatic and death may occur if the condition is recognised late. Affected babies have goitre, exophthalmos, feeding problems, pyrexia, tachycardia, failure to gain weight and may go into cardiac failure. The hyperthyroidism is self-limiting over a period of 2–3 months as the acquired maternal immunoglobulins disappear from the neonatal circulation, at which stage treatment can be withdrawn.

Diagnosis of hyperthyroidism

The diagnosis is usually made on clinical grounds initially but should always be confirmed by the appropriate biochemical tests (Table 4.4).

Treatment of hyperthyroidism

Satisfactory treatment of hyperthyroidism is achieved by one of three standard forms of therapy:

1. Medical
2. Radioactive iodine (^{131}I)
3. Surgical.

The decision as to which form of therapy to offer the patient may be somewhat arbitrary depending on such factors as patient or physician preference, age, employment and local circumstances, e.g. availability of ^{131}I, experience of surgeons. The majority of patients are, however, treated with antithyroid drugs, or radioiodine. Each method has its own indications and disadvantages and these will be discussed in general outline.

Medical treatment

All patients with hyperthyroidism will respond to antithyroid medication, but in certain instances medical therapy is positively recommended; in children and in pregnant women as well as in other young patients presenting with Graves' disease for the first time, medical therapy is the treatment of choice. Hyperthyroidism due to Graves' disease is self-limiting in some patients and thus long term medical treatment may enable the disease to be controlled until a spontaneous natural remission occurs. Patients with single toxic nodules or multinodular goitres should not be treated medically long-term in the hope of achieving cure, because relapse will almost invariably follow

Table 4.4 Diagnosis of hyperthyroidism

Serum thyroid hormones	Measurement of total and/or free T4 Measurement of total and/or free T3 essential in the diagnosis of T3-toxicosis)
Serum TSH	Undetectable in thyrotoxicosis
Radioisotope uptake tests	For specific indications only e.g. in suspected thyroiditis or thyrotoxicosis factitia
Microsomal and thyroglobulin antibodies	Of no diagnostic value but may indicate aetiology
TSH receptor antibodies	Not routinely available. May indicate aetiology of hyperthyroidism

drug withdrawal. The duration of treatment in Graves' disease is arbitrary but most patients are maintained in a euthyroid state for 9–12 months. The two most widely used drugs are carbimazole and propylthiouracil and they are administered in high dose initially (carbimazole 30–60 mg/day or propylthiouracil 300–600 mg/day). When the patient is euthyroid the dosage is reduced gradually to maintenance levels (carbimazole 5–15 mg/day or propylthiouracil 50–150 mg/day). Traditionally these antithyroid drugs have been administered in divided doses during the day but recent evidence suggests that a single dose of the full daily requirement is probably adequate and should lead to increased compliance. Carbimazole is converted in the body to its active metabolite, methimazole, which is the favoured drug in North America. The main disadvantage of medical therapy is that less than 40% of patients receiving an adequate course of antithyroid drugs remain in remission after drug withdrawal. It is possible that longer periods of high-dose treatment in combination with thyroid hormone replacement may improve remission rates, which may be related to inhibitory effects of the drugs on thyroid autoantibody synthesis. Some centres routinely use a blocking/replacement regimen of carbimazole 30 mg daily along with thyroxine 150 μg daily. Unfortunately there is as yet no reliable predictor of relapse of Graves' disease after discontinuation of antithyroid therapy.

Both groups of antithyroid drugs produce the same sensitivity and toxic side-effects. Skin rashes (maculopapular and itchy) are common and arthralgia, jaundice, lymphadenopathy, nausea, vomiting or pyrexia may occur. These effects are transient and usually respond to antihistamines without withdrawing the antithyroid drug. Sensitivity to one group of drugs is seldom shown to the other so if side-effects are troublesome the patient can be switched to the alternative drug. The only dangerous but uncommon toxic effect (1/1000 patients) is granulocytosis. The patient should be warned to discontinue the drug and to report at once should mouth ulcers or a sore throat develop. The suppression of granulocyte production is temporary and if the drug is stopped granulocytes reappear in the circulation within 1–2 weeks. Sensitivity and toxic effects of the antithyroid drugs are usually seen within 2 months of starting treatment after

which these drugs appear extremely safe. Monitoring of disease response to antithyroid drugs is normally achieved by measurement of circulating T4 or free T4. Serum TSH concentration may be undetectable and TSH response to TRH absent for some months after restoration of euthyroidism, therefore these tests may be misleading.

Many of the symptoms of hyperthyroidism are ameliorated by the use of β-adrenergic blocking agents. Propranolol (40 mg 3 or 4 times daily) is the most widely used agent and produces a fall in the pulse rate and a reduction of tremor, anxiety, heat intolerance and sweating in most patients. Propranolol optimally requires 6-hourly administration but there is now experience which demonstrates that longer acting β-blockers such as nadolol are also useful. Propranolol blocks the peripheral adrenergic effects seen in hyperthyroidism but has no direct effect on thyroidal secretion of thyroid hormones; although the drug reduces the peripheral conversion of T4 to T3 (with a consequent rise in reverse T3) this is not clinically relevant. Although β-adrenergic blocking drugs can be extremely useful in controlling symptoms, preparing patients for surgery and managing thyroid crisis, it must be emphasised that these agents are simply useful adjuncts to definitive antithyroid therapy.

Radioactive iodine therapy

Radioiodine therapy is an extremely effective method of treating hyperthyroidism and can be administered with the minimum of disruption to the patient's activities. Radioactive iodine acts by destroying functioning thyroid cells or by inhibiting their ability to replicate. The main disadvantage of radioiodine therapy is that too high a dose will render the patient hypothyroid and too low a dose leaves the patient hyperthyroid. Although the amount of radiation given to the gland depends on the dose of radioiodine given, the proportion of dose taken up by the thyroid, and the gland size, the radiosensitivity of the gland is variable and cannot be measured. Thus, most centres have now abandoned attempts to tailor the dose of ^{131}I to individual requirements and select an arbitrary dose of 3–8 mCi [131]I. It may take some weeks for the ^{131}I to produce a clinical effect and, in the interim, an antithyroid drug or propranolol may aid control. A period of about 6 months is usually allowed to lapse before a repeat dose is administered for uncontrolled hyperthyroidism.

The main consequence of ^{131}I therapy is the subsequent development of hypothyroidism. Ten to 15% of patients become hypothyroid within 2 years and thereafter a continued incidence of 2–3% a year is observed. As many as 30% of patients require a second dose because of uncontrolled hyperthyroidism and a few require a third or even fourth. It is therefore essential that all patients are followed indefinitely. Some groups prefer to give a standard large dose of 15 mCi of ^{131}I which results in control of hyperthyroidism in at least 80% of patients at 3 months, the majority of whom become hypothyroid within 6 months of therapy. Treatment with thyroxine can then be instituted on a planned basis and the patient rendered euthyroid and discharged from follow-up.

The use of radioiodine has been questioned on three grounds: carcinogenesis and leukaemogenesis, genetic damage and fetal damage; in the past many physicians have restricted the use of ^{131}I to postmenopausal women because of these questions. Forty years of use and two very large studies of the followup of patients (59 999 and 36 000 patients studied) have failed to produce any evidence of an excess of thyroid cancer, leukaemia or cancer in general. The genetic risk is theoretical and unsubstantiated but the fetal risks are potentially serious and pregnancy must be avoided by women who have just been treated with radioiodine, and radioiodine must not be given to pregnant women.

Indications for radioiodine treatment vary from clinic to clinic. Clear cut indications include relapse after partial thyroidectomy, severe disease in older patients and patients with toxic multinodular goitre or single toxic nodules. The latter patients may require a higher dose of [131]Iodine (15–30 mCi) to control hyperthyroidism. Radioiodine is now being administered with increasing frequency and in some centres is given routinely to young patients.

Surgical treatment

Partial thyroidectomy is the treatment of choice for hyperthyroid patients with large goitres. Surgical treatment may also be indicated for younger patients (less than 40 years) who have relapsed after medical therapy for Graves' disease, in centres with a cautious approach to radioiodine usage. Surgery aims to cure hyperthyroidism by removing the bulk of functioning thyroid tissue and offers prompt and effective control with little risk of complications.

At the end of the first year following surgery some 80% of patients are euthyroid, 15% are permanently hypothyroid, and 5% have relapsed. The incidence of postoperative hypothyroidism may reach 30% over a 10-year period but is not directly related to the amount of tissue removed. Thyroid function following thyroidectomy is difficult to assess and the incidence of postoperative hypothyroidism has been overestimated in the past because it was not appreciated that the thyroid failure might be temporary. Hypoparathyroidism or damage to the recurrent laryngeal nerve are rarely seen.

The patient should be rendered euthyroid before surgery and this has been achieved traditionally by the use of antithyroid drugs for 4–8 weeks followed by potassium iodine for 7–10 days. In recent years a number of studies have shown that propranolol alone is an effective alternative if administered regularly.

Treatment of thyroid crisis or storm

Emergency treatment is required consisting of standard antithyroid drugs in large doses, iodine in the form of Lugol's iodine or sodium or potassium iodide, propranolol given orally or intravenously and dexamethasone. General supportive measures include parenteral fluids, digoxin for cardiac failure, diuretics and oxygen therapy. The mortality from this condition remains high.

Treatment of Graves' ophthalmopathy

In most patients with Graves' disease no treatment is required for the eyes and lid retraction improves as the patient becomes euthyroid. In patients with symptomatic ophthalmopathy three lines of therapy are available:

1. Eye drops: methyl cellulose to counter grittiness of the eyes due to corneal drying, guanethidine

which may improve lid retraction and steroid for chemosis and periorbital oedema.

2. Oral corticosteroids in high dose (prednisolone 60–100 mg daily) when the ophthalmopathy is progressive; deterioration of vision due to optic nerve compression is an indication for immediate steroid therapy.

3. Surgery; tarsorrhaphy to protect corneal exposure resulting from lid retraction and proptosis and decompression of the orbit for severe progressive ophthalmopathy which is unresponsive to steroid therapy.

Treatment of localised myxoedema

No treatment is required if the myxoedema (usually pretibial) is asymptomatic. Nightly application of locally active steroid creams under occlusive dressings may relieve discomfort and pain, and occasionally local infiltration with steroids is required for resistant areas.

Treatment of hyperthyroidism in pregnancy and the neonatal period
See below.

Subacute thyroiditis (de Quervain's)

Subacute thyroiditis is an acute, subacute or chronic non-bacterial inflammation of the thyroid of unknown aetiology; an acute viral illness may be the cause. Characteristic histological findings include lymphocytic infiltration, giant cells and granulomas. The condition is thought to be uncommon in the UK and other parts of Europe, but is seen with greater frequency in North America. The characteristic early clinical presentation is with fever, malaise, anorexia, dysphagia and thyroidal pain. The thyroid gland is enlarged and tender with the pain typically radiating to the jaw or ear. In at least 50% of cases a transient hypermetabolic state suggestive of thyrotoxicosis occurs, resulting from release of thyroglobulin and excessive amounts of T4 and T3. Unlike classical thyrotoxicosis, however, the radioiodine uptake of the gland is very low. The thyrotoxic state soon remits spontaneously and a euthyroid state ensues. The thyroiditis should therefore be treated symptomatically with analgesics and β adrenergic blockade and not with antithyroid drugs. These are ineffective since the hyperthyroid phase is due to excessive release of stored hormone, with no change in hormone synthesis. In severe cases a reducing course of steroids may cause rapid symptomatic relief. In some patients transient hypothyroidism occurs, but complete recovery of normal thyroid function takes place in most patients over a period of weeks or months.

A 'silent' form of subacute thyroiditis has been recognised which may be responsible for up to 15% of all cases of hyperthyroidism in North America. The history is usually short and eye signs are absent, but otherwise it produces the clinical and biochemical picture of hyperthyroidism without local pain or tenderness, or pyrexia. This presentation can lead to diagnostic confusion and inappropriate treatment; since the condition usually remits spontaneously, destructive therapy of the thyroid is clearly to be avoided. This situation remains one of the few indications for a radioisotope uptake test of thyroid function. The nature of this condition and its relation to autoimmune thyroid disease is not understood. A mild transient increase in circulating thyroid autoantibodies is seen and some of the histological features (e.g. lymphocytic infiltration) are common to subacute thyroiditis, Hashimoto's thyroiditis and Graves' disease.

Jod-Basedow phenomenon

This refers to the occurrence of hyperthyroidism after iodine administration to a goitrous patient from an area of endemic iodine deficiency. This effect occurs more frequently in patients with thyroid autoantibodies or autonomous thyroid nodules.

Choriocarcinoma and hydatidiform mole

A small proportion of patients with choriocarcinoma or hydatidiform mole develop hyperthyroidism. The clinical features of the disease are similar to those of Graves' disease, although goitre and eye signs are usually absent. It has been shown that the thyroid stimulating factor in this condition is human chorionic gonadotrophin and treatment of the underlying disease by surgery or chemotherapy results in remission of hyperthyroidism.

Thyrotoxicosis factitia

This is thyrotoxicosis due to ingestion of excessive quantities of exogenous thyroid hormones; it usually represents a symptom of a personality disorder. The diagnosis should be suspected in patients with high serum thyroid hormone concentrations, in association with low thyroidal uptake of ^{131}I; it may be difficult to differentiate from silent thyroiditis.

Struma ovarii

Ovarian teratoma containing ectopic thyroid tissue are rare; hyperthyroidism due to function of such ectopic tissue is even more rare. The diagnosis may be indicated by the presence of ectopic thyroid tissue within the pelvis on ^{131}I scanning.

Metastatic thyroid carcinoma

Although cells of follicular thyroid carcinoma may concentrate iodine and synthesise thyroglobulin, thyrotoxicosis is rare. Thyrotoxicosis normally occurs in patients with metastatic disease.

Inappropriate secretion of TSH

Inappropriate secretion of TSH is rare and is diagnosed in patients in whom the basal and/or TRH-stimulated concentration of serum TSH is elevated in the presence of raised serum concentrations of free thyroid hormones. In conventional hyperthyroidism serum TSH levels are suppressed so that patients in whom free serum thyroid hormones are elevated, but in whom TSH is detectable, can be considered to have inappropriate TSH secretion. These patients should be classified depending on whether a pituitary tumour is present. Pituitary tumours associated with hypersecretion of TSH and hyperthyroidism have been rarely described. In general, neoplastic production of TSH is autonomous, i.e. unresponsive to TRH stimulation or thyroid hormone suppression. In this situation elevated circulating levels of a-subunit may help in the diagnosis of tumorous secretion of TSH. Hyperthyroidism responds to pituitary surgery. The syndrome of inappropriate TSH secretion caused by an autonomous thyrotroph adenoma can be easily distinguished from the 'thyrotroph feedback adenoma', which occurs occa-

sionally in the face of longstanding, severe primary hypothyroidism. In the latter both TSH levels and adenoma size respond appropriately to adequate T4 replacement therapy.

Hypersecretion of TSH from pituitary glands in which no neoplasm can be detected has been described in hyperthyroid and euthyroid subjects with elevated serum thyroid hormone concentrations. These patients have varying degrees of tissue resistance to the action of thyroid hormones. Several cases have been described in which inappropriate TSH secretion appears to be caused by a selective anterior pituitary resistance to the action of thyroid hormones; in these patients pituitary hypersecretion of TSH leads to overstimulation of the thyroid and overt hyperthyroidism. Treatment with dopamine agonists has been described. More recently a familial syndrome of hyperthyroidism caused by non-adenomatous TSH secretion has been described in which there may be defective intrapituitary monodeiodination of T4 to T3. Hyperthyroidism and TSH levels responded to T3 administration.

Differential diagnosis of hyperthyroxinaemia

Occasionally a raised serum T4 is found in a patient who appears clinically euthyroid. In clinical practice the commonest cause of falsely raised total T4 is a high serum concentration of TBG, most commonly seen in pregnancy, due to oestrogen containing contraceptive pills, or on a hereditary basis. The serum T3 will also be increased in these patients but the free T4 and free T3 measurements will be normal.

In true hyperthyroidism a raised serum T4 level is usually accompanied by a high serum T3 concentration, but so-called T4-toxicosis may occur in patients with associated non-thyroidal illnesses where serum T3 levels are normal or low, due to impaired conversion of T4 to T3.

A syndrome of familial dysalbuminaemic hyperthyroidism has been described. This is an autosomal dominant condition which causes a structural alteration in albumin, which has a high affinity for T4. Clinically the subjects are euthyroid and the TSH response to TRH is normal as are serum T3 concentrations. Occasionally the raised serum T4 is due to increased binding to TBPA.

Other causes of hyperthyroxinaemia include endogenous antibodies to T4 (which interfere with the radioimmunoassay of thyroid hormones), amiodarone therapy, and radiographic contrast reagents. Heparin causes a transient increase in free T4 and a lesser increase in total T4. The spontaneous occurrence of antibodies to T4 and T3 in man may not be a rare phenomenon.

HYPOTHYROIDISM

Aetiology

Hypothyroidism is divided into primary thyroid disease and disease secondary to abnormality of the pituitary or hypothalamus. Primary hypothyroidism is confirmed by the presence of an increase in serum TSH concentration. In clinical practice, primary hypothyroidism is most commonly caused by autoimmune thyroid disease (Hashimoto's thyroiditis) or by treatment of hyperthyroidism with radioactive iodine or partial thyroidectomy. The various causes of hypothyroidism are listed in Table 4.5. The prevalence of overt hypothyroidism in the UK, defined on clinical criteria and confirmed by low levels of serum thyroxine with raised TSH levels, is 14 per 1000 females and less than 1 per 1000 males.

Hashimoto's thyroiditis

Hashimoto's disease is characteristically found in

Table 4.5 Causes of hypothyroidism

Primary thyroid failure
  Autoimmune thyroiditis (Hashimoto's)
  Radioactive iodine, external irradiation
  Postoperative
  Antithyroid drugs
  Iodine deficiency
  Subacute thyroiditis
  Dyshormonogenesis
  Agenesis
  Infiltrative disease
  Idiopathic atrophy

Secondary to pituitary/hypothalamic disease

women aged between 30 and 60 who present with a small or moderate-sized goitre of 2–4 years duration and who have thyroid function tests which are normal or borderline hypothyroid. Histological examination of the thyroid reveals diffuse lymphocytic infiltration with lymphoid follicles and plasma cells and in some instances fibrosis and disruption of thyroid follicles. Patients have low levels of thyroglobulin antibodies detected by sensitive tests, but high levels of microsomal antibodies are invariably present.

Autoimmune thyroiditis is one of a group of organ-specific autoimmune diseases including pernicious anaemia, insulin-dependent diabetes mellitus, Addison's disease, idiopathic hypoparathyroidism, premature ovarian failure and

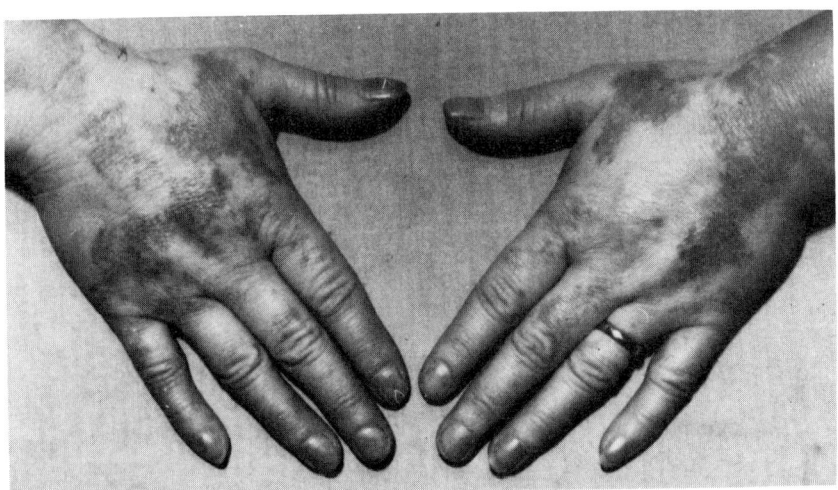

Fig. 4.4 Vitiligo of the hands occurring in association with Hashimoto's thyroiditis.

gravis. A feature of these conditions is the presence of specific antibodies directed against a constituent of the particular organ, e.g. antibodies to gastric parietal cells, adrenal cortex, ovary and pancreatic islets. Vitiligo, consisting of patchy areas of depigmentation of the skin surrounded by areas of increased pigmentation, is a common association (Fig. 4.4). In addition, thyroiditis is related to non-organ specific diseases with an autoimmune aetiology such as systemic lupus erythematosus, rheumatoid arthritis and Sjögren's syndrome. All of these diseases have a marked female preponderance.

Clinical features of hypothyroidism

Hypothyroidism has many different presentations and the patient is often unaware of any disorder. The symptoms, because of their non-specific and vague nature, are often attributed to non-organic causes and may be present for years before the diagnosis is made. A past history of treatment to the thyroid with radioactive iodine or surgery is important to elicit as is a family history of thyroid disease or autoimmune disorders. Symptoms characteristically include lack of energy, cold intolerance, dryness of skin and hair, weight gain, constipation, hoarseness of voice and generalised muscle aches and pains. Changes in facial appearance (Fig. 4.5), anaemia, bradycardia, and psychiatric disturbances may be apparent (Table 4.6). Anaemia is multifactorial in origin but the commonest abnormality is macrocytosis without evidence of folic acid or vitamin B_{12} deficiency. Autoimmune pernicious anaemia may coexist but true iron deficiency is rare.

Myxoedema coma

The most serious complication of hypothyroidism is myxoedema coma, which, although rare, has a mortality of about 50%. Older patients living in poorly heated houses are particularly at risk. Hypothermia is present in over 80% of patients, but myxoedema coma accounts for less than 20% of patients admitted to hospital with hypothermia. It may develop insidiously or be precipitated abruptly by drugs such as phenothiazines, narcotics and anaesthetics, as well as by infections. Myxoedema

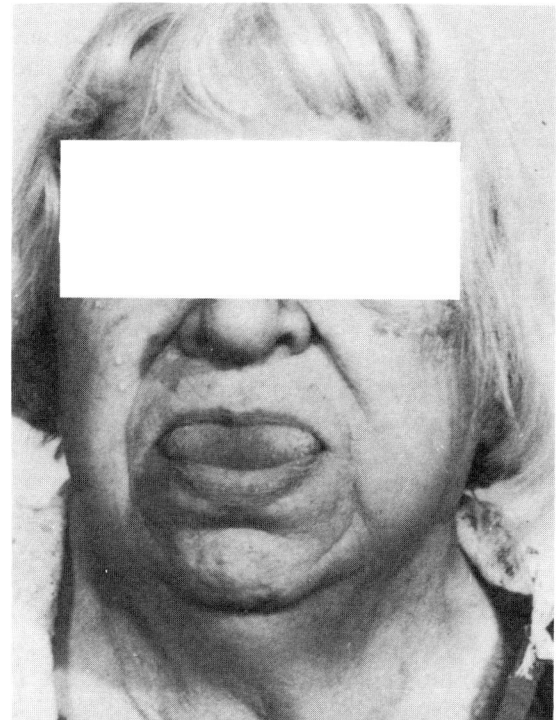

Fig. 4.5 Facial appearance in hypothyroidism.

Table 4.6 Clinical features of hypothyroidism

General	Tiredness
	Weight gain
	Cold intolerance
	Goitre
Cardiovascular	Bradycardia
	Angina
	Cardiac failure
	Pericardial effusion
Neuromuscular	Aches and pains
	Carpal tunnel syndrome
	Deafness
	Hoarseness
	Ataxia
	Delayed relaxation of tendon reflexes
	Depression, psychosis
Haematological	Anaemia — iron deficiency, pernicious, normochromic normocytic
Dermatological	Dry skin
	Myxoedema
	Erythema ab igne
	Vitiligo
Reproductive	Infertility
	Menorrhagia
	Galactorrhoea
Gastrointestinal	Constipation

Table 4.7 Diagnosis of hypothyroidism

Serum thyroid hormones	Measurement of total and/or free T4
	Measurement of total and/or free T3
	  not useful in routine investigation
	  may be normal in early hypothyroidism
	  may be reduced due to non-thyroidal illness

Serum TSH	A rise confirms primary hypothyroidism
Radioisotope uptake tests	Have no part to play
Thyroid antibodies	Of no diagnostic value but may indicate aetiology
Hypothalamic/pituitary function	If secondary hypothyroidism diagnosed proceed to skull X-ray, CT scan and combined pituitary stimulation test. (Enlargement of pituitary fossa may result from longstanding primary hypothyroidism

coma is a medical emergency requiring urgent treatment.

Diagnosis of hypothyroidism

The diagnosis of hypothyroidism may be clear on clinical grounds, but laboratory tests should be performed to confirm the diagnosis (Table 4.7).

Treatment of hypothyroidism

All patients with symptomatic hypothyroidism require therapy with thyroid hormone. This was originally administered in the form of thyroid extract containing a mixture of T4 and T3 but has now been superseded by pure synthetic T4. There is no indication for combined preparations of any sort. Although for many years the accepted dose of thyroxine for replacement therapy was in excess of 200 μg daily, the introduction of radioimmunoassays for thyroxine demonstrated that serum total T4 measurements in many patients were in the hyperthyroid range. At present the usual dose of thyroxine lies between 100 and 200 μg daily and the majority of patients are controlled on 150 μg per day. Patients with ischaemic heart disease may be unable to tolerate full replacement doses because of palpitations, angina, heart failure and even myocardial infarction. In such patients it is reasonable to start at a low dose (e.g. 25 or 50 μg daily) and increase slowly whilst monitoring the patient's symptoms. In most patients there is no obvious beneficial effect of a graded dose commencement of therapy. Because of the long half-life of T4 (7 days in the euthyroid subject), it is unnecessary to administer the tablets in divided doses.

Even on the conventional dose of 100–200 μg thyroxine per day, serum T4 concentrations (total or free) may still exceed the conventional upper limit of the normal range; this elevation is not an absolute indication for reduction in dose. Compliance with therapy and adequacy of dose should be checked by measurement of serum TSH which should be restored to the normal range.

Treatment of myxoedema coma

Myxoedema coma requires prompt treatment with thyroid hormone, but the correct method of hormone replacement is unclear. Thyroxine (400–500 μg) may be given as a bolus intravenous injection or by intragastric administration. Alternatively, small doses of T3 (20 μg twice daily intramuscularly) with 50 μg T4 daily orally may be used. Supportive therapy with steroids is recommended along with glucose infusions to correct the hypoglycaemia present in many patients. Assisted ventilation may be required, infection must be treated vigorously with antibiotics and rewarming should be undertaken cautiously by exposure to normal ambient room temperature.

Subclinical hypothyroidism

Thyroid failure is a graded phenomenon and the recognition of minor degrees of hypothyroidism may be difficult, since subjects with mild hypothyroidism may have trivial and generally non-specific symptoms. Subclinical hypothyroidism or 'compensated hypothyroidism' has been defined as an asymptomatic state in which reduced thyroid activity has been compensated by an increased TSH output to maintain a euthyroid state. Such patients have normal conventional tests of thyroid function with an elevated basal serum TSH level and/or an exaggerated rise in serum TSH following TRH administration. An alternative explanation for the finding of normal total (and free) thyroid hormone levels in combination with high TSH is that circulating thyroid hormone measurements may not accurately reflect intrapituitary hormone concentrations. Intrapituitary T3 is derived from both serum T3 and the deiodination of T4 to T3, and thus local regulatory mechanisms may play a part in the control of pituitary TSH secretion. The abnormalities of thyroid/pituitary function can be restored to normal by administration of thyroid hormone, although the need for therapy in these asymptomatic patients remains to be proved.

Neonatal hypothyroidism

In the newborn, thyroid hormone deficiency results in impaired brain development and mental retardation. This can be prevented if thyroid hormone therapy is initiated prior to two months of age. Maternal thyroid hormones and TSH do not cross the placenta, but many drugs including iodides, lithium and antithyroid agents do enter the fetal circulation and can induce goitre and hypothyroidism.

Neonatal hypothyroidism is a significant problem occurring in 1/3500–4000 infants in the UK (a prevalence 3–4 times that of phenylketonuria). Less than 5% of infants are diagnosed clinically and therefore neonatal screening is essential. Screening is carried out on the blood samples taken on the filter-paper strips which are used for the detection of phenylketonuria. Most screening programmes employ a T4 assay, followed by a TSH assay in patients with low-normal values (as in North America), or TSH assay alone (as in Europe). TSH concentrations in cord blood are significantly higher than in maternal blood; after birth there is a further sharp increase, reaching peak values within the first two hours of life which are many times higher than basal TSH levels. The rapid rise of TSH is followed by a relatively fast decline at first, approaching cord blood levels after 24 hours and normal adult basal values by the second day of life. TSH assay 5–7 days after birth has proved most satisfactory for mass-screening programmes. It does not, however, allow the detection of hypo-thalamo-pituitary hypothyroidism, TBG deficiency and other disorders associated with low T4 values, all of which are rare.

Alterations in tests of thyroid function in non-thyroidal illnesses

A number of abnormalities of standard thyroid function tests are seen in patients with a wide variety of non-thyroidal illnesses (NTI), amongst which a fall in serum T3 and an increase in reverse T3 (rT3) are the most common. This 'low T3 syndrome' has been estimated to be present in as many as 50–70% of hospitalised patients. The changes are due to a combination of reduced T3 production and decreased rT3 clearance rate apparently consequent on a reduction in activity of the enzyme 5'-monodeiodinase. In addition to these changes the serum T4 may also be altered in NTI. A low serum total T4 is especially common in severely ill patients and is correlated with the severity of the illness and subsequent mortality. Thyroxine secretion from the thyroid appears to be normal or only slightly decreased and several studies have suggested that the main cause of the low serum T4 is an abnormality in the binding of T4 by serum proteins. There is considerable uncertainty over what true free T4 levels are since the serum free T4 concentration measured by equilibrium dialysis is normal or high, the FTI and T4:TBG ratio give subnormal values in many cases, whilst commercial kits for measuring free T4 have normal or low values. In patients with NTI serum TSH concentration is typically normal but why this should be so in the face of markedly reduced serum levels and production rates of the most active hormone, T3, is not clear. It is apparent that many factors, including increased glucocorticoid levels and caloric deprivation, which are commonly present in NTI, may suppress TSH secretion and thus a normal serum TSH may not always be an entirely reliable index for euthyroidism in NTI.

Renal disease presents a particularly difficult problem since reduced serum T4 and T3 concentrations and an exaggerated but delayed TSH response to TRH may be seen in apparently euthyroid individuals. Reverse T3 concentrations are elevated, but measurement of rT3 is not routinely available. Euthyroid patients with hepatic cirrhosis may also have moderately elevated serum TSH values.

In view of these alterations in thyroid physiology and thyroid function tests in NTI, it is clear that the diagnosis of intrinsic thyroid dysfunction can be difficult. Until the condition is better understood and specific tests of tissue thyroid status become available, the low T4 state of illness should be differentiated from primary hypothyroidism by an elevated serum TSH in the latter. Hypothalamic and pituitary lesions may need to be excluded by a TRH test in those patients where there is a strong clinical suspicion of hypothyroidism and a low total or free T4 measurement, but a normal TSH level. The documentation of a high free T3 concentration and an absent TSH response to TRH should help establish the diagnosis of hyperthyroidism, although severely ill thyrotoxic patients may have normal serum T3 and T4 concentrations.

Drugs affecting thyroid function tests

Few of the drugs that affect transport, distribution and metabolism of thyroid hormones lead to permanent alteration in thyroid function or significant changes in metabolic status. The important mechanisms by which drugs affect thyroid function tests are 1. change in the concentration of serum binding proteins (oestrogens, androgens), 2. inhibition of hormone binding to serum proteins (phenytoin, salicylates, fenclofenac, clofibrate, heparin) and 3. alteration of peripheral thyroxine metabolism (phenytoin, carbamazepine, phenobarbitone, propranolol, glucocorticoids, amiodarone). Measurement of thyroid hormones in patients taking these and other drugs may not accurately reflect thyroid status. For example, both free T4 and free T3 measurements may be below the defined normal range in apparently euthyroid subjects taking phenytoin. Amiodarone, which is a potent antiarrhythmic agent, is also of interest because of its extensive use in the treatment of cardiac arrhythmias and angina pectoris, and because of the high incidence of associated abnormal thyroid function tests. The drug contains 37.2% iodine by weight. Doses of amiodarone between 200–600 mg daily increase total T4, free T4 and reverse T3; T3 levels are lowered but TSH secretion is unaltered. The mechanism of these changes is unclear but the drug would appear to block peripheral conversion of T4 to T3. Although uncommon, clinically overt hyperthyroidism and hypothyroidism may occur.

Thyroid disease and pregnancy

The changes in thyroid function during pregnancy are complex and difficulties in diagnosis and management may occur.

1. Goitre is common in pregnant women (up to 70% in some studies) and its frequency and severity are dependent on the iodine status of the community. A relative iodine deficiency state develops during pregnancy due to losses to the fetus and increased iodine clearance.

2. Oestrogens stimulate hepatic synthesis of TBG and cause a marked rise in serum TBG concentration in later pregnancy; thus serum total T4 and total T3 concentrations are increased. This rise in the levels of total hormones together with the increase in basal metabolic rate which is characteristic of pregnancy may lead to the inappropriate diagnosis of hyperthyroidism. Free thyroid hormone concentrations are normal during the first two trimesters of pregnancy and fall during the third. TSH concentrations are largely unchanged.

3. In normal pregnancy maternal IgG crosses the placenta and is detectable in the fetal and neonatal circulation. Antibodies to the TSH receptor may thus cross the placenta and stimulate the fetal thyroid causing intra-uterine and neonatal thyrotoxicosis. This is a rare condition, but it is important to recognise that such maternal antibodies may persist for many years even after thyroidectomy or treatment with radioiodine. Serum concentrations of thyroid-stimulating immunoglobulins should be checked in

the third trimester of pregnancy in women with a past history of hyperthyroidism.

4. Treatment of thyroid disease during pregnancy. Hypothyroidism is treated with replacement thyroxine along standard lines. Most hyperthyroid patients are treated satisfactorily with antithyroid drugs throughout pregnancy and definitive treatment delayed until after delivery. Antithyroid drugs cross the placenta and in high doses may cause fetal hypothyroidism or goitre. There is no increase in incidence of congenital malformations in infants born to mothers taking antithyroid drugs. Propylthiouracil does not appear to be concentrated in breast milk whereas significant amounts of methimazole are present in milk. If the mother has a large goitre and the hyperthyroidism is severe then surgery may be performed in mid-pregnancy after suitable medical control of the hyperthyroidism.

5. Treatment of neonatal hyperthyroidism. The baby should be treated with standard antithyroid medication for the first 2–3 months of life. After this hyperthyroidism remits as maternal thyroid stimulating immunoglobulins disappear from the circulation. Treatment of cardiac failure with digoxin and diuretics may be necessary.

Postpartum thyroid disease

The occurrence of transitory, or occasionally permanent, thyroid dysfunction following pregnancy is now widely recognised. The incidence of postpartum thyroid disease has been reported as 9% in the United States and 5.5% in Japan.

The characteristics of this postpartum thyroid dysfunction are 1. a high frequency of previous goitre, 2. early (less than 4 months) hyperthyroidism, 3. later (over 4 months) hypothyroidism, sometimes occurring in the same patient, 4. return to euthyroidism 5–10 months postpartum, 5. increasing titres of microsomal antibodies to a peak at 3 to 4 months, and 6. decrease in size but usually persistence of goitre. Whether this syndrome is autoimmune or viral is not known. A few patients with hyperthyroidism appear to have Graves' disease with increased radioiodine uptake by the thyroid, but most show suppressed uptake characteristic of 'postpartum painless thyroiditis with transient thyrotoxicosis' (PPTT syndrome).

Iodine and the thyroid

Variations in the amount of dietary iodine may affect thyroid function and the development and course of thyroid disease. Iodine deficiency is estimated to affect some 200 million people resulting in endemic goitre, cretinism or hypothyroidism. When iodine intake is consistently below the minimum daily requirement (50 μg/day) T4 synthesis is reduced with a compensatory rise in TSH secretion. This results in hypertrophy and hyperplasia of the thyroid followed by nodular transformation, as well as increased iodine trapping, increased T3/T4 ratio and goitre. Circulating T4 levels are reduced whereas serum T3 is normal or even raised. Autonomous nodules occur more frequently in areas where goitre is endemic. Iodine deficiency may be an aetiological factor in the development of follicular carcinoma, whereas papillary carcinoma is reported to be more common in iodine rich areas.

The effects of a high intake of iodine are complex. Thyrotoxicosis may develop after administration of iodine supplements (Jod-Basedow effect) in areas of endemic iodine deficiency. Affected patients may have nodular goitres or thyroid stimulating antibodies in the circulation indicative of subclinical Graves' disease. Similarly, patients with euthyroid 'hot' nodules given iodide may become overtly thyrotoxic. Hyperthyroidism has also been described in patients with apparently normal thyroid glands given iodine-containing drugs or radiodiagnostic contrast media.

Conversely iodide preparations have diverse suppressive effects upon the thyroid; an increase in intracellular iodide concentration in normal glands leads to interference with the iodination of tyrosine (Wolff-Chaikoff effect) thus inhibiting organification and reducing thyroid hormone biosynthesis. Prolonged administration of iodine-containing medicines therefore may induce hypothyroidism and goitre. In addition the short-lived inhibition of thyroid hormone release by iodine in thyrotoxicosis is well recognised.

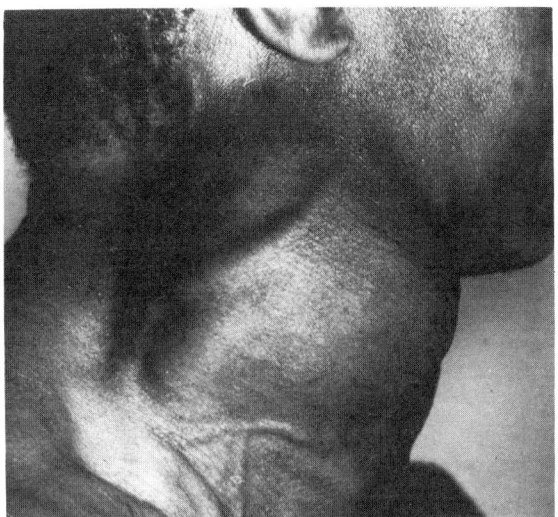

Fig. 4.6 Massive multinodular goitre.

Table 4.8 Causes of goitre

Endemic (iodine deficient)
Simple non-toxic (sporadic, colloid)
   diffuse
   multinodular

Physiological (puberty, pregnancy)

Dyhormonogenesis

Drug-induced

Thyroiditis
   autoimmune
   subacute (de Quervain's)
   Riedel's
   suppurative

Tumours
   adenoma
   carcinoma
   lymphoma
   metastatic

Others (sarcoidosis, tuberculosis etc.)

GOITRE AND THYROID NODULES

The term goitre is used to describe enlargement of the thyroid from any cause. Thyroid nodules may be solitary or part of a multinodular goitre (Fig. 4.6); many nodules which are thought to be single on clinical examination turn out to be multiple on further investigation or at surgery. Some goitres are due to deficient thyroid hormone secretion which leads to increased TSH secretion and enlargement of the thyroid which may or may not compensate for the deficiency. Some goitres, such as those due to subacute or suppurative thyroiditis, are due to inflammatory involvement, whereas in others, particularly the common simple non-toxic goitre, no cause for the thyroid enlargement can be found. There is an increased frequency of goitre in premenopausal women compared to men and, although the incidence of diffuse goitre falls with age, nodular goitres become more common in old age. Causes of goitre are outlined in Table 4.8.

Endemic goitre

Dietary iodine deficiency is the commonest cause of goitre worldwide and where its prevalence exceeds 10% the area is classified as endemic. Iodine deficiency is particularly prevalent in mountainous regions. Goitrogens may contribute to the prevalence and severity of endemic goitre but this is nearly always on a background of mild to moderate iodine deficiency. Clinically there is diffuse thyroid enlargement which usually progresses to nodule formation and occasionally to hypothyroidism. The most effective means of treatment is iodine prophylaxis via the introduction of iodised salt, bread and other foods. In isolated, less sophisticated communities injections of iodised oil are indicated. Occasionally hyperthyroidism may be induced (Jod-Basedow effect).

In these endemic areas it is apparent that a continuous spectrum of intellectual, neurological, physical and hormonal abnormalities may be seen. Endemic cretinism is characterised by 1. its association with endemic goitre and severe iodine deficiency, 2. the existence of mental retardation together with a predominant neurological syndrome, or predominant hypothyroidism and stunted growth, or a mixture of the two, and 3. its preventability with supplementary iodine.

Simple non-toxic goitre

This describes a benign enlargement of the thyroid gland which is diffuse or multinodular and for which there is no apparent cause. There is usually no clinical disturbance of thyroid function. The goitre occurs sporadically in non-endemic areas and may also be called sporadic non-toxic goitre, simple goitre or colloid goitre. It is often familial and invariably commoner in females. The most widespread hypothesis about the cause of the goitre formation is that thyroid enlargement is due to long-standing minor degrees of stimulation by TSH (perhaps consequent on incomplete dyshormonogenesis), although in most instances serum T4, T3 and TSH values are normal. In 30–50% of cases autonomy of nodules develops which is associated with suppressed TSH and impaired or absent TSH responses to TRH; occasionally hypothyroidism develops. If no pressure symptoms are present and there are no cosmetic problems treatment is not necessary. The evidence for the benefit of suppressive therapy with T4 is unconvincing. There is no good evidence that non-toxic goitre predisposes to thyroid carcinoma.

Dyshormonogenetic goitre

Thyroid enlargement occurs as a result of a compensatory response of the thyroid to its impaired ability to synthesise hormones. These familial conditions are rare, and are due to defects in various enzymes involved in thyroid hormone synthesis. Many patients are clinically and biochemically euthyroid.

1. Iodine trapping defects are least common and are characterised by low radioiodine uptake despite increased endogenous or exogenous TSH levels. Treatment is with large doses of potassium iodide, or thyroxine.

2. Organification defects are due to relative inability of the thyroid to bind iodide covalently to thyroglobulin. The defects are characterised by abnormal perchlorate or thiocyanate discharge tests.

    a. Pendred's syndrome: congenital nerve deafness and goitre. Patients are usually euthyroid and not mentally retarded.

    b. Defects of thyroid peroxidase system.

    c. Defective generation of hydrogen peroxide.

3. Defects in thyroglobulin synthesis which result in inadequate production of thyroglobulin

or synthesis of an abnormal thyroglobulin. Thyroidal radioiodine uptake is high and radioactivity of the gland remains high for several days.

4. Coupling defects result in a low ratio of iodothyronines to iodotyrosines in the thyroid, a high thyroidal radioiodine uptake and goitrous hypothyroidism.

5. Dehalogenase defect. Deficiency of the dehalogenating enzyme leads to a state of relative iodine deficiency since monoiodotyrosine and diiodotyrosine generated by the proteolysis of thyroglobulin are normally deiodinated and this iodine becomes the major source for new hormone synthesis.

Drug induced goitre

Goitrogens are substances that produce an increase in size of the thyroid by interfering with the synthesis of thyroid hormones. A fall in circulating thyroid hormones with rise in TSH results in hyperplasia but patients are usually euthyroid. A classification of goitrogens is shown in Table 4.9. Antithyroid drugs used in the treatment of hyperthyroidism are goitrogenic and overtreatment can lead to goitre and hypothyroidism. Goitre and hypothyroidism induced by lithium is an important problem. Lithium causes inhibition of thyroid hormone release probably due to an inhibitory effect on the action of cyclic AMP formed as a result of TSH stimulation. Thirty per cent of patients receiving lithium have an elevated serum TSH value at some stage and thus periodic checks of thyroid function

Table 4.9 Goitrogens

Antithyroid drugs
  carbimazole
  methimazole
  propylthiouracil
  perchlorate

Other drugs
  iodine-containing medicines
  lithium
  aminoglutethimide

Dietary factors
  iodine
  soya bean
  cassava

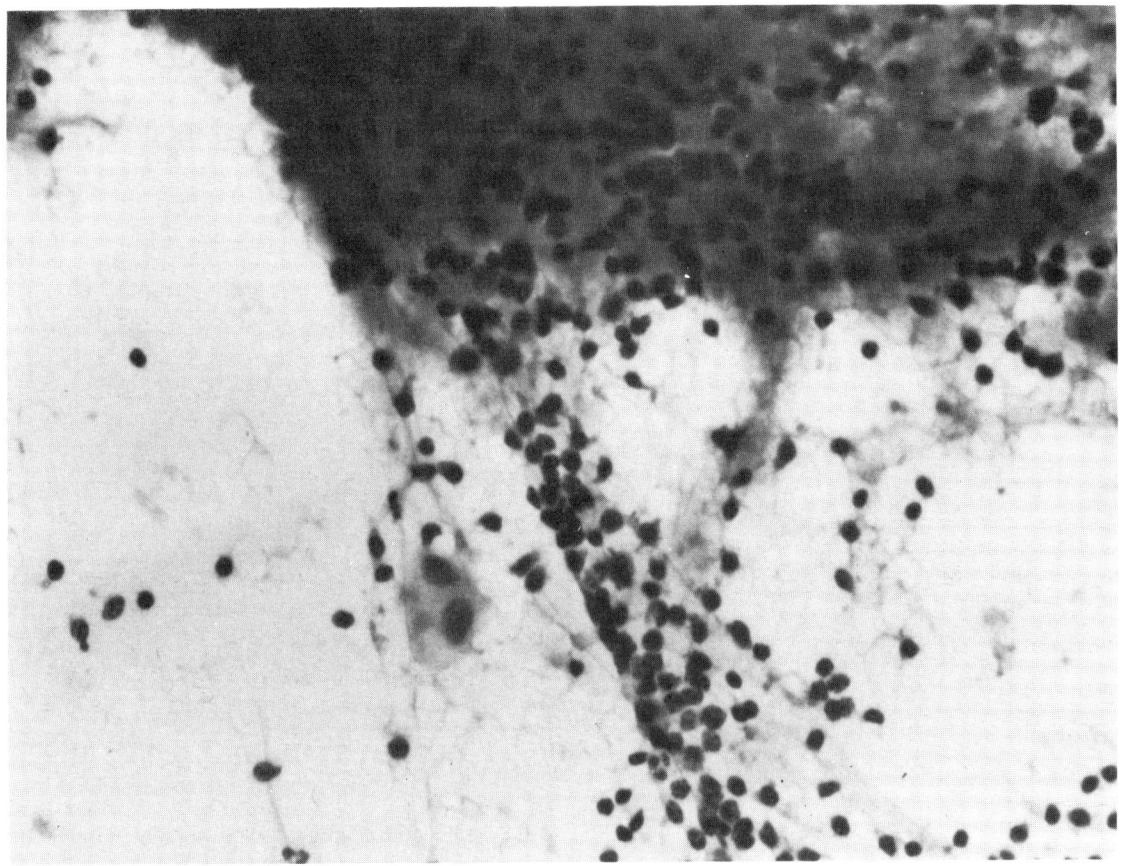

Fig. 4.7 Cytological appearance of lymphocytic infiltration in Hashimoto's thyroiditis.

should be performed. Occasionally irreversible hypothyroidism occurs.

Autoimmune thyroiditis

This is the group of conditions characterised by the presence of circulating thyroid antibodies, including Hashimoto's and Graves' disease.

Subacute thyroiditis

A palpable goitre is present in de Quervain's (sub-acute) thyroiditis and its variant 'silent' thyroiditis (see above).

Suppurative thyroiditis

An extremely rare condition due to bacterial infection of the thyroid. The gland is enlarged, painful and very tender; fluctuation and eventually discharge of pus may occur. Antibiotic therapy and possibly surgical drainage are indicated.

Riedel's fibrous thyroiditis

This is another very rare condition with symmetrical or asymmetrical enlargement of the thyroid. Normal tissue is replaced by dense fibrosis that may extend into mediastinal tissues. The thyroid is very hard and fixed, pressure symptoms are common, carcinoma is usually suspected and hypothyroidism may be a complication. Treatment is surgical although occasionally glucocorticoids may produce a dramatic response.

Solitary thyroid nodules

Single thyroid nodules are a relatively common

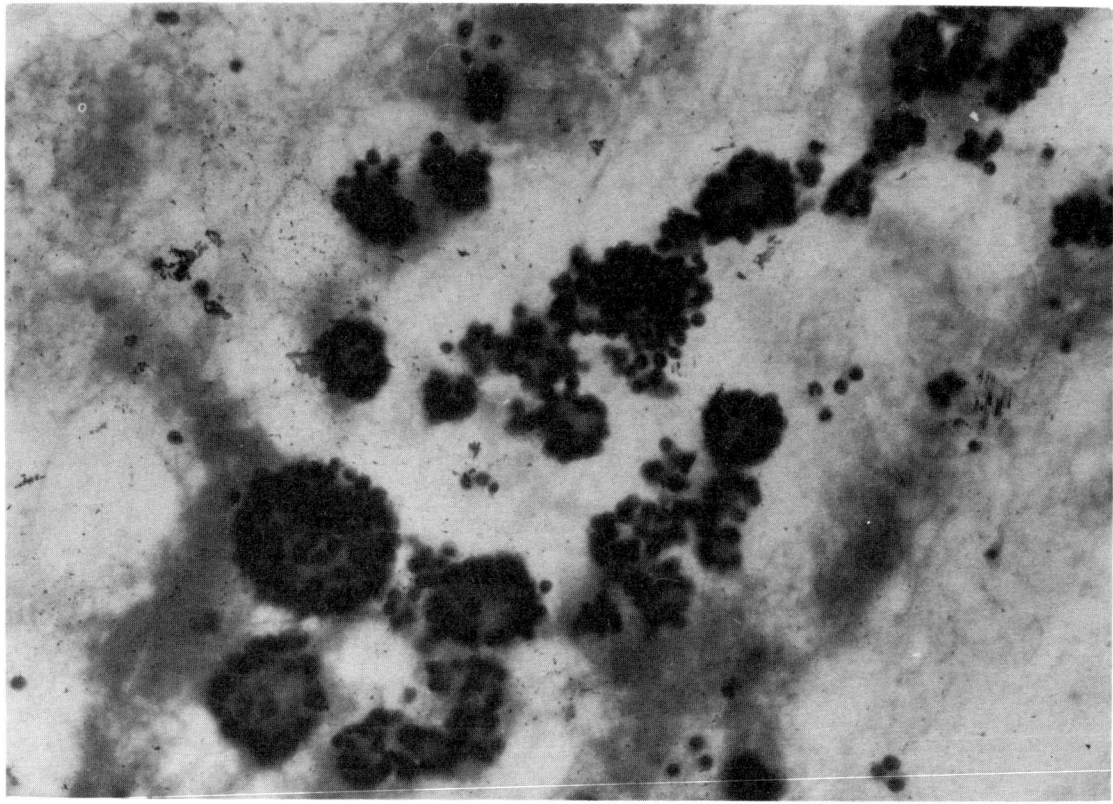

Fig. 4.8 Cytological appearance in a follicular adenoma.

finding in clinical practice with a prevalence of 3–4% of the general population. Higher rates are found in areas of iodine deficiency and they are more common in females. The nodules contain either functioning thyroid tissue or are functionless. Although the majority of functionless nodules are benign the major concern is to exclude malignant change. When a patient presents with a nodule in the thyroid the following questions need consideration:

1. Is the patient hyperthyroid, euthyroid or hypothyroid?

2. Is this a true single nodule or is it a palpable nodule in a multinodular goitre?

3. Is the nodule benign or malignant?

Management of thyroid nodules

Standard tests of thyroid function have been outlined and are important to determine the thyroid status of the patient.

Uptake scans of the thyroid using radioisotopes such as ^{131}I and $^{99}Tc^m$ have been used widely in the investigation of thyroid nodules. Hot nodules – characterised by a high concentration of radioisotope – are typical of autonomous nodules, often found in multinodular goitre. Non-functioning or cold nodules may represent zones of haemorrhagic or cystic degeneration within a nodular goitre, or, especially in the case of single nodules, are suspicious of malignancy. The reported prevalence of thyroid carcinoma in cold nodules varies between series but is approximately 10%, with a lower prevalence in hot nodules.

Ultrasound scanning of the thyroid is of value in distinguishing solitary nodules from a multinodular goitre and can easily define cystic lesions. Cystic lesions have a lower reported rate of malignancy than solid lesions.

The appropriate scheme for investigation of patients with solitary nodules remains controversial. In some centres, radioisotope and

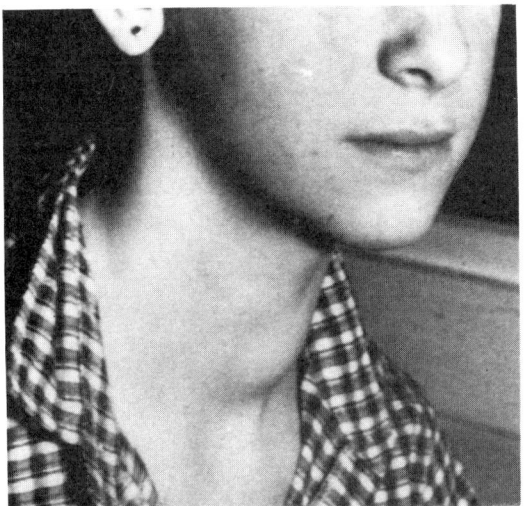

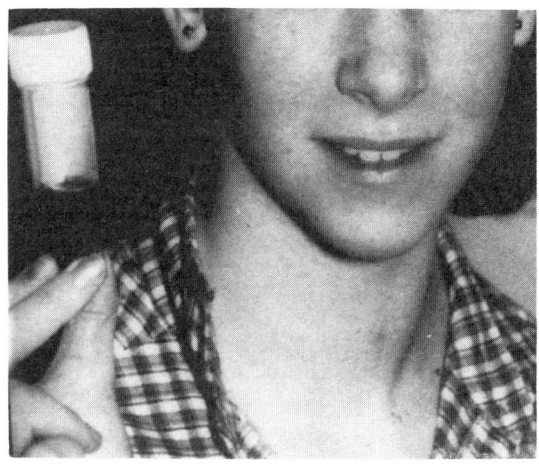

Fig. 4.9 Aspiration of fluid from a thyroid cyst.

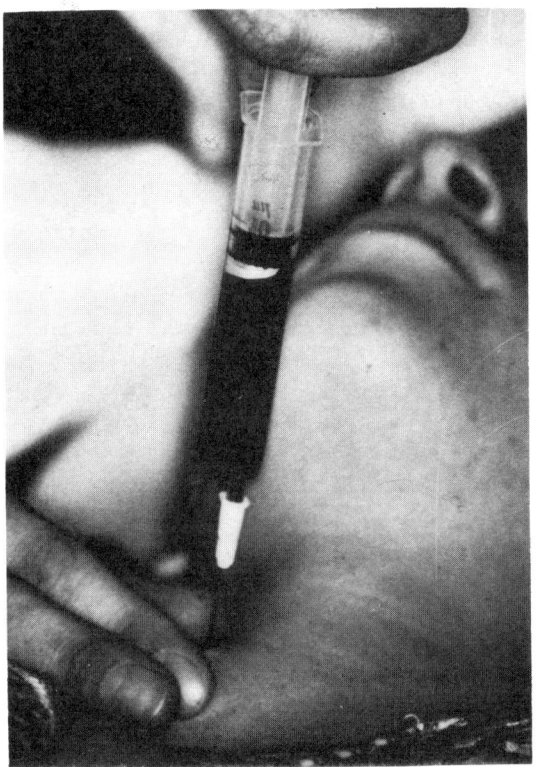

ultrasound scanning remain routine first line tests before proceeding to surgery in patients with solid, non-functioning nodules. In other centres cytological diagnosis of thyroid nodules is playing an increasingly important role, often obviating the need for surgical intervention.

Fine needle aspiration of the thyroid may provide diagnostic information in simple goitre, thyroiditis (Fig. 4.7), simple adenomas (Fig. 4.8) and carcinomas, anaplastic carcinomas and lymphomas. The diagnostic value of the investigation depends on the skill of tissue sampling, smear production, staining and cytopathologist. False negative diagnoses should occur in no more than 10% of cases. Fine needle aspiration of the thyroid may be of therapeutic benefit in simple thyroid cysts which may be cured by aspiration of cyst fluid (Fig. 4.9).

Thyroid adenoma

Thyroid adenomas are benign neoplasms of thyroid tissue which are classified according to their histological characteristics, the most important of which are follicular and capillary. Many nodules are asymptomatic and may be found at routine medical examination. The swelling is rarely large enough to cause pressure symptoms although occasionally sudden enlargement may be caused by haemorrhage. Examination reveals a nodule in the thyroid, the rest of the gland being impalpable. Most adenomas increase slowly in size over several years. Hyperthyroidism may occasionally develop ('toxic adenoma'). Thyroid hormone is prescribed routinely in some centres in an attempt to reduce the size of a benign nodule but in general results are unimpressive. If surgery is to be performed subtotal lobectomy is the preferred operation.

Thyroid carcinoma

Carcinomas of the thyroid gland are rare, comprising about 0.2% of all carcinoma deaths in men and 0.5% in women in the United Kingdom. Tumours derived from the thyroid follicular cell fall into two broad groups, the differentiated and the undifferentiated. The former group is subdivided into two types, papillary and follicular; undifferentiated tumours are designated anaplastic carcinomas. Carcinomas derived from the parafollicular cell are all referred to as medullary carcinoma, but show a wide gradation of malignancy. Malignant tumours of the thyroid can therefore be classified into papillary and mixed papillary/follicular (60–70%), follicular (12–20%), anaplastic (10–15%), medullary (3–6%), and lymphomas, sarcomas and metastatic (1–3%). The prognosis for well differentiated carcinomas is good and recent information suggests that, for patients under 40 years of age with papillary or follicular carcinomas, survival rates at 20 years are no different from unaffected individuals.

Aetiological factors include external irradiation to the heat and neck, high or low iodide intake, and a family history of multiple endocrine adenomatosis (type II). Clinical features depend on the type of tumour, its rate of growth, and the extent of metastases. Most patients complain of a lump in the neck that is increasing in size. It is usually impossible to be certain on clinical grounds whether the nodule is malignant or benign. The lump may, however, be very hard, tender or painful; invasion of local structures may result in paralysis of the recurrent laryngeal nerve with hoarseness, dysphagia and cervical lymphadenopathy. Occasionally the presenting feature is the result of a distant metastasis, e.g. bone pain or paraplegia. A tender gland which is hard, irregular and fixed to surrounding tissues is strongly suggestive of an anaplastic carcinoma.

The papillary carcinoma is the commonest type of thyroid carcinoma and is slow growing, non-encapsulated, multifocal, involves lymphatics and spreads to lymph nodes. The follicular carcinoma lacks papillae and may show a great resemblance to normal thyroid tissue. Characteristically it is encapsulated, solitary and spreads predominantly via the blood stream, especially to bone, brain and lungs. The majority of cases of anaplastic carcinoma show a spindle and giant cell pattern and largely lack evidence of follicular cell differentiation; secondary deposits may not be recognisable as originating from thyroid tissue.

Management of thyroid carcinoma

Thyroidectomy. Total thyroidectomy for differentiated capillary and follicular carcinoma is practised in many centres because the tumours may be bilateral (either because of the multifocal origin of the tumour or due to intrathyroidal lymphatic spread). However, since the progression rate of these metastases is low and because total thyroidectomy involves a greater risk to vital structures, there has been a gradual move to more conservative surgery, i.e. lobectomy.

Radioiodine therapy. [131]I ablation treatment is indicated in patients with differentiated papillary or follicular carcinomas where surgery is incomplete and tumour or normal thyroid tissue remains or where metastases have been detected. A dose of 30–50 mCi of radioiodine is administered to ablate any residual normal thyroid tissue; replacement therapy with T3, 20 μg tds, is then given for 2–3 months. Two weeks after withdrawal of T3 a therapeutic dose in excess of 100 mCi of ^{131}I is given. Residual or recurrent tumour tissue can be detected by subsequent ^{131}I scans or measurement of serum thyroglobulin.

External irradiation. This is the treatment of choice for anaplastic carcinomas and malignant lymphomas. In addition, this method of therapy is effective for metastases and relief of pain may be achieved rapidly.

Thyroid hormone therapy. Thyroid hormone replacement therapy is essential after total thyroidectomy or ^{131}I ablation. The growth of some tumours is dependent on TSH therefore most centres will treat all patients with suppressive doses of thyroxine.

Adrenal

The adrenal gland is a complex endocrine organ producing many hormones. The cortex differs from the medulla in many respects. All the hormones produced by the cortex are based on the steroid structure of the cyclopentanoperhydrophenanthrene nucleus, whereas the medullary hormones are derived from the amino acid phenylalanine. The release of cortical hormones is largely under the control of other trophic hormones, but the medullary secretions are under the influence of the sympathetic nervous system.

THE ADRENAL CORTEX

Histology

There are three well defined histological zones of cells: the zona glomerulosa, the zona fasciculata and the zona reticularis. The zona reticularis cells are described as 'compact' with very few lipid droplets in the cytoplasm, whereas the fasciculata contains 'clear' cells, so called because of the abundance of lipid droplets in their cytoplasm. The appearance of the glomerulosa cells is intermediate between the other two.

Secretions

The adrenal cortex secretes over 20 different steroids. They can be subdivided into three separate classes of compounds, namely, mineralocorticoids, glucocorticoids and adrenal androgens. They are all based on the same steroid ring (Fig. 5.1), but

they differ in the groups which are attached to the basic skeleton. Small chemical changes often lead to large biological differences between compounds. Examples of the structure of the main classes of steroids are also shown in Figure 5.1

It was thought originally that each histological zone of the cortex secreted its own unique class of steroids, but this has been largely disproved. It is true that aldosterone is only produced by the zona glomerulosa cells but both the zona fasciculata and the zona reticularis can produce glucocorticoids and adrenal androgens. In times of stress or ACTH stimulation lipid depletion occurs and the fasciculata cells are progressively replaced by compact reticularis cells.

Steroid biosynthesis

All steroids are synthesised from acetate via cholesterol. The pathway from cholesterol to pregnenolone is common to all steroid hormones, and it is here that ACTH has its effect in the adrenal cortex, stimulating the complex of enzymes resulting in 20 and 22-hydroxylation. The pathways of steroid biosynthesis are shown in Figure 5.2. In the human adrenal cortex the synthesis of cortisol is via the conversion of pregnenolone to 17-hydroxypregnenolone, to 17-hydroxyprogesterone, to 11-deoxycortisol and then to cortisol

Glucocorticoids

The principal glucocorticoid in man is cortisol. It is important in the maintenance of life and

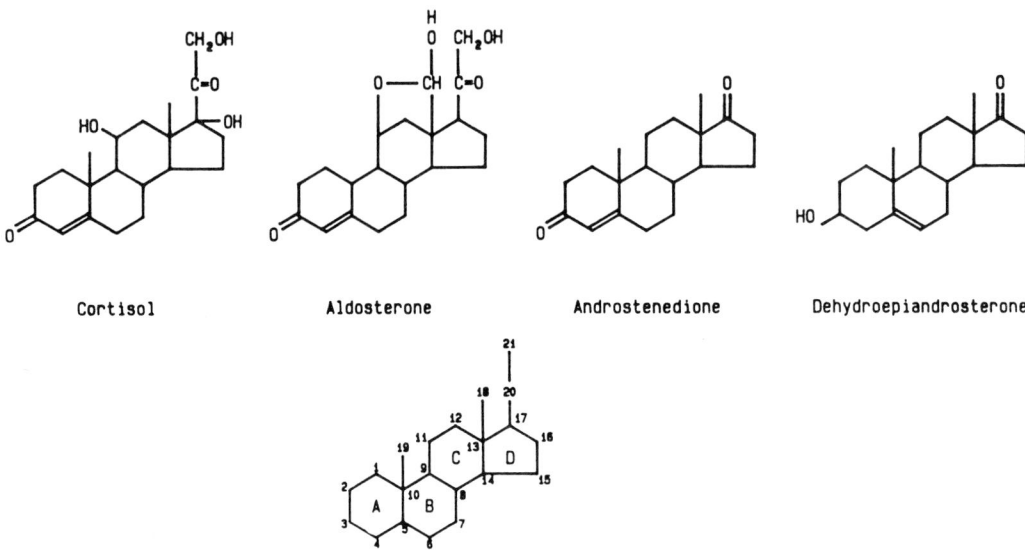

Fig. 5.1 The nomenclature of the basic steroid ring structure, and examples of the important steroid hormones.

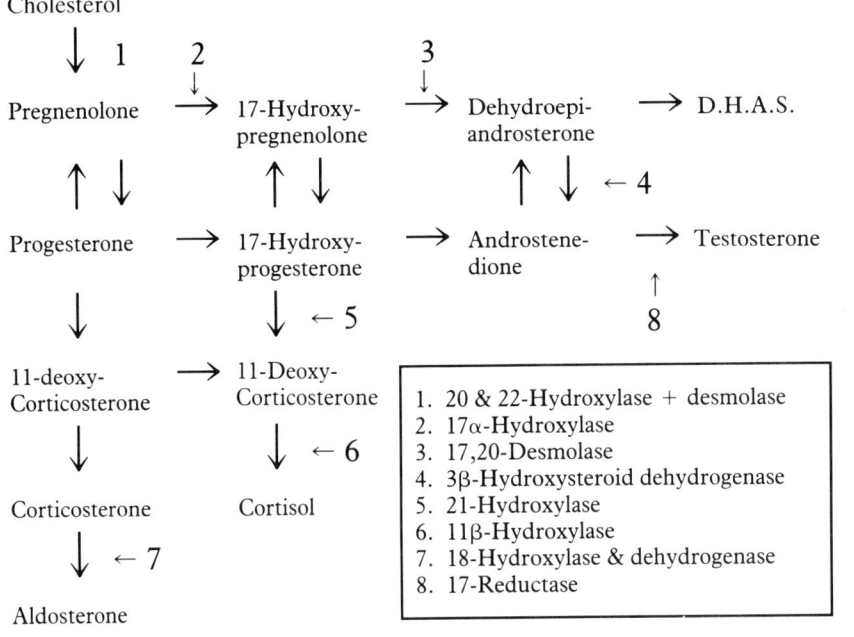

Fig. 5.2 The pathways of adrenal steroid biosynthesis.

in the protection against stress. It is the most potent and quantitatively the most important naturally occurring glucocorticoid. The effects of glucocorticoids are more widespread than any of the other steroid hormones. The 11-hydroxyl group is the essential feature of the steroid molecule for glucocorticoid action.

Synthetic glucocorticoids

A variety of chemical manoeuvres have been used to alter the glucocorticoid potency of synthetic steroids. These changes may increase glucocorticoid activity simply by increasing their half life or by altering binding affinity to receptors.

Prednisolone has increased anti-inflammatory and glucocorticoid activity. This is achieved by the removal of a double bond from the cortisol molecule. This activity is doubled in methyl prednisolone. The addition of a fluoride atom markedly alters function. 9 α-fludrocortisone is a potent mineralocorticoid, but further addition of either a hydroxyl group or a methyl group, as in triamcinolone and dexamethasone respectively, changes the main action back to glucocorticoid activity, abolishing nearly all mineralocorticoid effect.

Actions

As the name implies, glucocorticoids have considerable effects on carbohydrate metabolism, acting as insulin antagonists. The rise in glucose is a consequence both of stimulation of gluconeogenesis in the liver, and of a reduction in peripheral uptake of glucose. In addition, glucocorticoids profoundly affect protein metabolism. They stimulate catabolism, causing negative nitrogen balance, with loss of protein from muscle and bone. The anti-inflammatory action of glucocorticoids is mediated through a variety of effects. Stabilisation of lysosomal membranes, suppression of the formation of kinins, inhibition of the migration of polymorphs, inhibition of the mitotic activity of lymphocytes, and inhibition of the transformation of lymphocytes (by phytohaemagglutinin) are all thought to play a part in this aspect of their action. A fuller list of the actions of glucocorticoids is given below:

1. Stimulation of gluconeogeneis.
2. Reduced glucose utilisation.
3. Anti-inflammatory action.
4. Suppression of cellular and humoral immunity.
5. Enhancement of water diuresis.
6. Maintenance of extracellular fluid volume.
7. Reduction of eosinophil and lymphocyte count; increase in red cell and platelet count.
8. Increase in acid and pepsin secretion.
9. Sensitisation of arterioles to the action of noradrenaline.
10. Mineralocorticoid effect.
11. Reduction in growth hormone secretion.
12. Inhibition of cartilage and bone formation.
13. Reduction in calcium absorption from the gut.

Control of cortisol secretion

The basic control mechanisms involved in the regulation of cortisol secretion are summarised in Figure 5.3. Cortisol synthesis and release are stimulated by the pituitary secretion of ACTH. The secretion of ACTH is, in turn, under the control of the hypothalamus via the production of corticotrophin releasing factor (CRF). CRF, in common with other hypothalamic releasing hormones, is produced by neurones in the hypothalamus and secreted into the portal venous system which passes to the pituitary. Unlike most releasing hormones (but in common with GRF) it is a large peptide, being 41 amino acids in length. CRF secretion is under the control of higher centres in the brain. Control is mediated by a number of neurotransmitters, including serotonin and acetylcholine, which are thought to stimulate, and noradrenaline and gamma-aminobutyric acid, which are thought to inhibit its release.

The secretion of ACTH is episodic. The frequency and length of duration of secretory peaks increases between 04:00 and 09:00, and reduces between 21:00 & 24:00. This gives rise to the well known circadian rhythms of ACTH and cortisol secretion. As with other endocrine systems the secretory episodes are modulated by

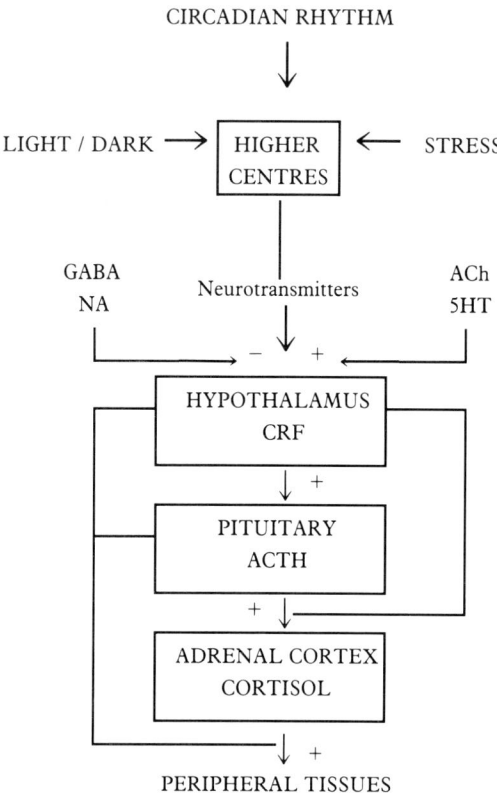

Fig. 5.3 Schematic diagram to show the control of cortisol synthesis. NA = Noradrenaline; ACh=Acetylcholine; 5HT= 5-Hydroxytryptamine (Serotonin); GABA=Gamma-aminobutyric-acid; + = stimulation; − = inhibition.

feedback systems acting at hypothalamic and pituitary levels.

Metabolism

The majority of steroid hormones are inactivated by the liver. The resulting compounds are then conjugated, mainly to glucuronide, and excreted in the urine. Measurements of urinary metabolites have been superceded by specific radioimmunoassays for individual steroids.

Approximately 0.5% of cortisol is secreted unchanged in the urine which is clinically important because it can be measured as 'urinary free cortisol'. It reflects the free plasma cortisol concentration, which is filtered by the glomerulus, and therefore the biologically active cortisol.

Mineralocorticoids

The most important and potent mineralocorticoid in man is aldosterone. Mineralocorticoids are so called because of their ability to promote active sodium transport across epithelial membranes. The most important site of this action is in the renal tubules where potassium and hydrogen ions are exchanged for sodium. Aldosterone and deoxycorticosterone exhibit this effect at physiological concentrations; other steroids (including cortisol) share this action but only at pharmacological concentrations.

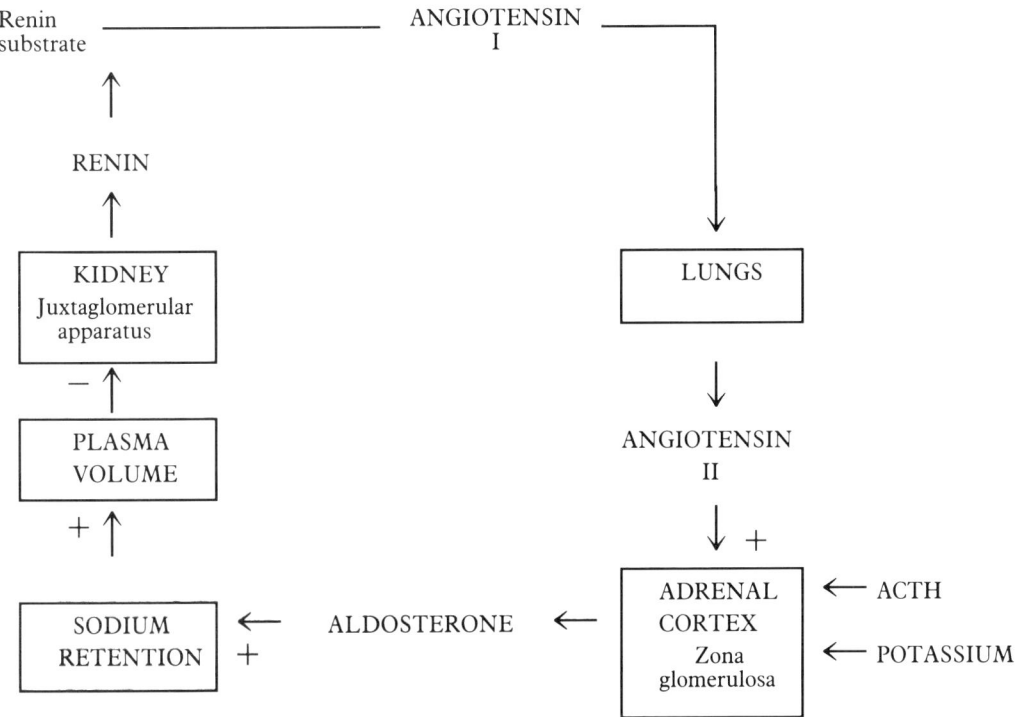

Fig. 5.4 The control mechanisms involved in the release of aldosterone.
+ = stimulation; − = inhibition.

Aldosterone is a unique steroid in that it possesses an aldehyde group at C18 (Fig. 5.1). The addition of a fluorine atom at position 9 in the B ring imparts potent mineralocorticoid activity and also prolongs its half-life. This is the basis of the clinically useful compound 9 α-fludrocortisone.

Actions

The effect on sodium balance is the most important action. The site of action is the distal tubule. This is quite distinct from the major sodium regulating site in the proximal tubule which is not controlled by hormonal factors and which may swamp the distal mechanism. This fact explains why patients with mineralocorticoid excess do not develop oedema. The aldosterone induced expansion of plasma volume is nullified by a diminished proximal tubular reabsorption of sodium. Aldosterone is also implicated in potassium homeostasis. There is a direct stimulatory effect of potassium on aldosterone secretion. Acid-base balance is also partially under the control of mineralocorticoid but

changes in acid-base status are only seen in severe mineralocorticoid depletion or excess.

Control of secretion

Unlike cortisol, which only has one main stimulatory mechanism, aldosterone secretion is influenced by several factors. The most important of these is the renin-angiotensin system which is summarised in Figure 5.4. Renin, an enzyme released by the juxtaglomerular apparatus in the kidney acts on renin substrate, a plasma globulin, to form the decapeptide angiotensin I. Two amino acids are split off angiotensin I, by a converting enzyme in the lung, to form angiotensin II. This is a very potent pressor substance which also stimulates conversion of cholesterol to pregnenolone in the zona glomerulosa, and thus aldosterone production. The action of angiotensin II is rapid in onset and the peptide has a very short plasma half life.

Renin secretion is influenced by many factors. Catecholamines can directly stimulate renin release as can the sympathetic nervous system. Most of the stimuli, however, are mediated through the common pathway of decreased perfusion pressure of the kidney. Examples of this are blood loss, dehydration, sodium depletion, renal artery stenosis, hypoalbuminaemia and sequestration of blood in the venous system such as in cirrhosis or congestive cardiac failure. In addition it has been shown that sodium flux in the ascending loop of Henle influences renin secretion.

As with cortisol, feedback loops again control secretion. Angiotensin II directly inhibits renin release. Aldosterone itself has indirect feedback in that the increase in plasma volume effected by sodium reabsorption increases renal perfusion and inhibits renin release. ACTH does stimulate aldosterone secretion, but this is a minor factor in its control. There is a diurnal rhythm of aldosterone secretion and this is partly mediated by ACTH, but there is also an intrinsic diurnal variation in renin secretion. Serum potassium concentrations affect the rate of aldosterone synthesis. High levels stimulate (even though they suppress renin release), and low levels suppress despite an increase in renin synthesis.

A smaller fraction of aldosterone (0.1%) is excreted unchanged in the urine, as compared to cortisol.

Adrenal androgen

The adrenal cortex secretes large quantities of weakly androgenic steroids. On a quantitative basis dehydroepiandrosterone (DHA) is the most important, half being excreted unchanged and half as the sulphated form. The most potent adrenal androgen is androstenedione, but even this has only one tenth the androgenic activity of testosterone.

In the adult male the adrenal androgen output is swamped by the large quantity of testosterone secreted by the testes, but in the adult female the adrenal cortex is the most important source of androgens.

Changes with age

The fetal adrenal produces a large amount of DHA which rises towards the end of pregnancy and acts as a precursor for the placental production of oestriol. After birth the output of DHA rapidly declines and thereafter remains low until a year or two before puberty. The rise before puberty is called the adrenarche and is responsible for the development of pubic and axillary hair. It has been postulated that the adrenarche is a trigger for the onset of puberty. It cannot be the only factor, however, since Addisonian patients have a normal puberty, albeit on average a year or two later than normal. Serum levels of DHA rise to a maximum in the third decade, and thereafter gradually tail off, falling to about a third to a half of the peak value by the age of 70.

Control of adrenal androgen secretion

The way in which adrenal androgen secretion is controlled is much less well understood than that of either cortisol or aldosterone. Both androstenedione and DHA peaks closely mimic cortisol peaks during the day and injections of ACTH increase their concentrations in serum. It has been proposed that different patterns of ACTH secretion, either different frequencies or different amplitudes of secretory episodes might favour the production of one or other adrenocortical product. There are a number of other observations which suggest that there must be other factors than ACTH which control their secretion. These observations point to the disparity between adrenal androgen and cortisol secretion at various times throughout life (the neonatal period, the adrenarche and later life). Oestrogens, prolactin and a pituitary factor with the eponym CASH (cortical androgen stimulating factor) have been proposed at different times as this alternative factor. Cortisol levels remain relatively constant throughout life, yet at these three times adrenal androgens alter markedly. Another difference is highlighted by adrenal suppression with exogenous glucocorticoids. Adrenal androgens show much more marked suppression and, at the same time, lower responses to ACTH stimulation than cortisol.

Metabolism

The most important feature of the metabolism of adrenal androgens, particularly in the female,

Table 5.1 Causes of Cushing's syndrome

Pituitary adenoma (Cushing's disease)

Adrenal tumour
  adenoma
  carcinoma

Ectopic ACTH

Exogenous admiinistration of glucocorticoids or ACTH

Alcohol-induced (pseudo-Cushing's)

---

is the interconversion which occurs after secretion. In the female, half of serum testosterone is derived from androstenedione, whereas, in the male, testicular secretions are by far the greater source.

The urinary metabolites of adrenal androgens are the 17 oxosteroids. Many other compounds which are either only very weakly androgenic or are not androgens at all also contribute to the 17 oxosteroids. This complexity of origin makes them less useful as markers of adrenal androgen production.

CUSHING'S SYNDROME (HYPERCORTISOLISM)

The term Cushing's syndrome encompasses all causes of hypercortisolism; the pituitary dependent variety is known as Cushing's disease. The causes of Cushing's syndrome are set out in Table 5.1. It is difficult to be certain of the relative prevalence of the different varieties, because of variation in the reported prevalence of the ectopic ACTH syndrome. The clinical entity of the ectopic ACTH syndrome is uncommon but elevated levels of immunoreactive ACTH are frequently encountered, e.g. in oat cell carcinoma of the bronchus. It is said that the first two causes encompass about 70% of cases and that 10% of all cases are due to adrenal adenomas. In children the commonest cause is an adrenal carcinoma.

The pathophysiological aspects of the ectopic ACTH syndrome are discussed in chapter 9 and no further mention will be made here except in the discussion of the differential diagnosis of Cushing's syndrome.

Cushing's disease

This variety of the syndrome is due to pituitary hypersecretion of ACTH. In the majority of cases the cause is a microadenoma, but occasionally there is hyperplasia of the basophil cells. The majority of microadenomas are too small to have any effect on the size of the pituitary fossa and pituitary radiography is normal. Large basophil adenomas are rare in adults but in children tumours may be more rapidly growing and present with symptoms of space occupation. Since in adults the tumours are small it follows that visual field defects are very uncommon.

There is still controversy about the pathogenesis of Cushing's disease. Hypersecretion of CRF from the hypothalamus causing secondary excess of ACTH is suggested by the finding of pituitary basophil hyperplasia in some cases. On the other hand a discrete pituitary adenoma is found in 80–90% of patients, at hypophysectomy. It remains to be seen whether, in the long term, those patients who have had selective microadenomectomies with preservation of normal pituitary tissue will develop the condition again.

Alcoholic pseudo-Cushing's syndrome

Both the clinical and the biochemical features of Cushing's syndrome may be found in patients with chronic alcohol abuse. There are no clinical distinguishing features apart from a history of alcohol intake. Consequently this aspect of the history should never be omitted in suspected Cushing's syndrome. The serum cortisol is elevated with loss of diurnal rhythm and there is resistance to suppression with dexamethasone.

The cause of this variety of Cushing's syndrome is unclear. In the few reported cases the plasma ACTH has either been normal or suppressed. The suggested mechanisms include impaired cortisol metabolism because of liver damage, or a direct effect of ethanol on either cortisol or ACTH secretion.

A sample of blood for ethanol estimation should be included in the investigation of any Cushingoid

Table 5.2 Percentage prevalence of symptoms and signs in Cushing's syndrome. (After Ross E J, Linch D C 1982 Lancet ii: 646–649.)

Symptoms	%	Signs	%
Weight gain	91	Obesity	97
		truncal	46
		generalised	55
Menstrual irregularity	84	Plethora	94
Hirsutism	81	Facial rounding	88
Lethargy/depression	62	Bruising	62
Thirst/frequency	44	Striae	56
Backache	43	Muscle weakness	56
Muscle weakness	29	Buffalo hump	54
Dyspnoea	26	Oedema	50
Recurrent infections	25	Acne	21
Abdominal pain	21	Pigmentation	4
Fractures	19		
Balding	13		

patient. Another biochemical distinction is that if the patient is admitted to hospital and denied alcohol then the biochemical abnormalities quite rapidly regress. Serial serum cortisol estimations or urinary free cortisol measurement would show this up.

Clinical features of Cushing's syndrome

The typical clinical features of the syndrome are well known and are listed in Table 5.2. The commonest symptom and sign is obesity. It is interesting to note that generalised obesity is as common as classically described truncal obesity with wasting of the limbs (Fig. 5.5).

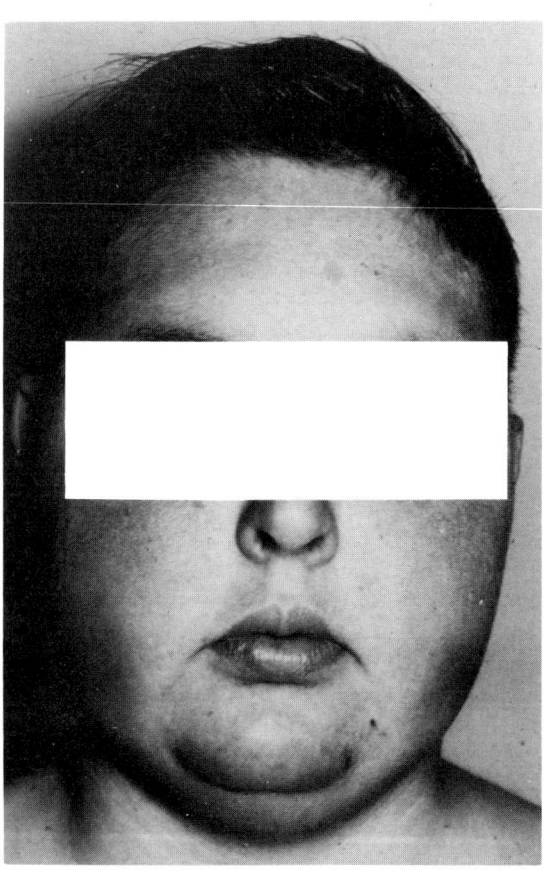
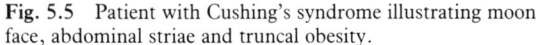

Fig. 5.5 Patient with Cushing's syndrome illustrating moon face, abdominal striae and truncal obesity.

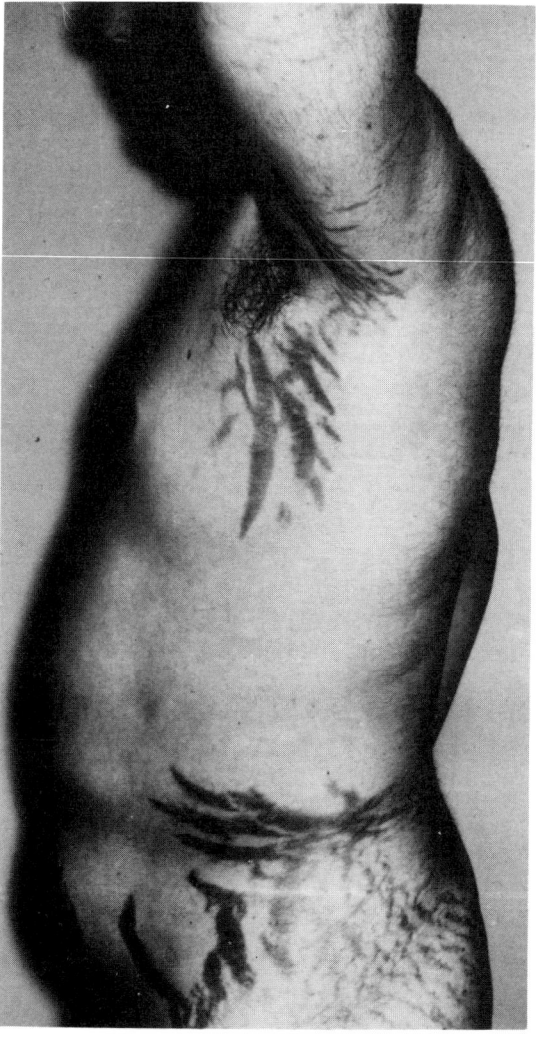

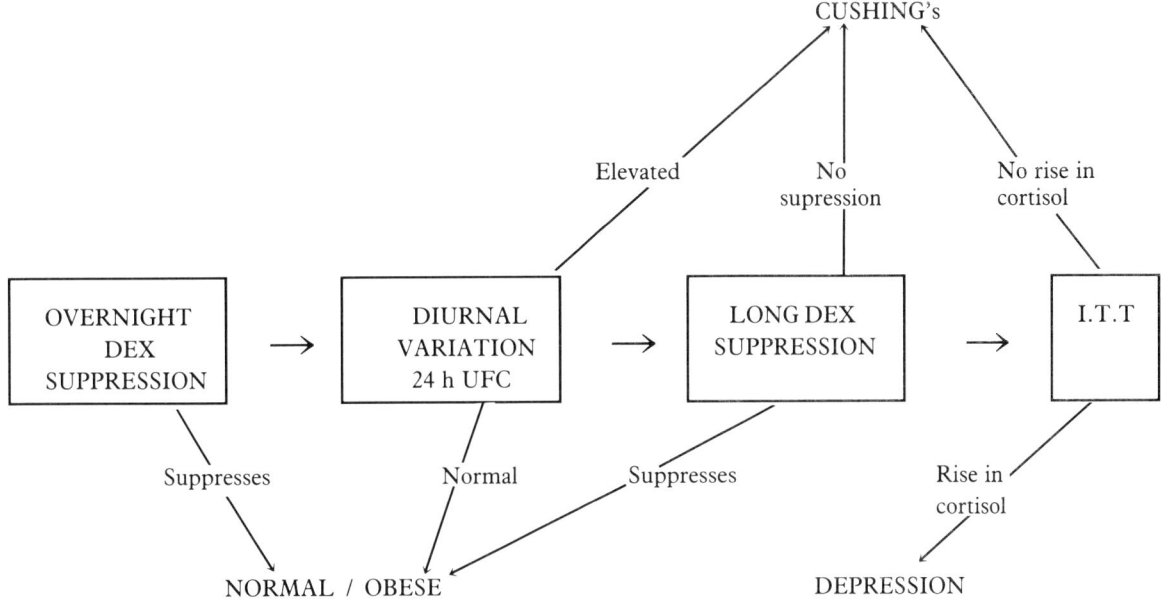

Fig 5.6 Scheme of investigation to establish the presence of Cushing's syndrome.
DEX = dexamethasone; ITT = insulin tolerance test.

The clinical syndrome in cases of ectopic ACTH syndrome may fall into two categories. Where a benign tumour is present, ACTH levels are not very high and the clinical picture is similar to that of Cushing's disease. The more common clinical presentation, with very high ACTH levels is quite different. The symptoms and signs are listed below and are due to the profound biochemical disturbances which occur because of the very high cortisol levels; there is insufficient time for the development of classical stigmata.

1. Weight loss
2. Weakness
3. Diabetes
4. Pigmentation
5. Hypokalaemic alkalosis
6. Oedema

The diagnosis of Cushing's syndrome

The investigation of patients with possible Cushing's syndrome falls into two parts. Firstly the presence of hypercortisolism has to be confirmed and if this is present then the differential diagnosis is sought.

Establishing the presence of hypercortisolism

The suggested scheme of investigation of a patient, to determine the presence of Cushing's syndrome is shown in Figure 5.6.

Short dexamethasone suppression test. The short dexamethasone suppression test is used as a simple outpatient screening test. 1 mg of dexamethasone (2 mg if the patient is very obese) is given at 23:00. The patient then attends at 09:00 the next morning to have blood taken for serum cortisol. The cortisol level in normal subjects will be suppressed to below 150 nmol/l. If this test is normal it is fairly certain that the patient does not have Cushing's syndrome. An abnormal result does not always mean that hypercortisolism is present, but further investigation is indicated.

Diurnal rhythm. If the short dexamethasone test is abnormal then the patient should be admitted for at least 48–72 h. An indwelling intravenous cannula is inserted and diurnal samples of blood are taken for serum cortisol (09:00 and 24:00). It is convenient at this time to take samples also for ACTH (though not necessary to measure them yet – see below). At the same time one or two 24 h urine samples are collected for urinary free cortisol measurement. Urinary free cortisol (UFC) reflects the free fraction of cortisol in the serum which is filtered by the glomerulus. It is independent of cortisol secretion rate unlike other urinary metabolites. In obesity there is an enhanced clearance of cortisol and therefore in order to maintain a normal serum cortisol there must be an increased production rate. UFC is therefore usually normal in obesity whereas metabolites such as 17 oxogenic steroids will be elevated. The only exception to this occurs when obese subjects are fasted: in this situation free cortisol levels are elevated. The first abnormality of serum cortisol is elevation of the midnight value with loss of diurnal variation. Eventually the morning cortisol concentration also becomes elevated. Levels over 1000 nmol/l are uncommon except in cases of ectopic ACTH.

If both these tests are abnormal then it is fairly certain that Cushing's syndrome is present and the differential diagnosis is then sought.

Long dexamethasone test. If there is still doubt about the diagnosis then a long dexamethasone test may be performed. The test falls into two parts: dexamethasone is given at 0.5 mg q.d.s for 48 h and then at 2 mg q.d.s for a further 48 h. The principle of the test is that normal subjects will suppress ACTH and therefore cortisol production completely and that serum cortisol concentrations will be less than 150 nmol/l or UFC will be less than 30 nmol/24 h at the end of the first part of the test. Patients with Cushing's disease will suppress partially on the low dose and completely on high dose, and patients with ectopic ACTH or an adrenal adenoma will not suppress at all. Unfortunately the test is not completely reliable. Sometimes suppression of Cushing's disease is variable and occasionally ectopic ACTH sources do suppress. Another exception is severe depression in which serum cortisol may not suppress even with 8 mg/day.

Insulin hypoglycaemia. In the event of still further doubt, such as in depression or extreme

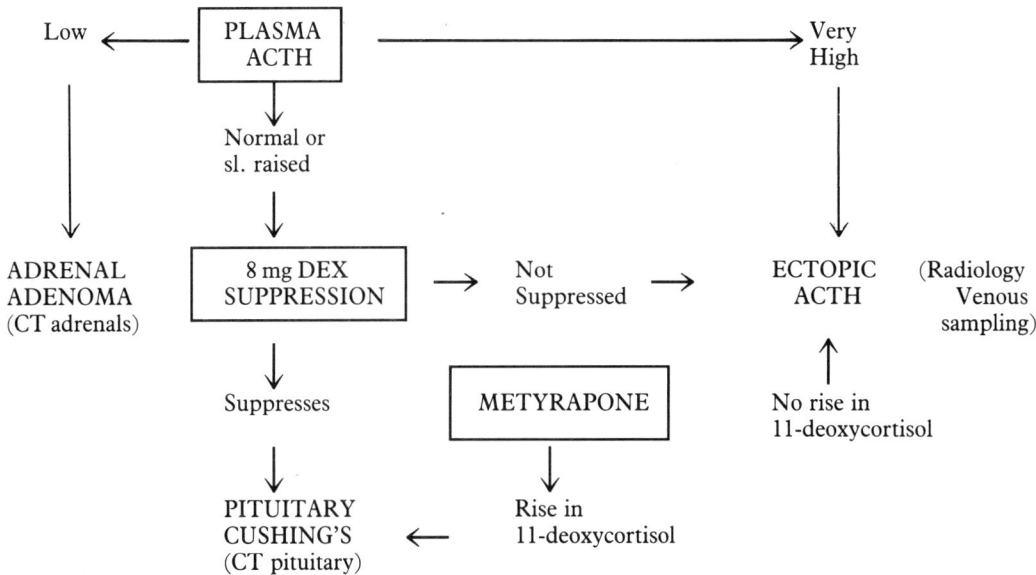

Fig. 5.7 Scheme of investigation to determine the cause of Cushing's syndrome.

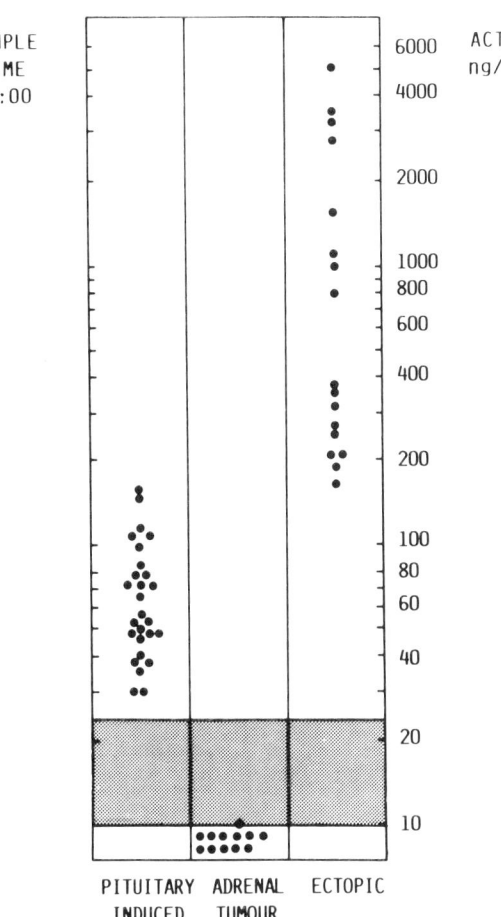

Fig. 5.8 Plasma ACTH values in the three different types of Cushing's syndrome. ACTH is measured in ng/l and plotted on a log scale. The timing of the samples is at 09.00. The shaded area is the normal range at 09.00.

obesity an insulin tolerance test may help to distinguish these conditions from Cushing's syndrome. The serum cortisol may initially be elevated but will rise even higher with hypoglycaemia. Patients with Cushing's syndrome will have a flat response of both cortisol and growth hormone.

The differential diagnosis of Cushing's syndrome

A scheme of investigation of the differential diagnosis of Cushing's syndrome is set out in Figure 5.7.

The single most important test is estimation of plasma ACTH. Figure 5.8 shows plasma ACTH levels at 09:00 in the three different types of Cushing's syndrome. The normal range

is also shown. Plasma samples taken at the time of determination of diurnal cortisol rhythm should be measured once the presence of hypercortisolism has been established.

If the plasma ACTH is very low, or undetectable (less than 10 ng/l in most assays) then the diagnosis is of an adrenal tumour. The autonomous production of cortisol suppresses normal ACTH production. The tumour may be localised either by CT scanning or by seleno-cholesterol scanning.

If the ACTH concentration is very high (>250 ng/l) then again the diagnosis is simple and an ectopic ACTH source is present. The tumour may be sought by conventional means or by selective venous catheterisation with multiple site sampling for plasma ACTH.

ACTH levels between 25–100 ng/l indicate that Cushing's disease is present. It is often stated that ACTH levels in Cushing's disease overlap with the normal range. The quoted morning normal range is 10-80 ng/l, but this range runs from 08:00 to 10:00. If the samples are taken at 09:00, only, then the normal range is much narrower (12 to 24 ng/l, see Fig. 5.8) and there is no overlap. CT scanning of the pituitary gland may be undertaken to try to demonstrate the presence of a pituitary adenoma.

Difficulty arises when the plasma ACTH lies between 100 and 250 ng/l. The diagnosis is either pituitary induced Cushing's disease or ectopic ACTH syndrome. This difficulty is compounded by the fact that the ectopic syndromes with relatively low ACTH levels are usually due to benign tumours (thymic carcinoids and bronchial adenomas), and the onset of the symptoms is much slower. There is therefore no clinical distinction between these two types of Cushing's syndrome. In this situation there are three possible avenues of further investigation.

The first of these is the high dose dexamethasone suppression test (8 mg/day for 48 h). Lack of suppression points to an ectopic source. Unfortunately cases of suppressible ectopic ACTH have been described where presumably functioning glucocorticoid receptors are present in the tumour cells. The second line of investigation is to perform a metyrapone test which tests the integrity of the pituitary adrenal axis. Metyrapone blocks 11-hydroxylation and lowers serum cortisol levels. This is sensed by a normal hypothalamic-pituitary axis which responds with an increase in plasma ACTH. A positive metyrapone response is therefore indicated by a rise in ACTH or a two fold rise in 11-deoxycortisol. Unfortunately, as with the long dexamethasone suppression test, cases of ectopic ACTH have been described that do show a positive response to this test. The third aspect of investigation is to search for a source of ectopic ACTH. With the necessary radiological expertise selective venous catheterisation is performed. Samples for ACTH are taken from high up in the jugular vein and from the venous drainage of likely ectopic sources. A gradient in ACTH concentrations from sample site to peripheral vein indicates the site of ACTH production.

Treatment of Cushing's syndrome

The treatment of adrenal tumours, like their diagnosis, is relatively straightforward. Laparotomy with removal of the tumour is indicated. If there is any doubt about the patient's fitness for operation they may be prepared medically.

Surgical control of disease in cases of ectopic ACTH would be most desirable, but often there are difficulties. The tumour may be so small (especially in the case of oat cell carcinomas of the bronchus) that it is impossible to localise it accurately. On other occasions there may be multiple secondaries present which make operation impossible. Again medical control of the disease is the treatment of choice.

Cushing's disease

The treatment of pituitary induced Cushing's syndrome may be by one of several methods, depending on the facilities available locally:
1. Transphenoidal hypophysectomy
2. Radiotherapy + medical management
3. Yttrium seed implantation.
4. Bilateral adrenalectomy + radiotherapy to the pituitary fossa.

Transphenoidal hypophysetomy. Transphenoidal surgery is probably the treatment of choice if an experienced surgeon is available. It is said that microadenomas can be found in 90% of cases and that two thirds of these are 2–5 mm in diameter. The cure rate is 70–80% in the best centres. The larger the tumour at operation the less the chance of cure. The advantage of transphenoidal hypophysectomy is the low morbidity (1–2% meningitis and cerebrospinal fluid rhinorrhoea) and the low mortality (1–2%). Few of the patients undergoing selective adenomectomy will require long term cortisol replacement therapy, although it may be necessary for several months after operation. The incidence of diabetes insipidus is low and is usually transient.

External radiotherapy. The reported results of external radiotherapy to the pituitary fossa are worse than for transphenoidal hypophysectomy. The best results are obtained in children where cure rates of 80% can be obtained with total doses of 4000–5000 rad. In adults the results appear to be age related. Remission rates vary between 50 and 70% but comparisons are difficult because of the different criteria used to define remission. Although the effect of radiotherapy to the pituitary fossa is usually slow in onset, most series report remissions occurring within 6 to 18 months, unlike acromegaly for instance, where improvement may continue for many years. Patients who are treated with radiotherapy also require medical management of the hypercortisolism until the treatment is effective (see below).

Yttrium implants. This form of treatment is available in very few centres. The technique involves the placement of yttrium-90 seeds in the pituitary fossa, via the transphenoidal route, using X-ray control. The isotope is a beta emitter and has the advantage of being able to deliver a high local dose of radiation without endangering other brain structures. The results of such treatment appear favourable, with 65% of patients in remission at 1 year and a further 16% being improved. As with other forms of treatment the success rate is dependent on the size of the pituitary tumour, larger tumours have a worse cure rate than that stated. Approximately 50% of patients require some form of replacement therapy. The mean time to remission is about 4 months. The incidence of c.s.f. leak is 5%.

Adrenalectomy. Bilateral adrenalectomy will cure the hypercortisolism, but there is a higher morbidity and mortality associated with the operation. Laparotomy in patients with Cushing's syndrome is more likely to be complicated by infection, problems of healing and venous thrombosis. The disease should be controlled medically before operation to try to minimise these risks.

A further possible complication of bilateral adrenalectomy is the occurrence of Nelson's syndrome. Feedback control is intact in Cushing's disease and reduction of the high serum cortisol by adrenalectomy leads to a further rise in ACTH levels; this is occasionally accompanied by a locally aggressive pituitary tumour. The patient presents with pigmentation, ocular nerve palsies and headaches. The incidence of this complication is variably reported to be 10–20% of bilateral adrenalectomies. Nelson's syndrome can usually be prevented by irradiation of the pituitary gland soon after adrenalectomy but cases have been described even after irradiation.

Medical management of Cushing's syndrome

Agents which act at the pituitary/hypothalamic level. Cyproheptadine is a serotonin antagonist which has been reported to lower ACTH levels in Cushing's disease and in Nelson's syndrome. Results in general, however, have been very variable, with as many reports of failure as success. Side effects of drowsiness and stimulation of appetite occur.

Bromocriptine has also been used in the treatment of both Cushing's disease and Nelson's syndrome. Many reports show an acute effect on ACTH levels but results in the long term have been poor. The occasional patient does appear to have a dramatic response. It has been suggested that response is more likely if the serum prolactin is also elevated.

Drugs acting on the adrenal cortex. Metyrapone and aminoglutethimide are the two drugs most commonly used to reduce cortisol synthesis. They both act by inhibiting one of the hydroxylation enzymes in the biosynthetic pathway.

Metyrapone blocks 11 β-hydroxylation and aminoglutethimide blocks the first step in the conversion of cholesterol to pregnenolone. Metyrapone is the better tolerated of the two drugs, with nausea being the main side effect. Aminoglutethimide in doses of more than 1 g daily produces drowsiness and ataxia. Skin rashes and pyrexial reactions are also not infrequent. Side effects may disappear spontaneously if the drug is continued.

The drugs may be used in one of two ways. The first method is to try to achieve complete blockade of cortisol synthesis. Using this method it will be necessary to provide replacement hydrocortisone and fludrocortisone. The second method is to tailor the dose to suit the individual and to give just enough of the blocking drugs to normalise cortisol production. The administration of smaller doses of both drugs together has been advocated in order to minimise the risk of side effects.

The dose of metyrapone which is required is very variable. A dose of between 250 mg twice daily and 1.5 g four times daily will be required. Initial monitoring of serum cortisol levels is required in order to tailor the dose to the individual patient. Since 11-deoxycortisol levels are very high on treatment, one has to be sure that the assay for cortisol does not cross-react with this compound giving a falsely high result.

A further compound known as o,p,DDD (1,1-dichloro-2-(o-chlorophenyl)-2-(chlorophenyl) ethane) has been used to treat adrenocortical carcinoma since it causes necrosis of adrenocortical cells. It commonly produces gastrointestinal side effects and also severe ataxia. It is, therefore, not used in the benign forms of Cushing's syndrome.

HYPOADRENALISM

There are several reasons why patients have loss of function of the adrenal cortex. Most of the conditions are acquired, but a few of the rarer causes are present from birth. The clinical features depend on which hormones are deficient. The most important deficit is that of cortisol, but the symptoms of cortisol deficiency may be very non-specific especially in the uncomplicated case.

The following is a list of the more important causes, and descriptions of the main conditions follow.

1. Addison's disease
2. Hypopituitarism.
3. Congenital adrenal hyperplasia.
4. Enzyme blocking drugs
   a. metyrapone
   b. aminoglutethimide.
5. Exogenous glucocorticoids.

Table 5.3 Percentage prevalence of symptoms and signs in Addison's disease. (After Ross E J 1984 In: Keynes W M, Fowler P B S (eds) Clinical endocrinology. Ch. 6. Heinemann, London.)

Symptoms or signs	%
Tiredness	100
Weakness	100
Anorexia	100
Weight loss	98
Pigmentation	94
Buccal pigmentation	68
Abdominal pain	32
Constipation	21
Diarrhoea	19
Muscle pain	16
Syncope	16
Vitiligo	9

ADDISON'S DISEASE

The causes of the disorder, in descending frequency of occurrence are:
1. Autoimmune adrenalitis
2. Tuberculosis
3. Adrenal destruction
   a. Malignant deposits
   b. Amyloidosis
   c. Sarcoidosis

very rarely:
   d. Histoplasmosis, blastomycosis, coccidio-mycosis, cytomegalovirus, SLE, haemo-chromatosis
   e. Infarction caused by thrombosis; haemorrhage due to anticoagulants.

It is said that 70% of cases are due to autoimmune disease, but it is often difficult to be certain whether tuberculosis is or has been the cause. The marker of autoimmune disease, adrenal antibodies, is not always positive and therefore the diagnosis is one of exclusion.

Autoimmune Addison's disease

This condition fits into the spectrum of destructive autoimmune endocrine disease, along with Hashimoto's thyroiditis, diabetes mellitus, hypopituitarism, hypoparathyroidism and premature ovarian failure. It is also associated with other autoimmune disorders such as pernicious anaemia, vitiligo and alopecia areata. The associations are not entirely with destructive conditions since the incidence of Graves' disease is also increased.

Clinical features

The majority of the symptoms and signs of adrenocortical insufficiency are non-specific (Table 5.3). The onset of the disease is usually insidious. A feeling of general malaise or tiredness and weakness is extremely common. Patients often have great difficulty in recovering from minor illnesses or operations. Even at rest the blood pressure is low in Addison's disease (systolic around 100–110 mmHg) and its reflex regulation is impaired resulting in postural hypotension. There are two reasons for this: firstly both cortisol and aldosterone promote sodium reabsorption, the sodium loss therefore contracts the extracellular volume; secondly, cortisol normally potentiates the action of catecholamines.

The pigmentation which occurs in 95% of cases is most prominent on light exposed areas. Indeed, the first symptom may be a failure of a summer tan to fade in the winter. It is also present in the mouth, on the inside of the lips and cheeks, around the nipples, in scars and pressure areas and also in skin creases. Pigmentation also increases in Negroid and Asian races but minor changes are much more difficult to detect. The reason for the pigmentation is the high level of both β-lipotrophin and ACTH which stimulate melanin production in melanocytes.

Gastrointestinal symptoms, apart from anorexia, occur late in the disease. Diffuse abdominal pain associated with diarrhoea are the commonest of these symptoms. Vomiting usually heralds the onset of an adrenal crisis. The extra fluid loss leads to vascular collapse and a vicious circle is entered. It is at this stage that patients may present as an apparent acute surgical emergency. The abdominal pain, vomiting, hypotension and history of diarrhoea pointing to an 'acute abdomen'. It is commonly felt that the patient is suffering from intestinal obstruction. Treatment with intravenous saline leads to a partial recovery, because it restores circulating volume and sodium deficit.

Women may suffer loss of body hair because of loss of adrenal androgens and it is very common for oligomenorrhoea or amenorrhoea to be present. This may be a functional abnormality of the pituitary ovarian axis, in which case recovery takes place with treatment of the Addison's, or it may be due to premature ovarian failure as previously discussed.

Cortisol is a gluconeogenic hormone and is one of the factors responsible for the correction of hypoglycaemia. Its loss may lead to fasting hypoglycaemia. In those cases where the Addison's disease is due to replacement or destruction of the adrenal gland, the loss of adrenaline also adds to this problem. A further factor in the aetiology of hypoglycaemia is that all cases show a degree of glucose malabsorption.

Adrenal crisis

This is an acute life-threatening event. It may be precipitated by a variety of different events. The common feature of them is that they would all normally induce an increase in cortisol production. The list of causes includes anaesthesia, surgical operations, blood loss sufficient to lower blood pressure, diarrhoea sufficient to reduce plasma volume, infections, pregnancy, thyrotoxicosis and hypoglycaemia (e.g. induced by an insulin stress test). The patient is shocked and, if the onset has been gradual, then he will be dehydrated and have the gastrointestinal symptoms listed above. Serum electrolytes will usually be abnormal with a low sodium, a high potassium, and an elevated urea. The treatment is documented below.

Diagnosis of Addison's disease

The biochemical abnormality which is first noticed is disturbance of urea and electrolytes. It is often this finding which provokes further investigation. It must be stressed, however that these abnormalities are not specific to Addison's disease and that early in the disease the electrolytes may be entirely normal.

The changes described are due to loss of mineralocorticoid action. Salt and water depletion leads to hyponatraemia and elevation of the serum urea. The subsequent potassium reabsorption produces hyperkalaemia. The problems of hyperkalaemia are made worse in patients who are also diabetic since insulin is involved in the control of the serum potassium. At times of insulin deficiency there may be life threatening hyperkalaemia.

As in the investigation of Cushing's syndrome, there are two aspects to the investigation of a patient with possible Addison's disease. Firstly, the presence of hypocortisolism must be established. Secondly, the cause should be investigated and, in particular, the distinction between primary and secondary adrenal failure made. In the latter case it is possible that other endocrine deficiencies may be present and require treatment. Once the diagnosis of primary adrenal failure has been made then a pathological cause should be sought.

The mainstay of investigation is the assessment of cortisol reserve. In the basal state a midnight cortisol is of no value at all. A serum cortisol at 09:00 is only helpful if it is extremely low. The same comment could also be made about urinary free cortisol measurement. The assessment of cortisol reserve by performing a stimulation test is mandatory.

Synacthen (CIBA Pharmaceuticals) is synthetic 1–24ACTH. Natural ACTH is 39 amino acids in length, but its biological activity resides in the N-terminal portion. The peptide which comprises the first 24 amino acids is the shortest one which retains full biological potency.

A short Synacthen test is the simplest assessment of adrenal reserve. Blood for serum cortisol is taken before and at 30 and 60 min after an intramuscular injection of 250 micrograms of soluble Synacthen. A normal test is characterised by a basal cortisol of greater than 140 nmol/l, an increment of at least 200 nmol/l and a peak response of over 500 nmol/l.

In order to distinguish primary from secondary adrenal failure a plasma ACTH measurement is necessary. In primary adrenal failure plasma ACTH will be elevated (usually over 300 ng/l) because of normal pituitary reserve. In secondary failure it will be less than 10 ng/l or undetectable. ACTH is rapidly degraded in plasma and care should be taken with the sample so that it is immediately separated and frozen at –20°C to avoid spuriously low values. If an ACTH estimation is not available the distinction between primary and secondary failure can be made by performing a long Synacthen test. This involves the injection of 1 mg of Synacthen depot on five successive days. If primary hypoadrenalism is present then there will be no rise in serum cortisol over this time. When secondary hypoadrenalism is present then there will be a stepwise increase in cortisol response over the five days, as adrenal enzymes are induced by ACTH. The rise in serum cortisol may be detected by successive day curves of serum cortisol, or more simply by a stepwise increase in serum cortisol taken each morning before the injection of depot ACTH.

There is often confusion about the method of investigation of a patient who presents in presumed adrenal crisis where it is necessary to treat before the results are available. A single sample of blood should be taken prior to giving steroids and stored for later estimation of cortisol and, if necessary, ACTH. It is often recommended that patients should be treated with prednisolone or dexamethasone because they do not interfere with later cortisol measurements. These are, however, very long-acting steroids which may well suppress the elevated ACTH. Alternatively, if the patient is normal, then they may suppress adrenal function leading to a mistaken diagnosis of Addison's disease. Hydrocortisone has the advantage that it has a short half life. At the end of a dose period cortisol levels are usually very low and certainly, once the patient is stable, a single dose may be omitted prior to performing the above tests. ACTH may be estimated on a sample taken before Synacthen is injected.

Once the diagnosis of primary adrenal failure has been established then further investigations into the cause may be undertaken. Adrenal antibodies may be measured in serum. The possibility of tuberculosis may be investigated by performing a chest X-ray, Mantoux test, and plain abdominal X-ray to look for adrenal calcification. A CT scan may show adrenal masses if metastases are suspected.

Treatment

This is dealt with in the section on steroid treatment (see below).

CONGENITAL ADRENAL HYPERPLASIA

Congenital adrenal hyperplasia encompasses a number of conditions each of which is caused by an inherited defect of one of the enzymes involved in the biosynthetic pathway of cortisol. Each one affects a different enzyme but each results in a reduced capacity to produce cortisol. The pituitary adrenal axis responds to the lack of negative feedback by increasing ACTH production, in an attempt to correct the situation. The result is hypertrophy of the adrenal cortex and overproduction of the steroids immediately before the enzyme block. The steroids which are produced in excess vary with the defective enzyme. The steroids which are most often produced in excess, with clinical consequences, are the adrenal androgens and occasionally mineralocorticoids.

In considering these disorders it would be wise to consult Figure 5.2, which is a representation of steroid biosynthesis. Note that the same enzymes are represented in one horizontal or vertical line. The following is a list of the enzyme defects, so far described, in order of frequency of occurrence:

1. 21-Hydroxylase
2. 11 β-Hydroxylase
3. 3 β-Hydroxysteroid dehydrogenase
4. 17 α-Hydroxylase
5. Cholesterol desmolase
6. 18-Hydroxylase

21-Hydroxylase deficiency

This is by far the commonest of these syndromes. The prevalence in Europe is thought to be 1 in 5000, and a screening programme in Alaska recently suggested 1 in 3000. It is inherited as an autosomal recessive disorder. The prevalence of the heterozygous form (or carrier state) is estimated at 1 in 37. Studies have shown a close genetic linkage with HLA antigens. The gene for 21-hydroxylase is located very close to the HLA-B locus. All affected members of one family share the same HLA genotype, but unaffected siblings are different. Carriers of the condition in the family will have one HLA haplotype identical to one of the haplotypes of affected members.

There are two subgroups of 21-hydroxylase deficiency. If the 21-hydroxylase in the zona glomerulosa is affected then aldosterone synthesis is impaired and the patients are 'salt losers'. If the aldosterone pathway appears to be intact then they are usually called 'simple virilisers'.

Cortisol deficiency is not an important clinical problem since the increased ACTH drive is able to overcome the block and cortisol production rates are low normal or normal. In times of stress, however, particularly in children, adrenal crisis may occur. The main adverse effects of 21-hydroxylase deficiency are seen in females because of the excess of androgen and progesterone production (Ch. 7).

Children with the condition may present either with ambiguous genitalia or in a salt-losing crisis. The excess androgen is mainly androstenedione, but some of this is converted to testosterone peripherally. In the female, a problem arises because the high androgens stimulate the Wolffian system with the development of a phallus and fusion of the labial folds. Because there is no testis, and therefore no Mullerian inhibitor, the internal female genitalia develop normally. Often these female infants are mistaken for males with partial or complete hypospadias. Milder forms may present with clitoromegaly. If the diagnosis is not made at birth, then they may sometimes present later as phenotypic males with 'bilateral cryptorchidism'; they are then discovered to be genotypically female.

Other problems which occur because of the increased production of sex steroids are primary amenorrhoea in girls and precocious puberty and short stature, due to premature fusion of epiphyses, in both sexes. In early years affected subjects are taller than their peers because of an early growth spurt, but their final height is less than would be expected because they miss out on the more prolonged phase of slow growth. Occasionally, females may present later in life because of hirsutism, virilism, and amenorrhoea (Fig. 5.9). This 'late onset' form of the disease is probably a different disorder from classical 21-hydroxylase deficiency.

Heterozygotes are usually asymptomatic. Occasionally they may present later in life with hirsutism or menstrual disturbance. In these people minor abnormalities of 17-hydroxyprogesterone secretion are found in response to ACTH stimulation.

Diagnosis

The two steroids which are most elevated are 17-hydroxyprogesterone (and its urinary metabolite

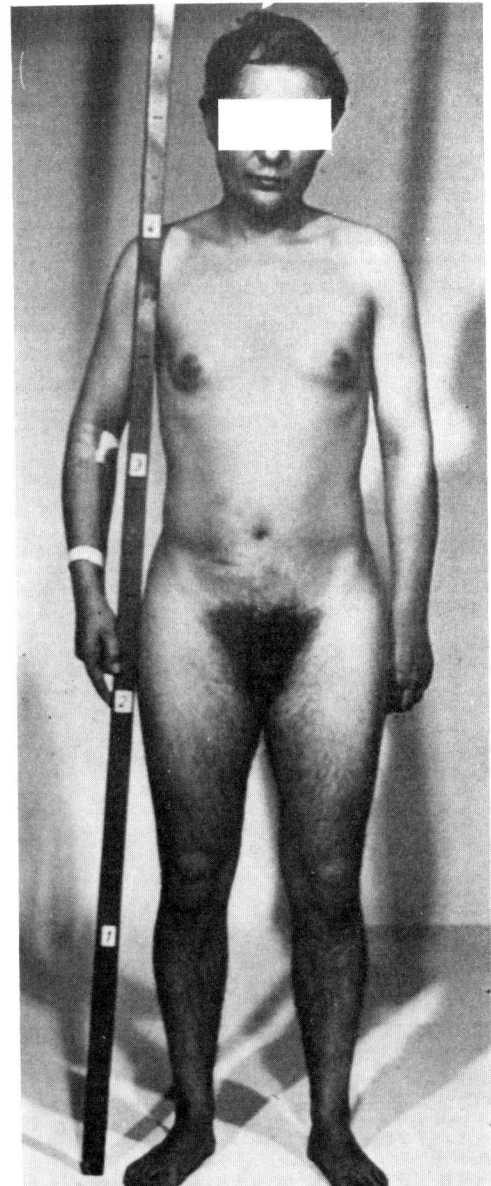

Fig. 5.9 Genotypic female with congenital adrenal hyperplasia. Note the short stature, frontal balding, virilisation and enlarged clitoris.

pregnanetriol) and androstenedione. Other steroids before the block will be elevated to a degree which is inversely proportional to their distance from the block. Both steroids may be measured in serum and 17-hydroxyprogesterone may be measured on a 24-hour urine. Serum testosterone is high as is DHA and DHAS. In the untreated patient ACTH is elevated as discussed above.

Treatment

The aim of treatment is to suppress harmful androgen production by replacement therapy with corticosteroids. Treatment needs to be carefully tailored to the individual and monitored closely. There is a fine line, especially in children, between oversuppression, which leads to a Cushingoid state with side effects such as growth retardation, and undersuppression with its already mentioned problems. There is much discussion about the correct agent to use. Dexamethasone has the advantage of being long acting and therefore of producing more uniform suppression over the whole 24-hour period. It is, however, more difficult to manipulate the dose, especially in children. Hydrocortisone, although providing adequate cortisol replacement, has a short half life and has to be given more frequently. This is a problem overnight because there is insufficient corticosteroid present in the early morning to suppress the ACTH surge. The dose is more easily manipulated, however. Salt losers should receive fludrocortisone in addition to hydrocortisone.

The adjustment of the dose of glucocorticoid must be made on the basis of the spectrum of clinical and biochemical data. The growth rate, pubertal status, degree of virilisation and clinical appearance should be assessed. 17-Hydroxyprogesterone, androstenedione and renin activity should be measured by the laboratory. In males, once the problems of growth and precocious puberty have passed, there are few clinical abnormalities to correct. In females, however, there are continuing problems throughout adult life. The pituitary-ovarian axis is very sensitive to poor control and oligomenorrhoea or amenorrhoea may lead to infertility. Hirsutism and acne are likely to be problems. In addition to the endocrine features there are often anatomical problems such as vaginal hypoplasia. Surgical treatment for this may be required but it is usually reserved until patients become sexually active.

11 β-Hydroxylase deficiency

This condition is much less common than 21-hydroxylase deficiency although there are no population studies to suggest its true prevalence. There is no known HLA association.

The main difference between 11- and 21-hydroxylase deficiency is the occurrence of hypertension in the former. This results from the accumulation of 17-deoxycorticosterone (Fig. 5.2). Even though it is a weaker mineralocorticoid than aldosterone high serum concentrations of 17-deoxycorticosterone produce hypertension. Just as there are salt and non-salt losers in 21-hydroxylase deficiency so there are hypertensive and non-hypertensive forms of 11-hydroxylase deficiency.

The presentation, apart from a salt losing state, is identical to that in 21-hydroxylase deficient patients. It may be difficult to distinguish the two if the patient is not hypertensive and specific measurements of 11-deoxycortisol are not made. Late onset forms are also said to occur. 17-Hydroxyprogesterone and androstenedione are again elevated.

3β-Hydroxysteroid dehydrogenease deficiency

The enzyme defect in this rare form of congenital adrenal hyperplasia leads to loss of production of cortisol, aldosterone and all the Δ-4 steroids. It is the weakly androgenic Δ-5 steroids, namely DHA and DHAS which accumulate. Because they are weakly androgenic, both sexes may have ambiguous genitalia. Males are incompletely virilised and females are mildly virilised. As with the previous types of the syndrome, there is a severe form presenting in childhood with salt and water loss and there is also a mild form presenting later in life in females with menstrual disturbance and hirsutism. This latter form may be more common than was previously recognised.

17 α-Hydroxylase deficiency

From inspection of Figure 5.2, it can be seen that this defect results in loss of cortisol and adrenal androgen production. The defect also affects steroid production by the gonad with absence of sex hormones. Males are not virilised at birth, whereas females have normal genitalia. Both sexes have delayed puberty and require treatment with either oestrogen or testosterone. Excess production of mineralocorticoids leads to hypertension and hypokalaemia.

Cholesterol desmolase deficiency

This condition is extremely rare and affects the first step in the conversion of cholesterol to pregnenolone. All adrenal and gonadal steroid synthesis is involved. The accumulation of cholesterol within the adrenal led to the description of 'lipoid adrenal hyperplasia'. As with 17-hydroxylase deficiency, the males are not virilised and females appear normal. Both have salt and water loss and both fail to show any pubertal development.

Long-term complications

Occasionally the diagnosis of congenital adrenal hyperplasia is missed, or the patient defaults from treatment. There are a number of complications which may occur in such patients as a consequence of prolonged undertreatment:

1. Short stature
2. Virilism and amenorrhoea in women
3. Azoospermia in men
4. Adrenal tumours
5. Pituitary feedback tumours (of ACTH cells).

MINERALOCORTICOID DEFICIENCY SYNDROMES

Some of these conditions have already been discussed but are listed here for the sake of completeness:

1. Addison's disease
2. Congenital adrenal hyperplasia
   a. 21-hydroxylase deficiency
   b. 3 β-hydroxysteroid dehydrogenase deficiency
   c. cholesterol desmolase deficiency
3. Bilateral adrenalectomy
4. Hyporeninaemic hypoaldosteronism
5. Normoreninaemic hypoaldosteronism
6. Hyperreninaemic hypoaldosteronism
7. 18-Hydroxylase deficiency
8. Pseudohypoaldosteronism (resistance to aldosterone action).

The first three conditions on the list also have cortisol deficiency and all are associated with high plasma renin activity. Of the selective aldosterone deficiencies number four is the most common.

Hyporeninaemic hypoaldosteronism

This condition usually occurs in elderly patients with either cardiovascular disease or diabetes mellitus. Patients usually present with moderate persistent hyperkalaemia (around 5.5–6.5 mmol/l) and they often have mild renal impairment. The hyperkalaemia is associated with a hyperchloraemic acidosis. The condition is probably due to an interstitial nephropathy with damage to the juxtaglomerular apparatus, but a degree of autonomic neuropathy (which is commoner with advancing age and in diabetes) might be implicated. The low renin is probably not the complete explanation. Normally hyperkalaemia directly stimulates the zona glomerulosa to produce more aldosterone. This fact has led to the suggestion that there is also an adrenal defect as well as the renin deficiency. Other people have argued that the presence of angiotensin II is required for potassium to exert its stimulatory effect.

Many of the patients are asymptomatic and do not require treatment. If the serum potassium is a problem (greater than 6 mmol/l) then fludrocortisone 100 μg daily may be required. Sometimes resistance to fludrocortisone is encountered and higher doses are needed. Since many of the patients are elderly, with cardiovascular disease, care should be exercised in case hypertension, oedema, or cardiac failure become problems, especially in the first few weeks of treatment.

SYNDROMES OF MINERALOCORTICOID EXCESS

It is convenient to classify these disorders into primary and secondary causes. (Tables 5.4 and 5.5) The secondary causes are all due to excessive aldosterone secretion in response to exaggerated or pathological stimulation of the normal renin-angiotensin system. The primary causes are due to the secretion of a variety of mineralocorticoid and mineralocorticoid-like

Table 5.4 Syndromes of mineralocorticoid excess. Primary hyperaldosteronism

Aldosterone

Adrenal adenoma — Conn's syndrome
Bilateral adrenal hyperplasia
Adrenal carcinoma
Dexamethasone supressible hyperaldosteronism

Other mineralocorticoids

Congenital adrenal hyperplasia
    11β-hydroxylase
    17α-hydroxylase
Cushing's syndrome

Drugs

Liquorice derivatives
Carbenoxolone

Table 5.5 Syndromes of mineralocorticoid excess. Secondary hyperaldosteronism

Redistribution of sodium

Congestive heart failure   ★
Cirrhosis with ascites   ★
Nephrotic syndrome
Idiopathic oedema

Abnormal electrolyte loss

Salt-losing nephropathy (chronic pyelonephritis)
Barrter's syndrome
Diuretic use or abuse   ★
Renal tubular acidosis
Vomiting or diarrhoea

Overproduction of renin

Renal artery stenosis
Malignant hypertension   ★
Renal ischaemia
Renin-producing tumour
Chronic renal failure

★ = common causes.

substances. The main distinction between primary and secondary hyperaldosteronism is the plasma renin activity, which is suppressed in primary and elevated in secondary causes.

Primary (low renin) hyperaldosteronism

Table 5.4 shows that there are a variety of causes of primary hyperaldosteronism. An excess of aldosterone may occur in association with an adrenal adenoma (Conn's syndrome). The same abnormalities have, however, been reported in the absence of an adenoma. In these cases the adrenal cortex is either normal or shows hyperplasia of the zona glomerulosa. Rarely, patients have been described in whom the same biochemical abnormalities have responded to suppression with dexamethasone. Usually, in these cases, hyperplasia of the cortex is present. The cases of adrenocortical carcinoma causing this picture are very rare.

Clinical

The commonest presentation of the condition is with hypertension. The discovery of hypokalaemia points to further investigation of adrenocortical function. Occasionally unexplained hypokalaemia itself is the first clue. The hypertension is not always mild, as has sometimes been stated. Patients may present with malignant hypertension, and

vascular complications occur in about a quarter of cases. There appears to be no difference in the severity of the hypertension between the three groups. Patients may be asymptomatic, but characteristic symptoms are headache, nocturia, muscle weakness, paraesthesiae, thirst and polyuria, and tetany. It can be appreciated that most of these are a consequence of the hypokalaemia.

Diagnosis and dfferential diagnosis

The factor which alerts the physician to the possibility of primary hyperaldosteronism is the serum potassium, which is a good screening test in hypertensive patients. Hypokalaemia is present in 90% of patients with an aldosterone-producing adenoma. However, it should be remembered that upright posture, exercise, haemolysis and thrombocytosis increase serum potassium.

The finding of hypokalaemia in hypertensive patients should prompt the measurement of both aldosterone and plasma renin activity. The interpretation of the results of the measurement of these two substances depend on three different factors. Firstly, there is no universal standard for plasma renin and results from different laboratories are not comparable. Secondly, the circumstances under which the samples are obtained must be defined. It is usual to take the blood sample between 08:00 and 10:00 with the patient supine (for at least an hour). The patient should be taking a diet containing not less than 100 mmol of sodium per day. Thirdly, both plasma renin activity and aldosterone fall quite markedly with age. It is vital, therefore, that each laboratory defines its own normal range for samples taken under a set of strictly controlled clinical conditions.

A combination of an aldosterone concentration and a plasma renin activity should allow the distinction between primary hyperaldosteronism (high aldosterone, low renin), low renin hypertension (normal aldosterone, low renin) and secondary hyperaldosteronism (high aldosterone, high renin). There is persistent elevation of aldosterone in 40% of cases of Conn's syndrome and intermittent elevation in 60%. Values are usually higher in those patients with an adenoma compared to those with no tumour. The consequence of the higher aldosterone in tumour patients is that the secondary biochemical disturbances are more severe. These include a lower potassium, a higher sodium, a lower renin, and a higher plasma CO_2.

The presence of a tumour may be sought by a number of methods of anatomical localisation. A CT scan of the adrenals is often valuable although sometimes the tumour is too small to be visualised. A high detection rate is found using selenocholesterol scanning. Selenium labelled cholesterol is taken up by actively synthesising adrenocortical tissue. A 'hot spot' on the scan is indicative of a tumour. The success rate of this technique is improved dramatically if the scan is performed during dexamethasone suppression. This effectively reduces the uptake of labelled cholesterol by normal adrenal tissue, thereby enhancing the uptake by the tumour. Arteriography and adrenal venography have been important, in the past, as localising techniques but they are being replaced by the two preceding methods. Adrenal venography does have the advantage that it may be combined with venous sampling, for aldosterone, to obtain functional localisation.

Anatomical localisation is the best method of determining the presence of a tumour. If no tumour is found then a trial of dexamethasone is warranted to look for the rare case of dexamethasone suppressibilty (see below).

Treatment

Spironolactone is the medical treatment of choice in these patients. Doses of 300–400 mg daily may normalise blood pressure, sodium and potassium levels. In patients without an adenoma it is the mainstay of treatment. If spironolactone is not tolerated, then amiloride may be substituted but the results of treatment are less successful (at doses up to 40 mg) in terms of blood pressure control.

In Conn's syndrome where an adenoma is present, surgical removal is successful in restoring blood pressure to normal in between 50 and 70% of cases. There is a positive correlation between the fall in blood pressure on spironolactone and the fall in blood pressure after the removal of the tumour. It is possible to state, therefore, that if the blood pressure is not controlled on spironolactone then there is unlikely to be any further benefit from surgery. Such patients should not be offered operation, but their hypertension should be controlled by conventional antihypertensive agents.

Patients in whom no tumour is found should undergo a trial of dexamethasone. If they are to respond, 1–2 mg is usually sufficient. The trial should continue for four weeks.

The management of primary hyperaldosteronism is summarised in Figure 5.10.

Secondary (high renin) hyperaldosteronism

The elevated levels of aldosterone in secondary hyperaldosteronism result from excessive stimulation of renin secretion and angiotensin II. The causes are set out in Table 5.5 and the commonest syndromes are marked with an asterisk. Most of the conditions are clinically obvious and the hyperaldosteronism forms a minor part of the pathology. Those conditions in which there is overproduction of renin are usually associated with hypertension. There are a few causes which are less obvious. Bartter's syndrome is one of these, but most are a result of patient manipulation (self-induced vomiting or diarrhoea and diuretic abuse). The clue

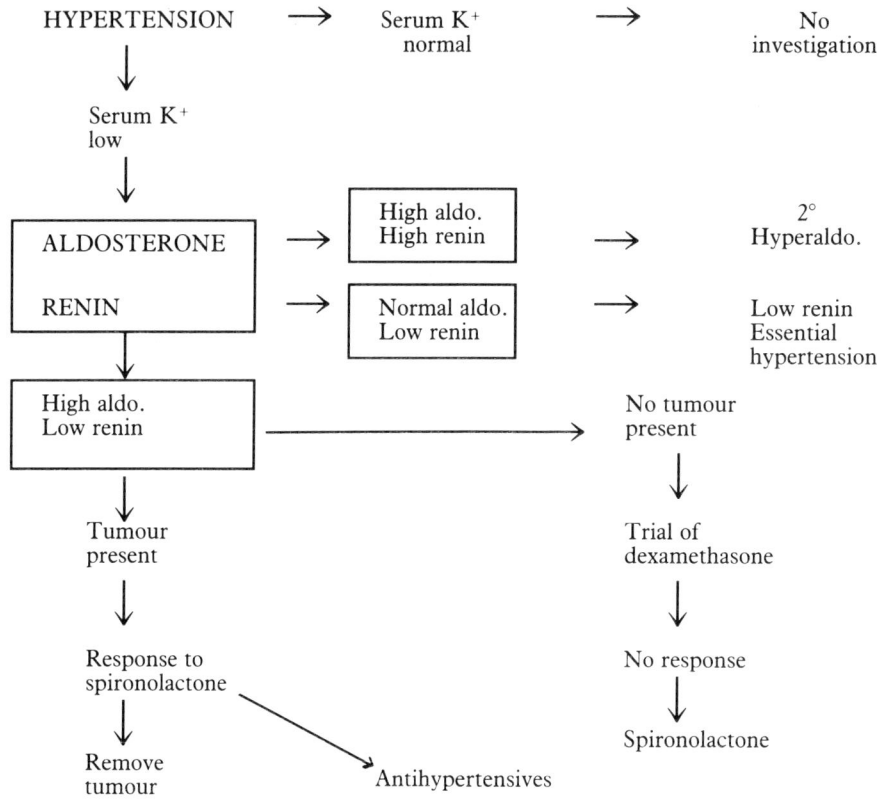

Fig. 5.10 The management of primary hyperaldosteronism.
Aldo = Aldosterone; K^+ = Potassium

to the secondary hyperaldosteronism is unexplained hypokalaemia, but often a high index of suspicion is required to make the diagnosis.

The treatment in most instances is to try to correct the underlying cause. If diuretics are required, as in congestive cardiac failure or cirrhosis, then spironolactone is of benefit.

Bartter's syndrome

This rare disorder is characterised by hypokalaemia, metabolic alkalosis and hyper-reninaemic aldosteronism. In addition, there appears to be a resistance to the action of angiotensin II, since patients have a normal or low blood pressure in the face of extracellular fluid expansion and

there is a reduced pressor response to infused angiotensin II.

The pathogenesis of the disorder is not completely understood. One of the findings, in the kidney, is hyperplasia of the juxtaglomerular apparatus, but this is not specific and is found in other disorders, such as protracted vomiting and chronic laxative abuse. Primary hyper-reninaemia is not, therefore, thought to be the cause of the syndrome. Some years ago, it was discovered that there was an increased excretion of urinary prostaglandins in Bartter's syndrome and it was wondered whether there was a defect in prostanoid production in the kidney. The consensus of opinion, however, favours the view that again this is a secondary phenomenon, since chronic hypokalaemia is itself an important stimulus to prostaglandin production.

basis of hypokalaemia.

The differential diagnosis of this condition includes diuretic abuse and protracted vomiting as they also share the features of hypokalaemia, metabolic alkalosis, and secondary hyperaldosteronism. Bartter's syndrome is distinguished from protracted vomiting by the finding of elevated urinary chloride levels; they are always low in protracted vomiting. Diuretic abuse can only be distinguished on the history.

Treatment of the condition is by giving potassium supplements and a prostaglandin inhibitor such as Indomethacin. The serum potassium may not be corrected completely, but symptoms are usually alleviated.

VIRILISING ADRENAL TUMOURS

The majority of the cases of hirsutism are idiopathic or due to the polycystic ovary syndrome (Ch. 6). The finding of virilisation, in addition to hirsutism, increases the chances of an androgen secreting tumour being present.

Adrenal tumours which secrete only androgens are rare. The majority secrete a combination of corticosteroids and androgens, and in these cases it is usually the Cushing's syndrome which dominates the clinical picture. In adults, most virilising tumours are benign adenomas, whereas in children a carcinoma is more likely. The age range of adult women with an adrenal adenoma is wide, stretching from the second to the eighth decade. Patients with a carcinoma tend to fall into the lower half of this range.

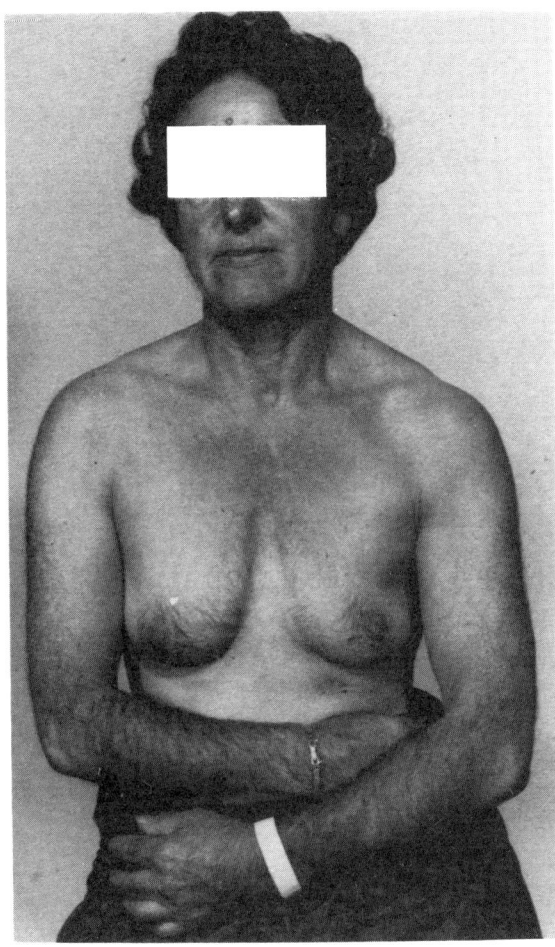

Fig. 5.11 Patient with a virilising adrenal tumour. Note the hirsutism, virilism, and frontal balding.

The presently favoured theory of the pathogenesis is that there is a primary defect in chloride transport in the ascending limb of the loop of Henle. This would explain why these patients are unable to excrete a low chloride urine regardless of dietary intake. All the other features of the disorder can be explained on this basis. In particular, the hyperaldosteronism results from the chronic volume contraction secondary to the defect in salt handling in the loop of Henle. The hypokalaemia is a result of impaired potassium reabsorption in the ascending loop of Henle plus the kaliuretic effect of the hyperaldosteronism. The resistance to the pressor effects of angiotensin II is explained on the

Clinical

It is usually stated that the duration of symptoms in women with a virilising adrenal adenoma is short, but in fact there is quite a wide range, varying between six months and many years. A rapid progression of symptoms, however, is a pointer to the presence of a tumour, as is the severity of the symptoms. Marked hirsutism, amenorrhoea and clitoromegaly are frequently present. Deepening of the voice, frontal balding, acne and atrophy of the breasts occur less frequently (Fig. 5.11).

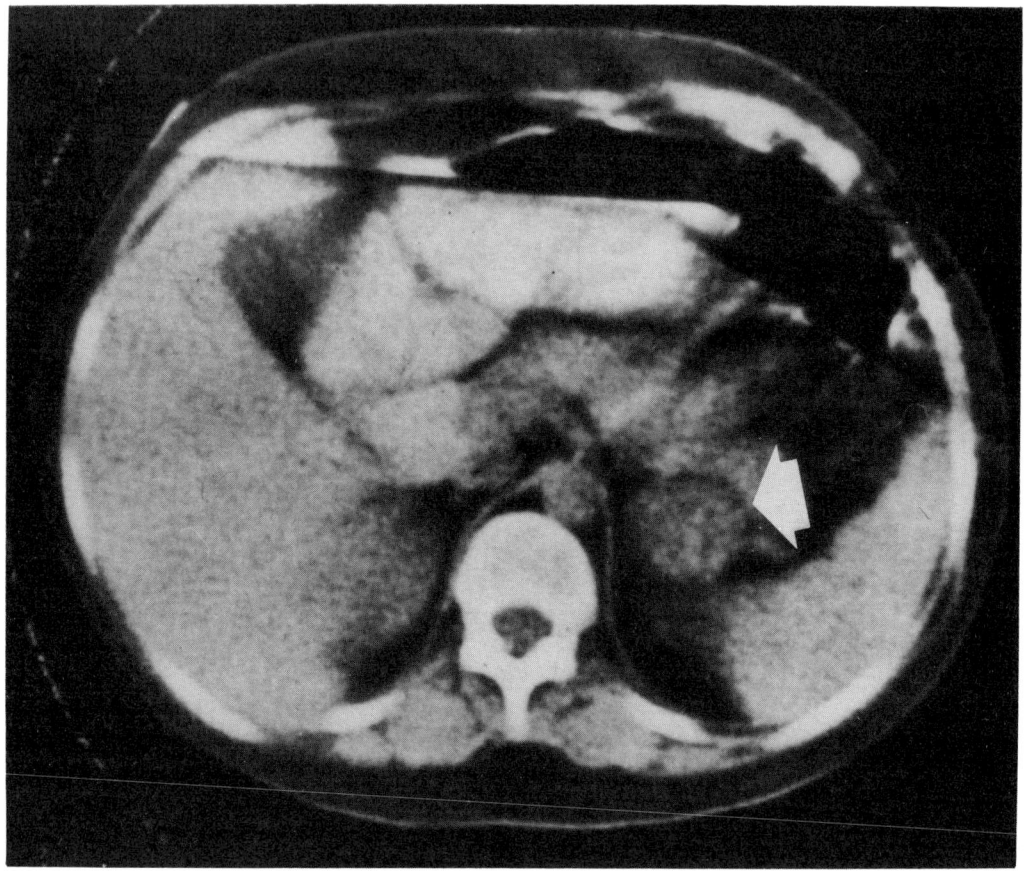

Fig. 5.12 An abdominal CT scan showing a left sided adrenal adenoma (arrowed).

In children the duration of symptoms is usually shorter since the virilising effects are more apparent. The common presentation is either with accelerated growth or with precocious puberty.

Diagnosis

The main clue to the presence of a virilising adrenocortical tumour is the level of serum androgens. A serum testosterone of greater than 6 nmol/l or a DHAS of greater than 20 μmol/l is suggestive of the diagnosis. In such cases the main differential diagnosis is that of an ovarian androgen secreting tumour. Adrenal tumours which secrete purely testosterone are extremely rare, but the serum testosterone is elevated along with DHAS and/or androstenedione in most cases. Arrhenoblastomas and hilus cell tumours of the ovary, on the other hand more commonly produce testosterone alone.

Dynamic tests, such as dexamethasone suppression tests or HCG stimulation tests, are of no value in determining the origin of the excess androgen secretion. Ovarian tumours have been described that suppress with dexamethasone and adrenal tumours may either suppress with oestradiol or be stimulated with HCG.

If the serum androgens are found to be high enough to suggest the presence of an adrenal tumour, the next step is anatomical localisation. Most adrenal tumours are over 1 cm in size and can be detected by CT scan (Fig. 5.12). An alternative method of localisation is either a dexamethasone suppressed seleno-cholesterol uptake scan (as described in the localisation of a Conn's tumour), or bilateral adrenal and ovarian vein sampling.

Table 5.6 Replacement steroid therapy

Steroid	Dose	Mineralocorticoid potency
Hydrocortisone	20mg + 10mg	1
Cortisone acetate	25mg + 12.5mg	0.8
Prednisolone	5mg + 2.5mg	0.8
Dexamethasone	0.5mg + 0.25mg	0
Fludrocortisone	50-200μg	125

CORTICOSTEROID TREATMENT

The therapeutic uses of corticosteroids fall into two categories :

1. Replacement therapy – adrenal failure
2. Pharmacological therapy – as an immuno-suppressive or anti-inflammatory agent.

It is beyond the scope of this chapter to deal with the latter aspect, except in terms of the complications of the treatment.

Replacement therapy

The replacement doses of the commonly used steroids are shown in Table 5.6. The steroid dose is usually split into two, with the largest amount in the morning to simulate the morning cortisol peak. A twice daily dosage regime is essential with hydrocortisone and with cortisone acetate, but not with prednisolone or dexamethasone.

Primary adrenal failure

All patients with adrenal failure, whether primary or secondary, require glucocorticoid treatment. Patients with Addison's disease also require mineralocorticoid treatment.

Hydrocortisone is the treatment of choice in adrenal failure. It has a rapid onset of action with peak serum levels being attained about an hour after an oral dose. One disadvantage is its short half life (more relevant in the treatment of congenital adrenal hyperplasia). In Addisonian patients the serum cortisol levels are low and plasma levels of ACTH are high just prior to the next dose of hydrocortisone. In practice therefore, the pattern of serum cortisol and ACTH is never normal. Nevertheless, patients' symptoms are alleviated.

The dose of hydrocortisone should be tailored to the individual patient (see section below on monitoring of treatment). The dose varies with the weight of the patient and is based on $24\,mg/m^2/24\,h$. For the average patient this means a dose of 20 mg in the morning and 10 mg at night.

Cortisone acetate has been widely used in the past, but it has to be converted to cortisol by the liver before it is biologically active. This does, however, give it a longer half life.

Fludrocortisone is the agent used as mineralo-corticoid replacement and this is started at a dose of 50 μg daily, increasing up to 200 μg if necessary. A once-daily dose only is required, because of the long half life.

Secondary adrenal failure

As with primary adrenal failure, hydrocortisone is the steroid most commonly used. The dosage is also identical. Since aldosterone is mainly controlled by the renin angiotensin system, most patients with hypopituitarism do not require mineralocorticoids. Sometimes, in long-standing hypopituitarism there is some atrophy of the zona glomerulosa and eventually mineralocorticoid therapy may be necessary.

Congenital adrenal hyperplasia

This topic has been covered in more detail above. Treatment here requires a different rationale. The main aim of the therapy is to suppress ACTH drive throughout 24 hours, in order to reduce the harmful effects of the elevated adrenal androgens. Hydrocortisone, because of its short half life, is less suitable for this purpose than the longer acting fluorinated steroids

Acute adrenal crisis

This condition presents an acute medical emergency. History, examination and investigations should be directed towards finding an under-lying cause. The precipitating stress should be vigorously treated. Immediate steroid therapy is with intravenous hydrocortisone at a dose of 100 mg.

Maintenance doses of 50 mg four times daily are required until the underlying cause has been adequately treated. The circulatory volume should be restored with intravenous saline to normalise the blood pressure. As the situation returns to normal the dose of hydrocortisone is gradually reduced back to replacement doses.

Monitoring steroid therapy

If patients are treated with one of the synthetic fluorinated steroids, then there is no method of monitoring treatment, except on a clinical basis. Hydrocortisone treatment may be monitored in one of two ways. A 24-hour urine may be collected for urinary free cortisol and this will give an average measure of the prevailing serum free cortisol throughout the day. The normal range for urinary free cortisol is used as an indicator of adequacy of treatment. Probably the best method of monitoring treatment is to take serial samples of blood at hourly intervals throughout the day in order to construct a day curve.

The monitoring of mineralocorticoid therapy is more difficult. The main clinical marker of efficacy is the blood pressure and the degree of postural drop. The biochemical marker which is most frequently used is the plasma renin activity. In cases of undertreatment this is elevated. The conditions under which the sample is taken should be carefully standardised (supine, no diuretics, sodium intake of at least 100 mmol/day).

Advice to patients

Replacement steroid therapy should be carefully explained to patients. Many patients have fears which are based on the well-publicised side effects of pharmacological doses. The nature of the treatment as physiological replacement needs to be stressed. The fact that the treatment, in most cases, needs to be life-long should be emphasised, as well as the fact that it needs to be taken regularly. All patients should know the name and dosage of their medication and should carry a steroid card in the same way that patients taking pharmacological doses do.

In the event of minor illness or infections patients

Table 5.7   The side effects of corticosteroids

Gastric ulceration	Infection
Pancreatitis	vaccinia
	varicella
Diabetes	herpes zoster
Weakness	herpes simplex
Hypokalaemia	tuberculosis
Myopathy	*monilia*
	aspergillosis
Osteoporosis	
Aseptic necrosis	Immunosupression
Neutrophil leucocytosis	Salt and water retention
Benign intracranial	
hypertension	Bruising
Cataract	Hirsutism
Raised intraocular pressure	Growth retardation
Adrenal atrophy	Weight gain

are advised to double the dose of steroids for the period of the illness. The same should apply in the case of prolonged diarrhoea. If they are vomiting persistently and unable to keep the medication down then they should seek medical advice.

Complications of steroid therapy

All drugs have side effects and treatment is usually a question of balancing the beneficial effects against the harmful ones. The side effects of most drugs occur because of allergy, idiosyncrasy, toxicity, or abnormal metabolism. The difference with corticosteroids is that their ill effects are due to sustained action of physiological substances in supraphysiological doses. Side effects should be expected in all cases. Corticosteroids have many physiological actions and therefore many adverse effects during treatment. The incidence of side effects is related to dose and duration of treatment, so that the aim should be to keep the dose down to the minimum required to control symptoms.

Table 5.7 lists the the main side effects associated with corticosteroid treatment. Adrenal suppression is one of the most serious and the reason why patients carry a steroid card.

Steroid withdrawal

The main factor which dictates the speed of steroid withdrawal is disease activity. Rapid withdrawal sometimes leads to rebound activity of the underlying disease. In addition, there does seem to be a degree of physical dependence on corticosteroids. A withdrawal syndrome of muscle pains and general malaise is recognised as a distinct entity. It is for these reasons that withdrawal is usually a slow process. Often, in the case of prednisolone, the dose needs to be reduced by as little as 1 mg/month, even at doses above the physiological replacement level. When replacement dosages are reached, reduction still needs to be slow in order to allow recovery of the pituitary adrenal axis, otherwise patients may be left in a hypoadrenal state. Recovery of adrenal function may take many months and often up to two years after prolonged therapy.

In cases where large doses have been used for a few days, such as in the treatment of an acute exacerbation of asthma, then the steroid may be stopped abruptly. Even so, abnormalities of adrenal function have been recorded. Usually they only last for a few days and do not present a clinical problem. If treatment has been for more than 10 days then some caution should be exhibited.

In cases of prolonged steroid therapy both the pituitary gland and the adrenal cortex have been suppressed. The usual pattern of recovery of the axis is that there is first a rise in ACTH. At this stage adrenocortical production of cortisol is still low. Eventually with continued ACTH stimulation the cortex begins to produce cortisol and ACTH levels go back to normal. This pattern of recovery is not constant. Occasionally there are abnormalities of ACTH release in response to different stimuli even when a Synacthen test is normal.

As the final stages of steroid withdrawal are reached adrenocortical function should be checked, especially when treatment has been prolonged. An insulin tolerance test measures the function of the whole system and should be the final arbiter of the stress response. However, insulin hypoglycaemia is not without hazard and serial tests are not justified. Initially assessment should be by repeated short Synacthen tests. When the cortisol response to ACTH is normal, a final insulin stress test may be performed. If this shows a normal response there is no further need for steroid cover in stressful situations.

ADRENAL MEDULLA

The chromaffin cells of the adrenal medulla secrete catecholamines. Of the catecholamine content, 80% is adrenaline and 20% noradrenaline. Usually the cells secrete either noradrenaline or adrenaline but not both. The release of catecholamines is by a process of exocytosis which is dependent on acetylcholine from sympathetic nerve endings.

Adrenaline is produced almost exclusively by the adrenal medulla. This is because of the presence of the enzyme phenylethanolamine-N-methyl transferase (PNMT – Fig. 5.13), which is not found in other sympathetic tissues. High concentrations of glucocorticoids are required for its synthesis and these are contained in the venous effluent from the cortex which passes through the medulla. Thus the adrenaline content is reduced in hypopituitarism and Addison's disease, and restored by ACTH and large doses of glucocorticoids.

Synthesis

Catecholamines are synthesised from tyrosine, which is taken up from the circulation. The sequence of events is depicted in Figure 5.13. The rate limiting step in the sequence is the first one and there is feedback inhibition on tyrosine hydroxylase by both catecholamines. In addition, release of catecholamines leads to an increase in the production of tyrosine hydroxylase. It can be seen, therefore, that the synthesis of catecholamines is controlled in a complex way by ACTH, glucocorticoids, feedback inhibition and release.

Secretion

The central nervous system has a great influence on the medullary secretions and this is the basis of the 'flight and fright' reaction. The hypothalamus receives fibres from the cerebral cortex and it is probable that the different cell types in the medulla are represented in different areas. Stimulation of different hypothalamic areas leads to alterations in the proportions of adrenaline and noradrenaline secreted. The central nervous system mediates catecholamine secretion in response to a wide variety of circumstances including emotional stress,

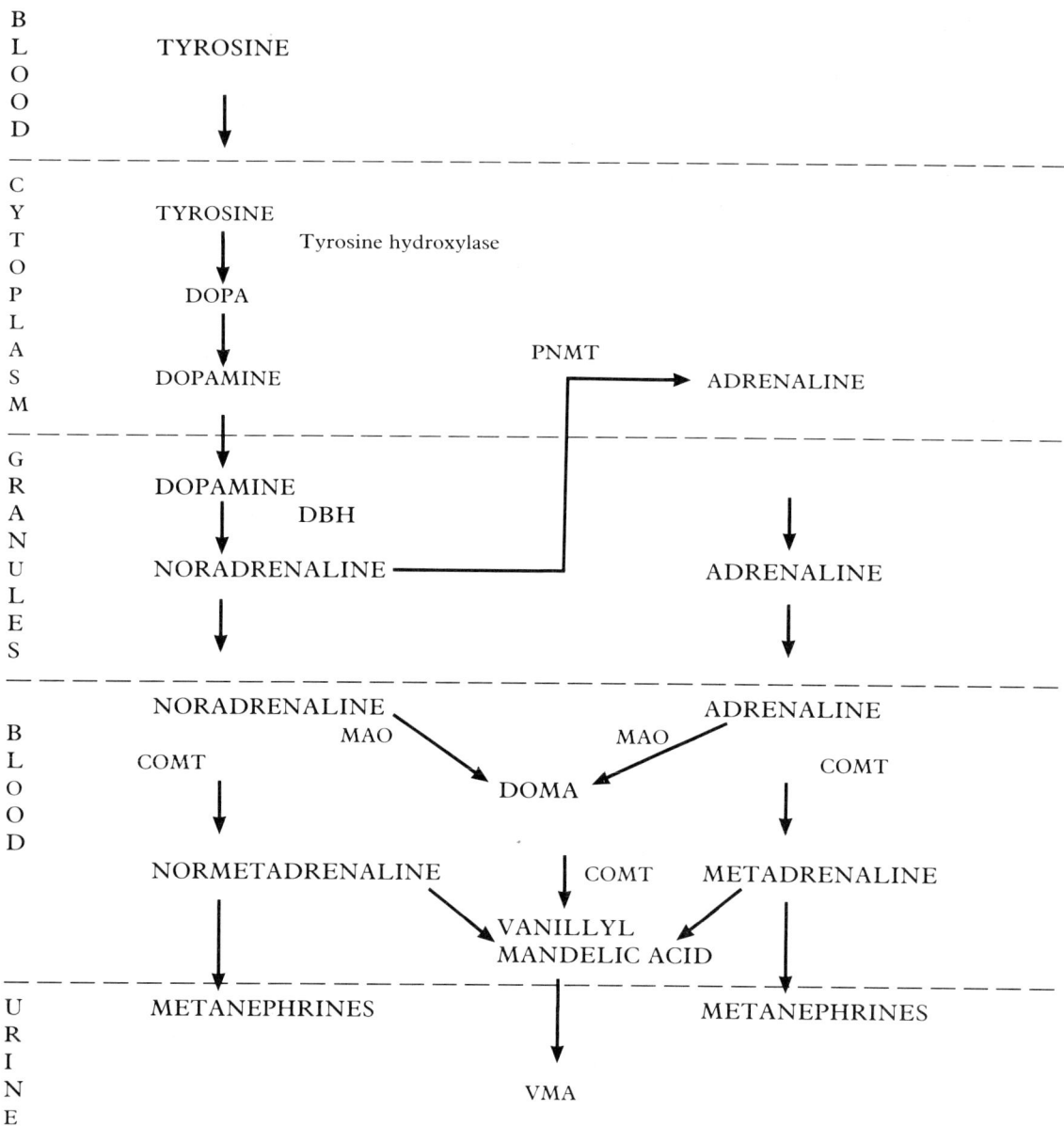

Fig. 5.13 The synthesis and degradation of catecholamines
DOPA = Dihydroxyphenylalanine
DOMA = Dihydroxymandelic acid
COMT = Catechol O-methyl transferase
MAO = Monoamine Oxidase
PNMT = Phenylethanolamine N-methyl transferase
VMA = Vanillyl mandelic acid
DBH = Dopamine β-hydroxylase

Metabolism

Monoamine oxidase (MAO) and catechol-O-methyl transferase (COMT) are the two main enzymes responsible for the breakdown of catecholamines. COMT is widely distributed throughout the body and is thought to be responsible for the disposal of exogenously administered catecholamines and also of adrenal catecholamines (Fig. 5.13).

The measurement of vanillyl mandelic acid (VMA) excretion is the most common estimation of catecholamine production in clinical practice, but the measurement of metanephrines, either individually or collectively, is thought to be better (see section on phaeochromocytoma). A very small amount of both noradrenaline and adrenaline are excreted unchanged in the urine.

PHAEOCHROMOCYTOMA

The popularity of entertaining a diagnosis of phaeochromocytoma far outstrips the finding of positive results. A tumour is the underlying pathology in only 0.1–1% (usually quoted as 0.5%) of a hypertensive population. It is, however, important to make the diagnosis early, because of the high morbidity and mortality in unrecognised cases and because it is one of the potentially curable causes of hypertension. The diagnosis is made difficult by two facts: firstly, the tumour may present in a wide variety of guises, hence its nickname 'the great mimic', and secondly the signs, symptoms and biochemical abnormalities may be intermittent.

The tumour may be found at any age, but there appear to be two peaks of incidence, one in childhood and the other in the 4th and 5th decades. It is rare in patients over the age of 60. There is no difference in incidence between the sexes.

The large majority of tumours are intra-abdominal (99%). 90% arise in the adrenal medulla, but they may also occur anywhere along the sympathetic chain. The majority of the extra-adrenal tumours present as a posterior mediastinal mass. Ten per cent of tumours in adults are bilateral (especially in MEA type II – see below), and 40% in children.

Phaeochromocytomas are found in association with a variety of diseases:

Table 5.8 Prevalence of symptoms in cases of phaochromotoma (% of cases) (After Gifford et al 1964 Mayo Clinic Proceedings 39:281–293)

	Paroxysmal	Persistent
Headache	92	72
Sweating	65	69
Palpitation	73	51
Pallor	60	28
Anxiety	60	28
Tremor	51	26
Nausea	43	26
Weakness	38	15
Chest pain	32	13
Abdominal pain	16	15
Weight loss	14	15
Dyspnoea	11	18
Flushing	11	8

Also: Visual disturbance, Raynaud's, constipation, fits, bradycardia, heat intolerance, paraesthesia in hands.

1. Multiple endocrine adenomatosis type II (a & b) (medullary thyroid carcinoma, phaeochromo-cytoma, parathyroid hyperplasia, and mucosal neuromas)
2. Neurofibromatosis
3. Von-Hippel-Lindau disease
4. Tuberose sclerosis.

The familial incidence is about 5–10% and many of the associated syndromes involve other tissues of ectodermal origin. In addition, many of the tumours are multicentric.

Clinical features

The fascination of this syndrome lies in the variety and often dramatic forms of presentation. Patients may be divided into those whose symptoms are paroxysmal and those whose symptoms are present all the time. The three commonest presenting symptoms (Table 5.8) are headache, sweating and palpitation. Sometimes the headache is characteristic, being sudden, severe, and of short duration, but often it is difficult to distinguish from tension headache. The frequency of paroxysms may vary from once every two months to many times per day. There is a tendency for attacks to become more frequent as time goes by. The typical attack presents the clinical picture of acute hypertension, palpitation, headache, sweating, facial pallor, and tremor. Paroxysmal attacks may be precipitated by

Table 5.9 Complications of phaeochromocytoma

Complication	Reason
Weight loss	Increased basal metabolic rate
Diabetes	Effect of adrenaline on carbohydrate metabolism: stimulation of glycogenolysis
Postural hypotension	Autonomic dysfunction
Cerebrovascular accident Left ventricular accident	Persistent hypotension
Myocardial infarct	Coronary artery spasm/hypertension
Cardiomyopathy	Catecholamine effect on myocardium
Cushing's syndrome	Ectopic ACTH syndrome
Hypoglycaemia	Non-supressible insulin-like activity
Cholelithiasis	Unknown
Abdominal pain Pseudo-obstruction	Effects of catecholamines on GIT

a wide variety of different circumstances. They are either a result of pressure, or of pharmacological agents.

The hypertension in this syndrome is characterised by a high degree of variability, with paroxysmal changes of differing degree and frequency. Between attacks 75–80% of patients will, however, be hypertensive. It should be noted that a paroxysm may be followed by an episode of hypotension, and that some patients may present with postural hypotension.

Most of the signs that are found in patients with phaeochromocytoma are predictable on the basis of the known actions of catecholamines and on the effects of hypertension:
1. Hypertension – intermittent or sustained
2. Postural hypotension
3. Tachycardia or reflex bradycardia
4. Sweating
5. Tremor
6. Pallor
7. Pupillary dilation
8. Raynaud's phenomenon
9. Fever

There are a variety of complications of phaeochromocytoma (Table 5.9) and patients may sometimes present with these as the primary problem. In addition to the listed complications, sudden death may occur during an attack, presumably related to an arrhythmia. However, the majority of deaths in untreated patients, as might be expected, are due to cerebrovascular disease (19%) and heart failure (15%).

Diagnosis

Biochemical tests

The traditional screening test for phaeochromocytoma is urinary VMA (Fig. 5.13). The methylated urinary derivatives, the metanephrines, are generally regarded as more reliable in distinguishing proven phaeochromocytoma from normals in whom the diagnosis has been suspected. This is probably because O-methylation is the predominant metabolic pathway.

Two factors should be borne in mind when assessing catecholamine derivative results. Firstly, the secretion of catecholamines is intermittent and urinary metabolites may be normal in between attacks. Secondly, there are several drugs which may alter urinary values. Methyl dopa and l-dopa may give false elevation in free catecholamines, monoamine oxidase inhibitors may increase metanephrines and decrease VMA estimations and clofibrate and nalidixic acid lead to a false increase in VMA.

It is now possible, using sensitive radioenzymatic assays, to measure the minute quantities of plasma catecholamines, and this seems to be a more reliable method of diagnosing phaeochromocytoma. Plasma levels of noradrenaline and adrenaline are almost always elevated in patients with phaeochromocytoma, irrespective of the level of blood pressure, and even between attacks. It is important to standardise the conditions under which the blood samples are taken, since many emotional and physical stresses may augment plasma catecholamines. The patient should be lying quietly for an hour before the sample is withdrawn. Again drugs interfere with the measurements; clonidine, methyl dopa, ganglion blockers and guanethidine decrease levels and alpha blockers increase them.

Tumour localisation

In the majority of cases an adrenal tumour is sought. An intravenous pyelogram is useful only in delineating large tumours, but is relatively safe. Arteriography, either flush aortography or selective renal arteriography, is more successful at locating tumours, but pressor crises are commonly precipitated and the patient should always be pharmacologically prepared (see below). Computerised tomography (CT), on the other hand, has a low morbidity and is the investigation of choice. In those cases where other methods to localise the tumour have failed, inferior vena caval catheterisation, with multiple site sampling for plasma catecholamines, may be successful.

More recently, a further technique for tumour localisation has become available; this test utilises radiolabelled ^{131}I-meta-iodobenzylguanidine (MIBG), which is taken up by cells which are actively synthesising catecholamines. As with CT scanning, the test is non-invasive and does not precipitate paroxysmal release of catecholamines. Isotope uptake scanning may visualise tumours which are too small to be found by other radiological techniques and should prove helpful in detecting extra-adrenal tumours.

Treatment

The aim of diagnosis and localisation is surgical removal of the tumour. In addition, there remains the problem of controlling blood pressure and preparing the patient medically either for arteriography or operation.

Acute crises

Acute rises in blood pressure are usually controlled by intravenous bolus injection of the alpha blocker, phentolamine. This drug has a very short half life (3–5 min) and the dose may have to be repeated as required. It may also be given by infusion, alternatively sodium nitroprusside may be used. If an arrhythmia occurs then intravenous practolol or propranolol should be given.

Routine control of blood pressure

Blood pressure should be controlled using a combination of alpha and beta blockers. Beta blockade alone may be dangerous leaving the patient with unopposed alpha mediated vasoconstriction and, therefore, a rising blood pressure. It may also produce severe Raynaud's phenomenon.

Labetolol, a combined alpha and beta blocker has been used in the treatment of phaeochromocytoma, but in some cases there has been a rise in blood pressure. This is probably because of the relatively weak alpha-blocking effect of the drug. The most successful alpha-blocking drug in current use is phenoxybenzamine. It has a long half life and only needs to be given once daily. Its effect may last several days after discontinuation. The dose range starts at 20 mg/day and it should be gradually increased until blood pressure is controlled. The maximum dose needed is usually 100 mg.

There is little to choose between the different beta-blocking agents. Relatively small doses of propranolol are effective in controlling symptoms (40–80 mg daily). Care should be taken in those patients with cardiomyopathy as cardiac failure may be precipitated. Raynaud's phenomenon may be a problem in those patients who are not adequately alpha blocked.

Operative management

Severe pressor crises and cardiac arrhythmias may arise during surgery. This is a result of the sudden surge of catecholamines, which occurs when the tumour is handled. Both alpha and beta blockade should be continued up to the day of operation. Careful perioperative monitoring with intra-arterial measurement of blood pressure and continuous ECG recording are essential. The entire abdominal cavity should be inspected and the tumour removed with the minimum of handling. Failure of the blood pressure to fall may be an indication of the presence of a further tumour. A precipitous fall in blood pressure may follow removal of the tumour. This phenomenon is probably due to the marked expansion of the vascular space. It may be necessary to infuse additional blood or plasma at the time of clamping of the tumour circulation. Very occasionally, hypoglycaemia is a problem. This is a result of excessive insulin secretion.

If the blood pressure remains elevated in the postoperative period there may be several reasons:
1. Overtransfusion
2. Incomplete removal
3. Coexistence of essential hypertension
4. Secondary renal vascular disease
5. Multiple tumours.

In the majority of cases, however, the hypertension is cured.

Reproductive endocrinology

FEMALE REPRODUCTIVE ENDOCRINOLOGY: A. THE MENSTRUAL CYCLE

The endocrinology of the menstrual cycle

The human menstrual cycle lasts approximately 28 days. There is little variation between subjects in the length of the luteal phase (usually 14 days) but the follicular phase is more variable. In the majority of women, the cycle length varies little from month to month, but the variation is more marked at either end of reproductive life (i.e. during adolescence and approaching the menopause), when anovulatory cycles are more frequent. The cyclical changes in pituitary and ovarian hormones are shown in Figure 6.1. By convention, the cycle starts on the first day of menstruation; at this stage there is an increase in circulating concentrations of follicle stimulating hormone (FSH) and, to a lesser extent, luteinising hormone (LH). This increase in gonadotrophins is triggered by a fall in progesterone and oestradiol concentrations resulting from luteolysis. FSH acts on the granulosa cells of the follicle and stimulates production of oestrogens (predominantly oestradiol) from androgen precursors in the theca interna. This initiates a chain of events within the follicle whereby the interaction of oestradiol and FSH leads to an increase in the number of granulosa cells and their sensitivity to FSH.

In the early follicular phase, several follicles ranging from 0.5 to 5 mm in diameter are 'recruited' from a pool of antral follicles which undergo a limited amount of growth, but which, without adequate FSH stimulation, would otherwise become atretic. From this group of follicles recruited in the late luteal to early follicular phase only one, or at the most two, are destined to reach maturity and ovulate. The process by which the 'dominant' follicle is selected is not entirely clear, but it seems likely that the fall of serum FSH concentration which occurs in the mid-follicular phase is important (Fig. 6.1). This decline in FSH secretion is brought about by the negative feedback action of increasing levels of serum oestradiol and probably also by the secretion of a non-steroidal ovarian hormone which selectively inhibits FSH – inhibin. The largest follicle at this stage has a full complement of FSH receptors on the granulosa cells and is able to withstand this decline in serum FSH concentrations, whereas the subsidiary follicles lose the capacity for further growth and oestrogen production and become atretic.

The dominant follicle grows rapidly from 10–20 mm in diameter within 5 days in the late follicular phase. This is associated with a sharp rise in serum oestradiol concentrations (Fig. 6.1) and, when optimum growth of the follicle has been achieved, oestradiol stimulates a mid-cycle surge of LH and (to a lesser extent) FSH. This positive feedback mechanism is unique among endocrine systems. Its precise mechanism is not clear but it in part involves increasing oestradiol mediated sensitivity of the gonadotrophs to gonadotrophin releasing hormone (GnRH). Ovulation occurs approximately 36 hours after the start of the LH surge. The follicle then involutes, becomes haemorrhagic and forms the corpus luteum. Granulosa cells by this time have acquired LH receptors and have the capacity to produce large quantities of progesterone as well as oestradiol. Gonadotrophin levels during most of the luteal phase are at their

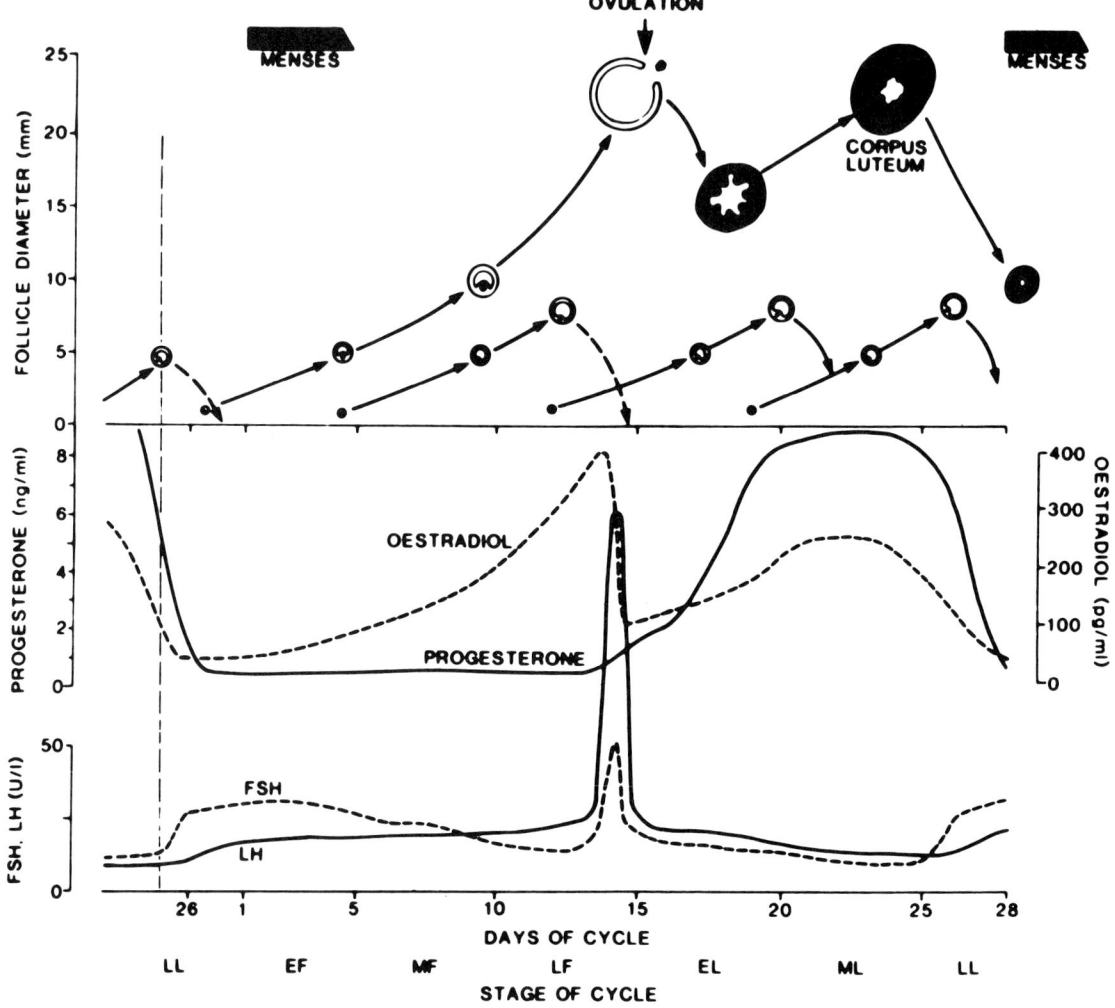

Fig. 6.1 Endocrine and follicular changes throughout the menstrual cycle. The vertical dotted line indicates onset of luteal regression. (From Baird D T 1983 Prediction of ovulation; biophysical, physiological and biochenmical coordinates. In: Jeffcoate S L (ed) Ovulation: Methods for its prediction and detection. Wiley: Chichester, with permission of the author and publisher.)

lowest under the negative feedback action of gonadal steroids. Unless sustained by secretion of human chorionic gonadotrophin (HCG) following conception, the corpus luteum has a limited lifespan. Luteolysis occurs, serum levels of progesterone and oestradiol fall, the negative feedback signal to the pituitary is removed and gonadotrophin concentrations increase, thereby initiating the next cycle.

The control of these events is dependent on the pulsatile secretion of the gonadotrophins LH and FSH, secondary to pulsatile release of GnRH from the hypothalamus, which has been discussed previously (Ch. 2). The physiological importance of the pulsed GnRH signal to the pituitary can be demonstrated by the finding that changing from a pulsatile to a continuous mode of GnRH delivery results in a steady fall in LH and FSH concentrations; a process referred to as pituitary 'desensitisation'. In patients with anovulation due to GnRH deficiency (see below) the administration of pulsatile GnRH is able to restore normal ovulatory menstrual cycles.

Changes in the genital tract during the menstrual cycle

The structure of the endometrium comprises two components, the glandular epithelium and the supporting stromal cells. The follicular or proliferative phase of the cycle is marked by mitotic proliferation in both endometrial and stromal cells which occur as a result of oestrogen stimulation. The mucosa therefore increases in thickness and the glands lengthen although at this stage they are still straight. Following ovulation and due to production of progesterone as well as oestradiol the stroma becomes oedematous and more vascular and the epithelial glands become coiled. There are also morphological changes in the epithelial cells which include a reduction of mitosis and marked vacuolation of the cytoplasm. When luteolysis occurs and serum concentrations of progesterone and oestradiol fall the spiral arteries which supply the endometrium undergo intense vasospasm leading to necrosis of the endometrium and menstrual loss. The biochemical mechanisms by which the process of endometrial degeneration occurs remain uncertain, but it is clear that prostaglandins have an important role.

There are also cyclical changes in the epithelium of the cervix and vagina, which are likewise hormone dependent. Proliferative changes occur in both the cervical and vaginal mucosa as a result of oestrogen production and there are marked changes in the secretory ability of the cervical cells so at the time of ovulation the cervical mucus is characteristically abundant and stringy and provides optimum conditions for the passage of spermatozoa.

Endocrine disorders of the menstrual cycle

Endocrine disorders of the menstrual cycle are usually related to failure of ovulation. Anovulation is the cause of infertility in 20–30% of couples presenting with this problem. The patient may present with infertility and/or menstrual disturbance associated with amenorrhoea, or irregular and infrequent periods (oligomenorrhoea). Anovulatory menstruation is often characterised by prolonged, heavy or painful periods. Another endocrine disturbance of the cycle is luteal phase insufficiency. In this case ovulation occurs but progesterone secretion in the luteal phase is inadequate and the cycle may be short.

Amenorrhoea

Amenorrhoea (usually defined as no periods for 6 months or more) is a common symptom in women

Table 6.1 Causes of primary amenorrhoea

Gonadal dysgenesis
Genital (Müllerian) tract abnormality
Intersex disorder
Isolated deficiency of gonadotrophin releasing hormone
Any of the causes listed under 2° amenorrhoea

Table 6.2 Causes of secondary amenorrhoea

Primary ovarian failure	Premature menopause Resistant ovary syndrome (ovarian follicles present)
Deficiency or disordered regulation of gonadotrophins	*Specific* Hyperprolactinaemia Structural lesions of pituitary or hypothalamus Polycystic ovary syndrome
	Functional Weight-loss, exercise Psychogenic Chronic illness Idiopathic
Genital tract abnormality	Aschermann's syndrome (intrauterine adhesions)

of reproductive age. It occurs in 10–20% of patients complaining of infertility and is one of the commonest reasons for referral to a gynaecological endocrine clinic. Investigation and management of patients with amenorrhoea, although often straightforward, is best performed in gynaecological endocrine clinics with direct access to an endocrine laboratory and facilities to select, initiate and monitor programmes for induction of ovulation.

Classification

Although it is conventional to subdivide patients into those with primary and those with secondary amenorrhoea, this is not always a useful distinction since many of the commonest causes of anovulation may present as either primary or secondary amenorrhoea. Nonetheless, it is important to realise that about 60% of cases of primary amenorrhoea result from congenital abnormalities in the development of the ovaries, the genital tract or external genitalia (Table 6.1). Gonadal dysgenesis (accounting for half this group) is the most common of these (a third of all cases of primary amenorrhoea), followed by abnormalities of genital development (one sixth). The underlying diagnosis in the 40% of women without developmental abnormalities of the reproductive tract includes any of the causes listed under secondary amenorrhoea, as shown in Table 6.2.

Clinical assessment (Fig. 6.2)

In women with primary amenorrhoea it is important to assess pubertal development. Delayed puberty is often constitutional (i.e. these girls will eventually enter puberty spontaneously) but may indicate primary ovarian failure or hypothalamic deficiency of GnRH. A disparity in the signs of puberty such as breast development without pubic hair or vice versa, suggests the possibility of male or female pseudohermaphroditism. Careful examination of the external genitalia is important in such cases (Ch. 7). Short stature is a feature of gonadal dysgenesis.

Patients with weight loss related amenorrhoea are underweight at the time of presentation or have a recent history of weight loss. It may not be immediately apparent that the patient is underweight. The most reliable way to assess this is to use the body mass (or ponderal) index in which the weight is corrected for height ($BMI = kg/m^2$). The normal range is 20–25. Although most of the women with weight loss related amenorrhoea (WRA) are not seriously underweight, the distinction between these patients and those with anorexia nervosa is not clear cut. The underlying psychopathology is often similar and psychological assessment may be indicated as part of management. Vigorous exercise is becoming an increasingly important cause of amenorrhoea and history should include an assessment of the amount of exercise taken. The reproductive abnormality in such women has much in common with that in WRA. A history of psychological disturbance ranging from 'normal' stress (such as taking 'A' levels, or moving house) to frank psychosis may be an important pointer to the cause of amenorrhoea. In women with weight- and exercise-related or psychological amenorrhoea, there is a disturbance in gonadotrophin regulation due to abnormal patterns in the secretion of GnRH. As a result oestrogen deficiency is common. It may present as loss of interest in sexual intercourse, vaginal dryness and occasionally hot flushes. These symptoms, however, are not specific to WRA and may occur in any other cause of gonadotrophin deficiency such as hyperprolactinaemia as well as in primary ovarian failure. Galactorrhoea occurring in women with amenorrhoea is highly suggestive of hyperprolactinaemia, but most women with hyperprolactinaemic amenorrhoea do not have inappropriate milk secretion. Hirsutism or persistent acne are indicative of androgen excess and make the diagnosis of polycystic ovary syndrome (PCOS) very likely. Pelvic examination is not often helpful, but it is possible to define certain developmental abnormalaties of the lower genital tract, to assess oestrogenisation of the cervix and to palpate polycystic ovaries which are often, but not always enlarged.

Endocrine assessment

The endocrine assessment of amenorrhoea is illustrated in Figure 6.3. Initial investigations include measurement of FSH, LH and prolactin and assessment of oestrogen production. A positive response to a progestogen challenge (i.e. vaginal bleeding occurring following a short course of exogenous progestogens) is a useful biological marker of oestrogen activity and predicts induction of ovulation with antioestrogens. Measurement of serum oestradiol concentrations is unreliable because of the wide variability of oestradiol levels in the normal menstrual cycle and in amenorrhoeic women.

Pelvic ultrasound

Modern ultrasound is a useful and non-invasive means of visualisation of the ovaries and uterus, but its clinical value is dependent on the skill of the ultrasonographer. At best it is possible to define accurately ovarian size and morphology (e.g. definition of PCOS) and to make precise measurement of uterine dimensions, which may provide useful information about endogenous oestrogen levels.

Management

Management of patients with amenorrhoea should be directed towards correction of any underlying pathology (e.g. weight-loss, hyperprolactinaemia), replacement of cyclical ovarian hormones (particularly important in women with oestrogen

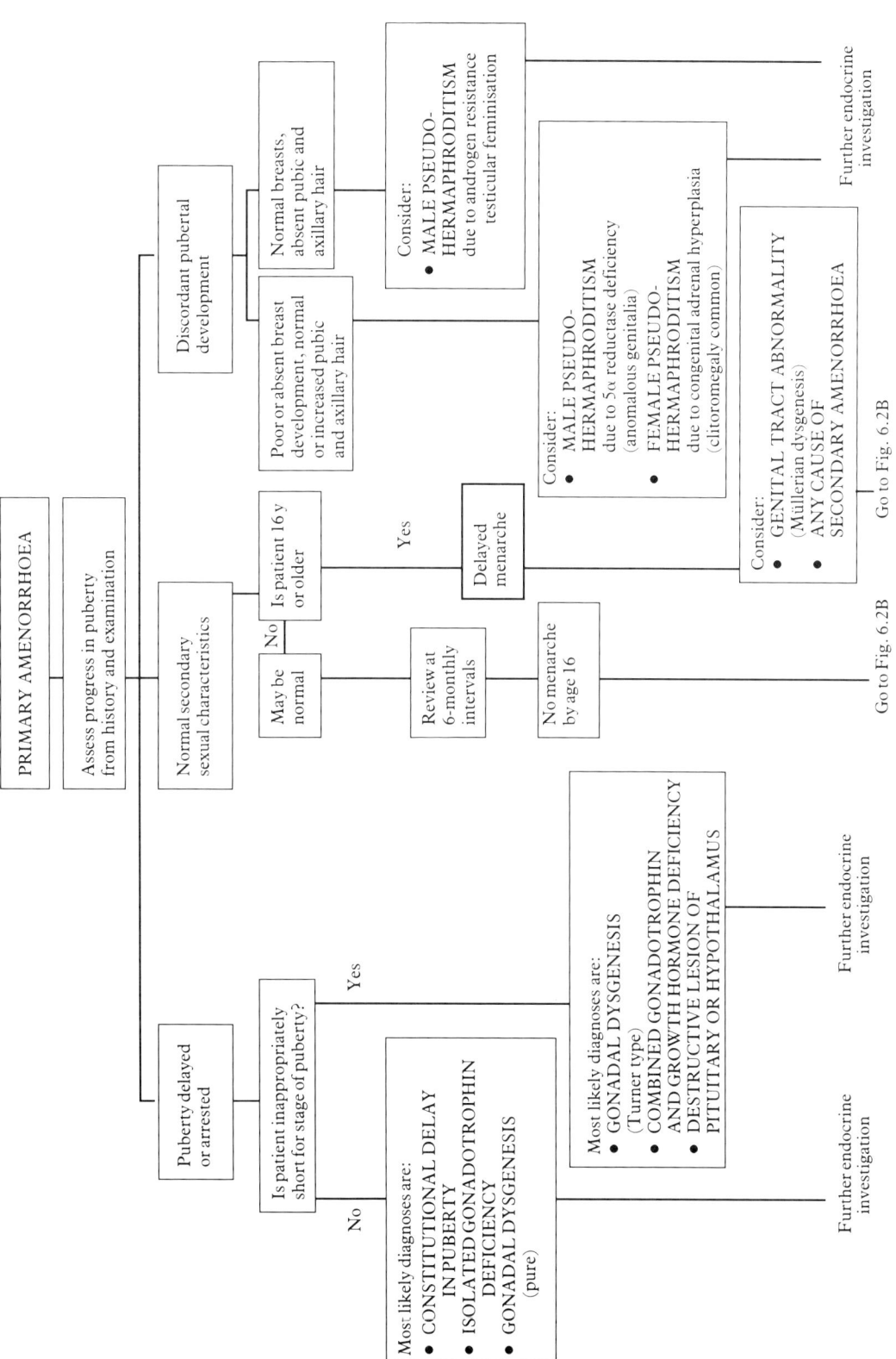

Fig. 6.2A Clinical assessment of patients with primary amenorrhoea. (Adapted from Franks S 1987 Primary and secondary amenorrhoea. Clinical algorithms. British Medical Journal 294: 815–819.)

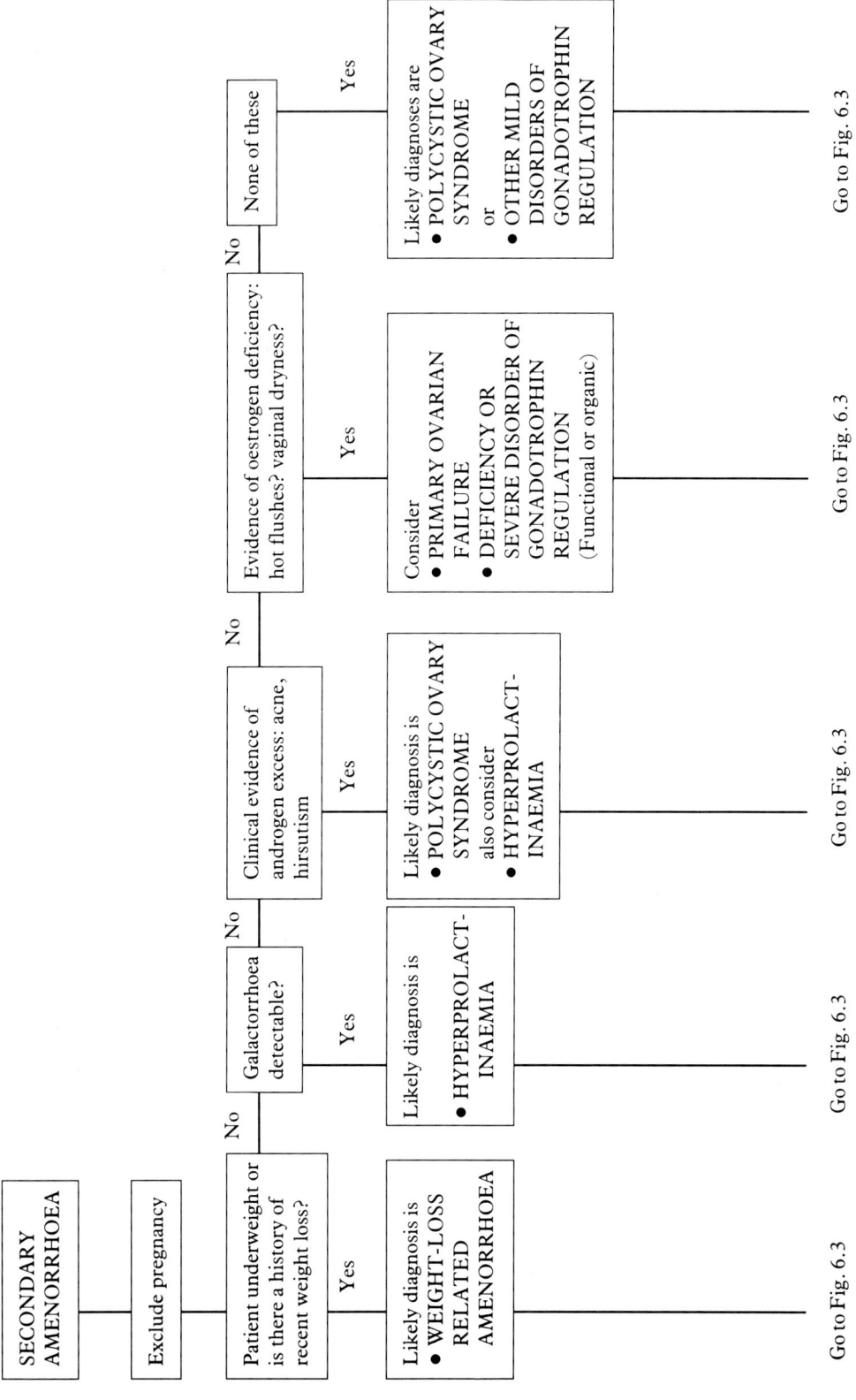

Fig. 6.2B Clinical assessment of patients with secondary amenorrhoea. (Adapted from Franks S 1987 Primary and secondary amenorrhoea. Clinical algorithms. British Medical Journal 294: 815–819.)

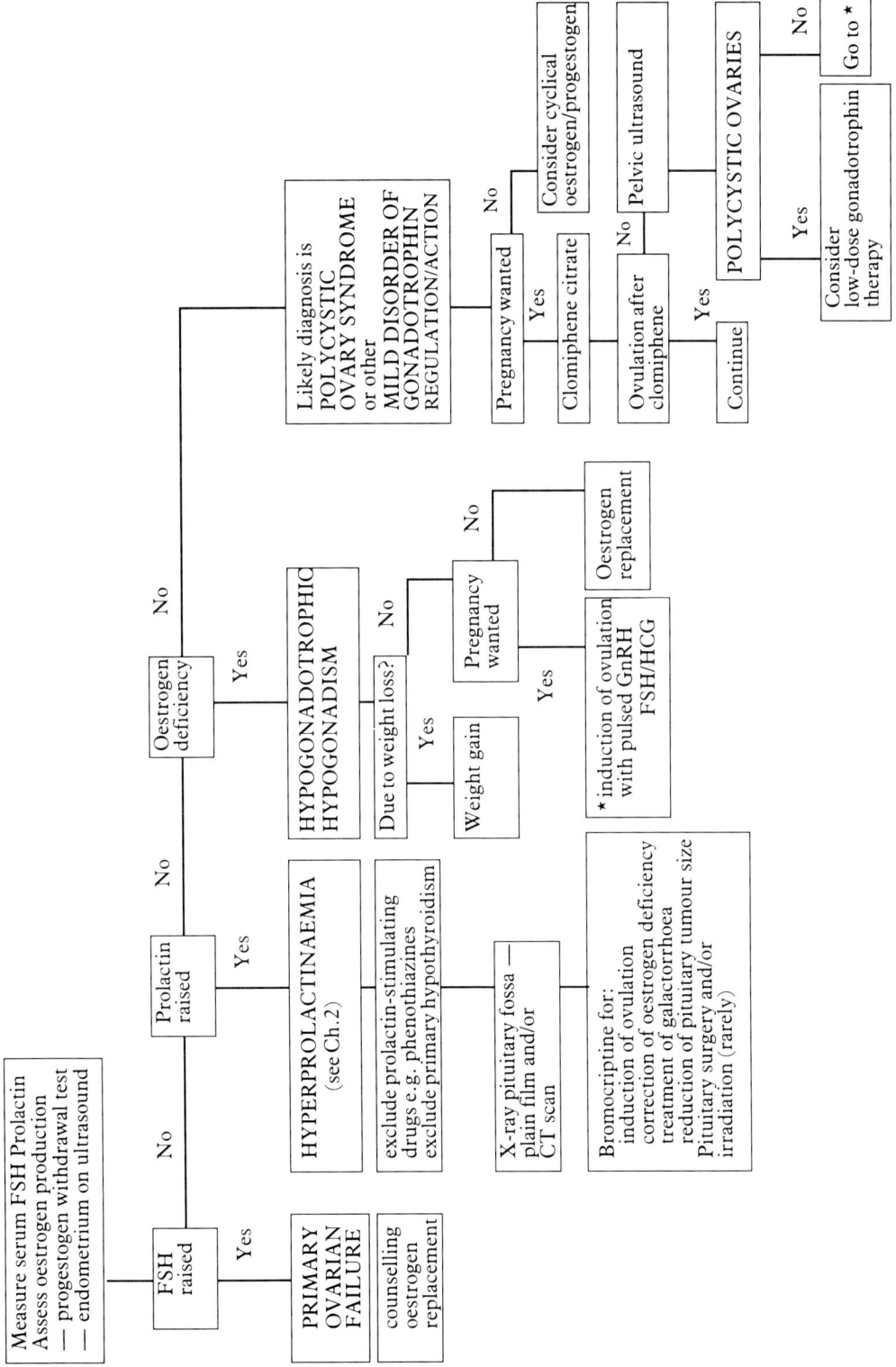

Fig. 6.3 Endocrine assessment and management of amenorrhoea. (Adapted from Franks S 1987 Primary and secondary amenorrhoea. Clinical algorithms. British Medical Journal 294: 815–819.)

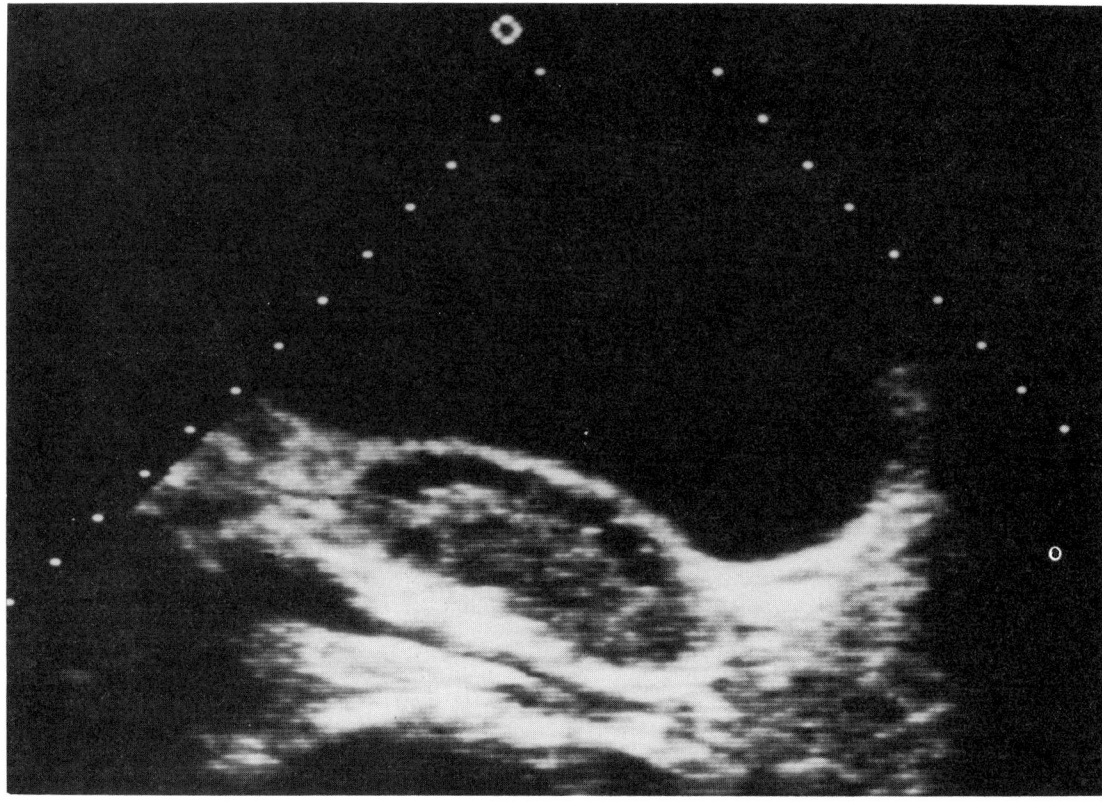

Fig. 6.4 A pelvic ultrasound scan showing the typical appearance of a polycystic ovary. The ovary is enlarged and contains many follicles distributed peripherally around an increased core of stroma. The white dots are 1 cm markers. (Picture by courtesy of Miss J. Adams and the Editor of the *Lancet*. From Adams et al 1985 Lancet 2: 1375–1378.)

deficiency) and, when required, induction of ovulation. In those patients who do not wish to become pregnant immediately, it is important to offer counselling about the chances of future fertility or about contraception. The choice of treatment for induction of ovulation depends on the results of investigations as indicated in Figure 6.3. Clomiphene is an antioestrogen, which, in well oestrogenised patients, stimulates endogenous secretion of LH and FSH, promoting follicular development and ovulation. Patients with normal oestrogen production who fail to respond to clomiphene are usually those who have PCOS and treatment of this group is often difficult. The treatment of hyperprolactinaemic amenorrhoea is bromocriptine (Ch. 2), but other forms of hypogonadotrophic amenorrhoea can be managed by administration of exogenous gonadotrophins or more physiologically by pulsatile GnRH therapy. Subcutaneous intermittent administration

of GnRH is proving to be a highly successful means of inducing ovulation and fertility in patients with functional or organic impairment of GnRH secretion. It is important to note that although women with WRA will ovulate in response to GnRH or exogenous gonadotrophins, the mainstay of treatment in this group is to encourage weight gain. This may involve the participation of the psychiatrist as well as the dietician.

Oligomenorrhoea

In many women with anovulation, follicular activity is not completely suppressed and oestrogen production may be sufficient to cause intermittent and usually irregular menstrual bleeding. Bleeding may be heavy and prolonged (dysfunctional uterine bleeding) and may well be the reason for presentation. The most common cause of anovulatory cycles is polycystic ovary syndrome, but they also occur commonly after the menarche and in perimenopausal women.

Polycystic ovary syndrome

The classical description of polycystic ovary syndrome includes anovulatory menses and amenorrhoea, hirsutism and obesity associated with the finding of bilateral sclerocystic ovaries. If polycystic ovaries are identified by laparoscopy or (as in recent studies) by pelvic ultrasound (Fig. 6.4), it is clear that the spectrum of clinical and biochemical features of PCOS is wide, but in most patients there are clinical and biochemical signs which point to the diagnosis. Typically, serum levels of the androgens, testosterone and androstenedione are elevated. The major source of excess androgen appears to be the ovary although there is evidence for excessive secretion of adrenal androgens in some cases. There is an increase in serum LH concentrations in the face of normal or low FSH giving rise to a raised LH to FSH ratio (greater than 2.5). The pathogenesis of PCOS is not yet clear, but it is possible to explain failure of follicular maturation and persistent anovulation by the low (or at least unvarying) FSH concentrations. Follicular development and ovulation can be induced by either antioestrogens (raising endogenous FSH levels), or by administration of exogenous FSH.

Management of patients with PCOS and other causes of oligomenorrhoea

NB. In those patients who do not require induction of ovulation, treatment is directed towards regulation of the menstrual cycle. Menorrhagia related to anovulatory cycles can usually be controlled by high dose progestogens given for 7–10 days (e.g. norethisterone 5–10 mg daily). Following this, cycle control can be achieved by giving a combined oestrogen-progestogen preparation and the low dose birth control pill is often satisfactory. Many patients with PCOS require treatment for hirsutism and their management is discussed below.

Luteal phase insufficiency

Luteal phase insufficiency has been reported to occur in up to 30% of ovulatory cycles in women with otherwise unexplained infertility, but it is still not clear whether there is a causal relationship between the inadequate luteal phase and infertility. The diagnosis is based on the finding of suboptimal mid-luteal serum progesterone concentrations. The pathogenesis of luteal phase insufficiency is variable. It has been reported to occur in disorders as different as hyperprolactinaemia and polycystic ovary syndrome, either during spontaneous cycles or following induction of ovulation. Luteal phase insufficiency usually reflects inadequate follicular development rather than a specific defect during the luteal phase.

The menopause

Cessation of menstruation in the fifth or sixth decade of life (mean age 52) is related to primary failure of the ovaries. The rate of atresia of ovarian follicles is high and the process which begins during intra-uterine life continues until there are few functional antral follicles. Premature menopause in most cases represents an acceleration of this process.

Clinical problems

The menopause rarely occurs abruptly. The perimenopausal months are typically associated with infrequent and irregular menstruation which reflects a higher proportion of anovulatory cycles. This may result in menses of varying duration and severity. Heavy bleeding is not uncommon in such cycles. When oestrogen deficiency ensues, the patient may complain of hot flushes and vaginal dryness. The vascular disturbance associated with menopausal flushes has been well documented, but the mechanism remains unclear. The flushes are relieved by oestrogen and also by infusion of the opiate receptor antagonist naloxone, suggesting that endogenous opiates may mediate the hypothalamic response to oestrogen deficiency. Other symptoms typically occurring in the menopause, such as forgetfulness, irritability, loss of libido and depression, are not specifically related to oestrogen deficiency, although they too may improve with hormone replacement therapy.

Endocrinology of the menopause

The onset of the menopause is heralded by a rise in serum FSH when LH levels remain normal. This is thought to be due to diminished production of ovarian inhibin, symptomatic of failing follicular function. Eventually both LH and FSH become chronically raised. Oestrogen production by the ovary is, of course, low after the menopause, but both oestradiol and oestrone are measurable in the circulation and are derived from non-FSH dependent conversion of adrenal androgens to oestrogens in peripheral tissues, principally the fat. This extraglandular conversion of adrenal androgen to oestrogen is, therefore, more marked in obese patients and explains the tendency towards postmenopausal bleeding in such women and, more seriously, their increased risk of endometrial cancer.

Hormone replacement therapy

Oestrogen replacement in the menopause is an effective treatment for flushes and vaginal dryness and, as indicated above, may also improve changes in mood and behaviour. There is also clear evidence that oestrogen replacement will delay the onset of postmenopausal osteoporosis, a serious cause of morbidity in elderly women. Despite these benefits, hormone replacement therapy has been viewed with caution and this is mainly because of the reported adverse effects. Exogenous oestrogen treatment, like excess endogenous oestrogen production in obese postmenopausal women, is known to increase the risk of endometrial carcinoma. However, endometrial cancer has occurred almost exclusively in women receiving unopposed oestrogen (i.e. oestrogens without progestogens), often at high doses for prolonged periods. Addition of cyclical progestogens sharply reduces the chance of endometrial hyperplasia and malignancy and recent studies have shown that it only requires small doses of progestogen (e.g. 350 μg of norethisterone, or 75 μg of norgestrel) to keep the endometrium suppressed. There remains some controversy about whether synthetic or 'natural' oestrogens are preferable but many physicians prefer to prescribe the latter. A typical regimen would therefore be Premarin (conjugated equine oestrogens) 0.625–1.25 mg daily for 28 days with norgestrel 150 μg for 12 days of each cycle.

Side effects of low-dose hormone replacement therapy (HRT) include headache, abdominal bloating and breast tenderness but these are rarely troublesome when low doses are used. Treatment is contraindicated in women with a history of breast cancer or other hormone-dependent carcinoma, chronic liver disease, thrombotic episodes or significant cardiovascular disease. Mild hypertension is not an absolute contraindication to treatment. The optimal duration of treatment is controversial. With increasing use of low dose regimens, there are many physicians who feel that both the short- and long-term benefits (e.g. on bone) outweigh the possible disadvantages. There is some concern about the effects of sex steroids, particularly progestogens, on glucose and lipid metabololism. However, preliminary studies in women on low-dose progestogens suggest that these effects are minimal with such treatment schedules. More problematical is the long-term risk of cardiovascular disease, but despite large scale epidemiological studies there is still no clear cut answer as to whether there is an increased risk of cardiovascular problems in women receiving HRT. This area remains to be clarified.

B. HIRSUTISM

Hirsutism, or excessive hair growth, is a common symptom in women presenting to a gynaecological endocrine clinic. In the vast majority of cases there is a benign cause. In this section the various causes of hirsutism and the management of the disorder are discussed.

Androgen production in women

Adrenal androgen production has been discussed in Chapter 5. The two main circulating androgens in women are androstenedione and testosterone. In premenopausal women, 60% of androstenedione is derived from the ovary and 40% from the adrenal. Sixty per cent of circulating testosterone is produced by extraglandular conversion of androstenedione, the remaining 40% by direct secretion of the ovary or adrenal. Dehydroepiandrosterone (DHA) and dehydroepiandrosterone sulphate (DHAS) are quantitatively important but weak androgens, produced primarily by the adrenal. Testosterone and its 5α-reduced metabolite dihydrotestosterone (DHT) are the most biologically

Table 6.3 Causes of hirsutism. (After Morris D V 1985 Clinics in Obstetrics and Gynaecology 12:566)

Ovarian
Polycystic ovary syndrome
Hyperthecosis
Hilus cell hyperplasia
Gonadal dysgenesis
Virilising tumours
   arrhenoblastoma
   hilus cell tumour
   lipoid cell tumour

Adrenal
Congenital adrenal hyperplasia
Adrenal adenoma/carcinoma

Table 6.4 Investigation of hirsutism

Mild-moderate hirsutism	LH, FSH, testosterone (SHBG) Pelvic ultrasound scan
Severe hirsutism ± virilisation or short history of hirsutism and/or serum testosterone > 6 nmol/l	Above tests +: 17-Hydroxyprogesterone — ? congenital adrenal hyperplasia Assessment of cortisol secretion — ? Cushing's syndrome (Ch. 5) Dehydroepiandrosterone sulphate (DHAS) — ? adrenal source Imaging of ovary and adrenal — ultrasound, CT scan

active androgens. Most (about 95%) of testosterone and DHT in the circulation is bound to plasma proteins, principally sex hormone-binding globulin (SHBG). This is important, since it is thought that only non-bound or 'free' androgens are available to tissues and therefore biologically active.

Causes and presentation of hirsutism

Hirsutism can be attributed to increased production of androgen, increased biological availability (i.e. increased free androgen levels), increased metabolism of testosterone to the more potent 5α-reduced metabolites in the periphery, or increased sensitivity of the target tissues to testosterone. In practice, excessive hair growth probably results from a combination of these factors, but the most important of these is almost certainly increased production of androgen. The source may be ovarian or adrenal. A list of the more common causes of hirsutism is shown in Table 6.3. The most common diagnosis is so-called 'idiopathic' hirsutism, i.e. hirsutism occurring in women with regular menstrual cycles who have no evidence of adrenal or ovarian disease. Recent studies suggest that this diagnosis may in fact represent one part of the spectrum of polycystic ovary syndrome. Cushing's syndrome, congenital adrenal hyperplasia and tumours of the adrenal or ovary are uncommon but important diagnoses to bear in mind, particularly in patients with severe hirsutism or with a short history of unwanted facial hair (Ch. 5). Virilisation (i.e. male pattern hair distribution, temporal balding, breast atrophy, deepening of the voice and clitoromegaly) may occur in women with severe hirsutism and is an index of greatly elevated testosterone production. Certain drugs other than testosterone itself may cause hirsutism, notably danazol which has androgenic properties, neuroleptics such as phenytoin and the H_2 receptor antagonists cimetidine and ranitidine.

Investigation of hirsutism (Table 6.4)

In women with mild, long-standing hirsutism and regular cycles, testosterone concentrations are often at the upper limit of normal, or only slightly raised, as is the ratio of testosterone to SHBG (an index of free testosterone). LH and FSH levels and pelvic ultrasound will help to define patients with polycystic ovary syndrome. If the serum testosterone level is very high (greater than 6 nmol/l), if there is a short history of hirsutism, or if there are signs of virilisation, more extensive investigations are required to exclude, for example, tumours of the adrenal or ovary.

Management of hirsutism

When excessive hair growth is well localised, e.g. to the upper lip or chin, local cosmetic treatment is often the most effective means of management. This may include shaving, bleaching, use of depilatory creams and electrolysis. When the hirsutism is not easily controlled by these means then hormonal treatment should be considered. The three forms of endocrine therapy are glucocorticoids, oral contraceptive treatment and antiandrogens. Glucocorticoids suppress the pituitary-adrenal axis and therefore inhibit adrenal secretion of androgen. This is very effective in congenital adrenal hyperplasia where the primary source of androgen excess is the adrenal, but much less effective in other forms of hirsutism. Oral contraceptives suppress ovarian androgen secretion and may be beneficial to some patients, but it should be noted that most of the currently available combined oral contraceptives contain either norethisterone or norgestrel, which have endogenous androgenic properties. By far the most effective form of treatment is the antiandrogen cyproterone acetate. Its primary action is as an androgen receptor blocking agent, but it also suppresses androgen production. The combination of cyproterone acetate and ethinyl oestradiol provides good cycle control and effective contraception. Cyproterone acetate has progestogenic properties; it has a long half life and is usually given for the first 10 days of the cycle, with ethinyl oestradiol being given for 21 days, the so-called 'reverse sequential' regimen. The incidence of side effects varies from series to series, but although lethargy, breast tenderness and weight gain are common, they usually last only one or two cycles and the drug is generally very well tolerated at doses of 50–100 mg daily. There have been reports that spironolactone (usually in combination with a combined oral contraceptive) provides effective control of hirsutism. Like cyproterone it is thought to act as an androgen receptor blocking agent.

MALE REPRODUCTIVE ENDOCRINOLOGY

Despite important advances in the last 15 years in knowledge of the endocrine mechanisms controlling male reproductive function, the major clinical problem in male reproduction – that of the infertile man – seems no nearer resolution. This contrasts strongly with female reproduction in which application of recent knowledge of hormonal control of the menstrual cycle has enabled successful treatment of the majority of infertile patients with ovulatory failure. The reason for the disparity is clear; endocrine disorders manifesting as anovulation account for 20% or more of women with infertility, whereas clear-cut endocrine abnormalities are uncommon in subfertile men. Nevertheless, hormone measurements do have

a part to play in the management of the infertile man.

A. HORMONAL CONTROL OF TESTICULAR FUNCTION

Leydig cell function

Leydig (interstitial) cells of the testis occupy the well-vascularized connective tissue stroma between the seminiferous tubules; they synthesise and secrete testosterone. Gonadal testosterone secretion begins as early as the seventh week of intrauterine life (under the influence of human chorionic gonadotrophin, HCG). Leydig cell function diminishes after birth, but is reactivated during puberty in association with 'maturation' of the hypothalamic-pituitary axis. Testosterone secretion is primarily under the control of LH, for which there are specific cell-surface receptors. FSH appears to increase the sensitivity of the Leydig cell to LH, but there are no specific receptors for FSH on the Leydig cell and the precise mechanism of this action remains unknown.

Despite the finding of prolactin binding sites in Leydig cells it is not clear what, if any, role prolactin has in normal human Leydig cell function. There is little doubt that hyperprolactinaemia can cause gonadal dysfunction, but it is unlikely that this is due primarily to a direct effect of prolactin on the Leydig cell.

The biological activity of testosterone may be altered by peripheral conversion to 5α-reduced metabolites (dihydrotestosterone and the androstenediols) or by aromatization to oestradiol, a mechanism which is probably important in sexual differentiation of the brain and which may play a part in feedback control of gonadotrophin secretion. Oestradiol, however, may be secreted directly by the testis and direct glandular secretion probably accounts for about 25% of circulating oestradiol levels. The cellular origin of testicular oestradiol remains controversial, but there is evidence that both the Leydig cell and the Sertoli cell (see below) can synthesise it. The possible role of oestradiol in local regulation of Leydig cell function and in abnormalities of spermatogenesis is discussed later. The main actions of testosterone and its metabolites are effected by binding to specific

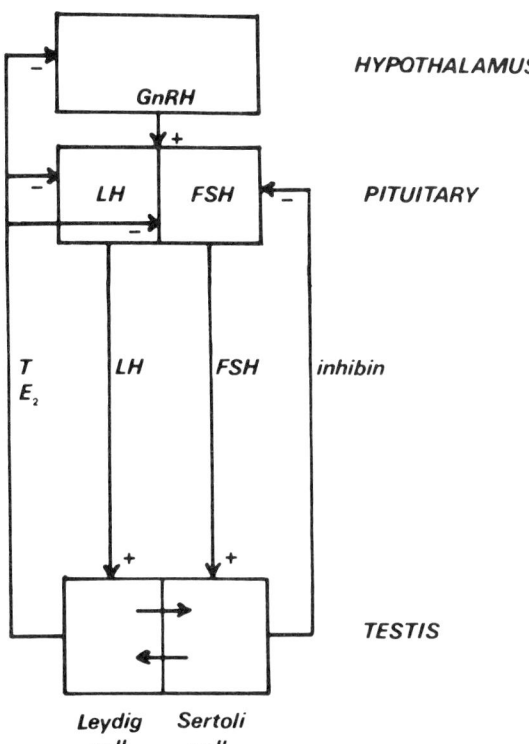

Fig. 6.5 The hypothalamic-pituitary-testicular axis showing stimulatory (+) and negative-feedback (−) mechanisms. The relative importance of the hypothalamus and pituitary as feedback sites for testosterone (T) and oestradiol (E₂) remains to be determined. From Franks S 1981 Male reproductive endocrinology. Clinics in Obstetrics and Gynaecology 8:549-569. With kind permission of the publisher, W B Saunders.

intracellular receptors. Disorders of the peripheral metabolism of testosterone or of androgen binding to its receptor – the so called 'androgen-resistant states' – may lead to hypogonadism or infertility and are discussed below.

Seminiferous tubule function

The seminiferous tubule comprises the germ cells at various stages of the spermatogenic cycle, supported by interspersed Sertoli cells. The Sertoli cell is responsible for the synthesis and secretion of androgen-binding protein and inhibin and is a site for aromatization of testosterone (probably derived from the Leydig cell) to oestradiol. These actions (at least in the immature testis) are under the influence of FSH, which has specific receptors in the Sertoli cell. The precise role of FSH in adult

Table 6.5 Causes of hypogonadism. (After Franks S 1981 Male reproductive endocrinology. Clinics in Obstetrics and Gynaecology 8: 555.)

Leydig cell failure
Primary hypogonadism — hypergonadotrophic hypogonadism
    Klinefelter's syndrome
    Genital infection
    Chronic illness, e.g. chronic renal failure
    Disorders of testosterone biosynthesis
Secondary hypogonadism — hypogonadotrophic hypogonadism
    Constitutional delayed puberty
    Isolated gonadotrophin deficiency (Kallman's syndrome)
Hyperprolactinaemia
Hypopituitarism
Anorexia nervosa
Laurence-Moon-Biedl syndrome
Prader-Labhardt-Willi syndrome

Impaired androgen action
Defects in androgen binding to target organ, e.g. Reifenstein's syndrome
Defects in testosterone metabolism
    5α reductase deficiency

Sertoli cell function and indeed in spermatogenesis remains unclear.

The humoral control of spermatogenesis in man appears to involve both testosterone and FSH. High intratesticular concentrations of testosterone can initiate spermatogenesis in the absence of FSH in rats and in boys with testosterone-producing testicular tumours. FSH appears to be important in completion of spermatogenesis, since maturation is arrested at the spermatid stage in its absence. However, the evidence that it is necessary for the maintenance of established spermatogenesis in man is controversial.

Regulation of gonadotrophin secretion by the hypothalamus and testis

The fundamental concept of negative feedback control of gonadotrophins by testicular hormones (i.e. a rise in testosterone leading to a fall in LH) remains valid, but needs qualification particularly in view of knowledge of the important role of GnRH in control of gonadotrophins. Gonadotrophin-releasing hormone stimulates synthesis and secretion of both LH and FSH but this action may be influenced, at both hypothalamic and pituitary level, by gonadal hormones (Fig. 6.5). Luteinising hormone is secreted in a pulsatile manner in men as well as in women, as a result of episodic secretion of GnRH. As in women there have been many studies in men supporting the existence of selective control of FSH by inhibin.

B. ABNORMAL GONADAL FUNCTION

Disorders of gonadal function in men may present in two ways: 1. hypogonadism, which results from failure of Leydig cell function (or rarely from impaired androgen action) and is usually associated with seminiferous tubule failure, and 2. infertility, due to impairment of seminiferous tubule function (usually with normal Leydig cell function). In the infertility clinic hypogonadism is uncommon, but can often be treated successfully (when due to defective secretion of gonadotrophins), whereas impaired germ cell function is common but is seldom amenable to treatment. In the following sections the clinical features, diagnosis and management of these disorders will be discussed.

Hypogonadism

The major causes of hypogonadism are listed in Table 6.5. Hypogonadism may be due to primary testicular dysfunction (hypergonadotrophic hypogonadism) or secondary to hypothalamic-pituitary disease (hypogonadotrophic hypogonadism).

Clinical features

When gonadal dysfunction has delayed the onset of puberty the patient may complain of failure of sexual development in comparison with his peers. In adult life, and particularly when hypogonadism ensues after previously normal sexual function, the complaint may be of loss of libido, impotence, diminished facial and body hair and muscle weakness. Gynaecomastia, particularly if painful, may be a presenting feature in patients with hypogonadism (see below). Galactorrhoea is rare, even in men with hyperprolactinaemia. Visual impairment or symptoms associated with other endocrine deficiencies, such as hypothyroidism, may lead one to suspect the presence of a space-occupying lesion of the pituitary or hypothalamus.

Mumps, torsion of the testes, injury or surgery can result in hypogonadism and any relevant history should be noted. Sometimes the patient may notice a change in size of the testes following such an insult. Systematic questioning may reveal the presence of chronic diseases, particularly chronic renal failure and hepatic cirrhosis, which may be associated with hypogonadism.

A careful family history may be helpful in the differential diagnosis of delayed puberty: late onset of puberty in parents or siblings favours the diagnosis of constitutional delayed puberty.

Examination of the man with hypogonadism should include a thorough general examination, as well as careful assessment of the genitalia, breasts and hair distribution. Anosmia suggests Kallman's syndrome; some of the rarer syndromes of hypogonadotrophic hypogonadism may include intellectual impairment and congenital abnormalities of the face and hands. The height of the patient may be an important pointer to the diagnosis. Growth in patients with associated growth hormone deficiency may be markedly retarded. Abnormally tall stature and eunuchoid proportions are suggestive of testicular failure due to Klinefelter's syndrome or its variants.

Poor muscle and laryngeal development and abnormal distribution of body fat resembling the female habitus may be found in men with hypogonadism. Gynaecomastia is usually obvious in the thin patient, but it may be difficult to palpate breast tissue in obese men and the presence of subcutaneous fat can be misleading. Facial hair is typically sparse or absent, but in those men who have gone through puberty, loss of pubic and axillary hair is variable. Staging of the pubic hair using criteria of Marshall and Tanner is helpful in assessing delayed puberty.

A small penis, suggesting prepubertal androgen deficiency, may be a feature of any type of hypogonadism. The rare finding of hypospadias or ambiguous genitalia in the hypogonadal male indicates an abnormality of sexual differentiation, which may be due to androgen insensitivity (Ch. 7).

Testicular size should be assessed with an orchidometer, which is simply a string of graded ovoids for comparison. Since the greater part of the mass of the testis is made up of the seminiferous

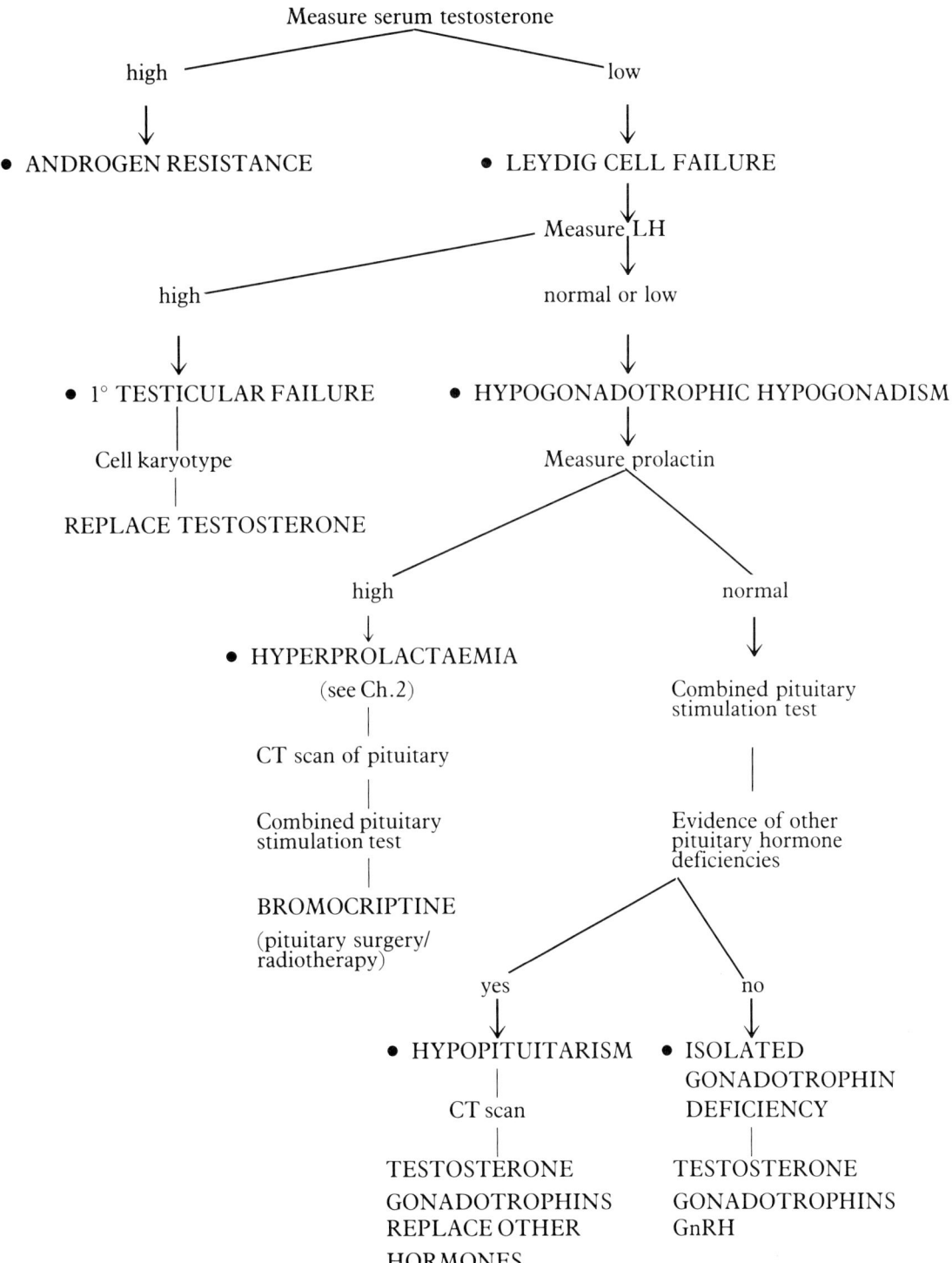

Fig. 6.6 Investigation and management of hypogonadism in men.

tubules, small testes indicate lack of development or atrophy of the germ cells. If one or both testes are absent from the scrotum, the inguinal canal should be carefully palpated. True cryptorchidism (one or both testes in the inguinal canal or intra-abdominal) occurs in both primary Leydig cell failure and hypogonadotrophic hypogonadism.

Differential diagnosis of hypogonadism

The differential diagnosis of hypogonadism can be made on the basis of clinical features and endocrine tests, occasionally helped by radiological investigations (Fig. 6.6). Low serum testosterone confirms Leydig cell failure in suspected hypogonadism; a higher than normal level suggests an androgen-resistant state. The syndromes of androgen resistance occurring in a male phenotype are of two types: those due to disorders of the androgen receptor (including incomplete testicular feminisation and Reifenstein's syndrome) and, more rarely, those due to 5α-reductase deficiency.

Measurement of serum gonadotrophin concentrations differentiates hypergonadotrophic from hypogonadotrophic causes. If gonadotrophin concentrations are high, chromosome analysis will define Klinefelter's syndrome (XXY karyotype) or its variants. Normal or low basal gonadotrophin levels with low testosterone indicate a hypothalamic or pituitary cause.

Measurement of serum prolactin can be performed at this stage. Hyperprolactinaemia in men with hypogonadism is usually associated with a radiologically evident pituitary tumour.

Assessment of gonadotrophin response to exogenous GnRH by means of a standard 50 or 100 μg intravenous GnRH test is occasionally useful in differentiating constitutional delayed puberty from isolated gonadotrophin deficiency, but this distinction may be difficult to make since a normal LH response to GnRH can be seen in isolated gonadotrophin deficiency, and an impaired response is occasionally observed in constitutional delayed puberty prior to testicular development. The clinical picture may help, anosmia and eunuchoidal proportions suggesting isolated gonadotrophin deficiency. It is often difficult to decide how far to investigate a teenage boy who has not progressed beyond Tanner stage 1 of puberty. Reasons for further investigation include a testicular volume of less than 4 ml, no family history of delayed development and psychological factors.

In the patient with gonadotrophin deficiency it is important to exclude more extensive disease of the hypothalamus and pituitary. This may be clinically apparent, but a combined pituitary stimulation test (Ch. 2) should be performed in order to assess the pituitary reserve of growth hormone, ACTH and TSH. A serum thyroxine measurement can be made on the baseline sample. PA and lateral X-rays of the pituitary area, and if necessary further radiological investigation, such as CT scanning, may be performed to visualize the suprasellar area.

Treatment of hypergonadotrophic hypogonadism

Patients with primary testicular failure or androgen resistance usually have untreatable dysfunction of the seminiferous tubules and are likely to remain infertile. Thus the aim of treatment is to replace testosterone. Testosterone replacement is conventionally given in the form of intramuscular injection of a long-acting testosterone ester (e.g. testosterone enanthate 250 mg every 2–4 weeks). Subcutaneous depot implants of crystalline testosterone (100–200 mg) are available; these are a little more difficult to administer, but their effect may last for up to six months. Oral preparations of testosterone have been generally unsatisfactory because absorption from the gastrointestinal tract is poor. Methyltestosterone, which is better absorbed, is rarely used because of the danger of cholestatic jaundice; however, good results have been reported with oral testosterone undecanoate. The recommended dose is 120–160 mg daily. Testosterone can also be given by the sublingual route but its absorption tends to be variable.

Treatment of hypogonadtrophic hypogonadism

Hypogonadism due to hyperprolactinaemia can be managed successfully by treatment which lowers serum prolactin levels. Bromocriptine, a long-acting dopamine agonist, will reduce prolactin levels to normal even in men with pituitary tumours, resulting in a rise in serum testosterone and improvement in sexual function (Ch. 2).

Constitutional delayed puberty usually needs no specific treatment, but if active therapy is considered necessary because of psychological difficulties, testosterone (see hypogonadotrophic hypogonadism above) is recommended. Treatment is continued for three months in the first instance and repeated if necessary after a three month period of assessment without treatment.

Low testosterone levels due to gonadotrophin deficiency, whether isolated or associated with hypopituitarism, can, in most cases, be treated with human chorionic gonadotrophin (HCG), but it is more convenient and much cheaper to treat the androgen deficiency with testosterone (see hypergonadotrophic hypogonadism). Treatment with testosterone does not appear to affect the response to exogenous gonadotrophins in men who subsequently require treatment for infertility.

For induction of spermatogenesis a combined regimen of HCG and human menopausal gonadotrophin (FSH and LH) is successful in producing complete spermatogenesis in about 85% of cases, but the data on pregnancy rates are limited. HCG is given intramuscularly 2000 units once or twice a week, the dose determined by reaching a normal testosterone level checked initially after 3 and 5 days and then monthly. Semen analysis is done every three months and if spermatogenesis is not fully restored in 6 months human menopausal gonadotrophin is added.

If gonadotrophin deficiency is due to impaired synthesis or secretion of GnRH (Kallman's syndrome), it has been shown that treatment with pulsatile GnRH may induce spermatogenesis, but prolonged treatment is required.

C. GYNAECOMASTIA

The definition of gynaecomastia is controversial. It is usually taken to mean palpable breast tissue in men, but it is not always easy to differentiate clinically between fatty changes and true enlargement of breast (glandular) tissue. It may occur physiologically, as in puberty, but may indicate an underlying endocrine disturbance. In addition, a variety of drugs, hormonal and non-hormonal, can cause gynaecomastia either by disturbing the endocrine environment or by a more obscure direct

Table 6.6 Causes of gynaecomastia. (After Frantz A G, Wilson J D, 1985 Endocrine disorders of the breast. In: Wilson J D, Foster D W eds Williams Textbook of endocrinology. Saunders: London, p412)

Physiological	Adolescent gynaecomastia
	Gynaecomastia of the elderly
Pathological	Testosterone deficiency
	Klinefelter's syndrome
	Androgen resistance
	Mumps orchitis
	Excess oestrogen production
	Testicular tumours
	Liver disease
	Thyroid disease
Drug induced	Oestrogens
	Gonadotrophins
	Spironolactone
	Cimetidine
Idiopathic	

effect on the breast. In general, the pathogenesis of gynaecomastia may be seen to represent an increase in the exposure of breast tissue to oestrogen, either by an increase in oestrogen production or (as in Klinefelter's syndrome) by a decrease in testosterone production. A classification of the causes of gynaecomastia is shown in Table 6.6.

The physiological gynaecomastia of the newborn or adolescent usually resolves spontaneously. Common causes of pathological gynaecomastia include Klinefelter's syndrome, liver disease and drugs, notably stilboestrol, spironolactone, cimetidine and α methyl-dopa. Despite its lactogenic action, prolactin is not directly involved in the pathogenesis of gynaecomastia. Patients with hyperprolactinaemia may have breast enlargement but this is related to testosterone deficiency rather than elevated serum prolactin concentrations per se.

The cause of gynaecomastia is usually apparent from history and examination; detailed endocrine investigation is rarely required. Measurement of testosterone and gonadotrophins may be helpful and assessment of adrenal androgen secretion is sometimes useful, but there is little place for routine estimation of serum oestradiol concentrations. Treatment should be directed at the underlying pathology. Testosterone is not always successful even when serum testosterone concentrations are low and this is principally because the structural changes in the breast may not be reversible. Consequently cosmetic surgery remains the only consistently effective means of management.

D. FERTILITY

In considering the causes of infertility, it is useful to categorize patients according to sperm density. Sperm density of less than 5 million per millilitre in a subfertile man may be associated with either seminiferous tubule dysfunction, ductal obstruction or partial androgen resistance (see below). Causes of acquired germ cell damage include genital infections, irradiation, cytotoxic drugs and trauma. Other common causes of oligospermia or azoospermia are Klinefelter's syndrome and varicocoele, but in about 50% of cases there is no obvious cause. Patients with oligospermia (5–20 x 10^6/ml) and low sperm motility (less than 60% motility with a normal sperm count) account for 75–80% of subfertile men and in most cases there is no definable cause for the poor semen quality. About one-third of men with oligospermia or poor sperm motility have a varicocoele and in a few patients there is history of genital infection, trauma or treatment with drugs such as sulphasalazine.

In addition to seminal analysis, clinical assessment and selected endocrine tests will enable most of the diagnostic subgroups to be identified, and treatment can be assessed on this basis. In fact, specific treatment can be offered in only a small minority of patients; the place of drugs and surgical treatment in the majority of men, i.e. those with idiopathic oligospermia and/or low sperm motility, will be discussed below.

Clinical features

Although it is important to take a careful history from the patient with infertility this is not usually helpful in diagnosis. Enquiries about sexual intercourse may reveal a small group of patients in whom coital difficulties are the cause of infertility and may also bring to light symptoms of androgen deficiency. A few patients will have a clear history of genital infection, trauma or irradiation of the testis. Chronic illness may also be associated with infertility. A recent drug history may be helpful:

cytoxic chemotherapy may be associated with a low sperm count and it has been suggested that sulphasalazine may cause oligospermia and that this is reversible when the drug is withdrawn. The true significance of oligospermia is so often doubtful that thorough investigation of the female partner is always essential as well.

Physical examination of the man will reveal no abnormalities in perhaps 50% of patients. Evidence of androgen deficiency is rare in men presenting with infertility, but is important to define because of therapeutic implications. Whilst general physical examination is not often helpful, examination of the genitalia is important. Testicular size should be assessed with an orchidometer as described previously. The finding of small testes in the patient with severe oligospermia or azoospermia suggests serious impairment of seminiferous tubule function, whereas normal testicular size favours the diagnosis of ductal obstruction. A large varicocoele is usually obvious, but it may be necessary to ask the patient to stand and to perform a Valsalva manoeuvre in order to demonstrate its presence. Varicocoele is commonly associated with infertility, although it also occurs in a significant proportion (approximately 10%) of normal fertile men. The precise mechanism by which this causes abnormalities of spermatogenesis is not known.

Investigation of the infertile male

The most important investigations of the male with infertility are semen analysis and hormone measurements. These tests may be supplemented when indicated by other investigations such as karyotype (e.g. when Klinefelter's syndrome is suspected) and measurement of sperm autoantibodies. Testicular biopsy is rarely helpful in management except perhaps in association with surgical exploration for ductal obstruction. The importance of reliable semen analysis cannot be overemphasised. Because of the considerable temporal variation in sperm density, even in normal men, it is rarely sufficient to obtain a single semen sample; preferably three to six samples should be obtained over the course of at least one month. There are many factors responsible for the variability of sperm count and it is important to remember acute febrile illness which may be associated with transient azoospermia.

Endocrine tests are most likely to be helpful in the management of the patient with severe oligospermia or azoospermia. Serum FSH is an important marker of seminiferous tubule function, FSH levels being consistently elevated in men with small testes and sperm counts below one million per millilitre and showing a strong negative correlation with the degree of spermatogenic activity on testicular biopsy.

When ductal obstruction is suspected on the basis of history, normal sized testes or normal FSH levels, testicular biopsy may be considered in order to confirm normal spermatogenesis before proceeding to vasography and exploration of the scrotum. However, the prognosis for fertility following reconstructive surgery is poor. It may, therefore, be argued that, even if an obstructive lesion seems likely on clinical and endocrine grounds, no further investigations or treatment should be considered until the prognosis has been explained to the patient.

Testosterone and LH concentrations are useful in men with sperm counts of less than 5×10^6/ml; a low testosterone level indicating Leydig cell failure may occasionally occur in the absence of clear-cut signs of androgen deficiency and the finding of a normal testosterone and elevated LH concentration indicates a state of compensated Leydig cell failure. In both cases the patient may require androgen replacement at a later date. Since impaired Leydig cell function is particularly common in Klinefelter's syndrome it is useful to perform chromosome analyses in patients with this hormone profile.

Endocrine investigations are seldom of value in men with sperm counts of between 5 and 20×10^6/ml or in those with poor sperm motility and it is doubtful whether measurement of FSH, LH and testosterone should be made routinely. Serum prolactin levels should not be measured routinely in men with infertility who have no evidence of hypogonadism.

Management of the infertile male

Specific treatment is possible in only a small proportion of infertile men. Those who have hypogonadotrophic hypogonadism (less than 1% of men with infertility), those with coital difficulties (less than 1%) and those with ductal obstruction (6–7%). Hypogonadotrophic testicular failure can be treated successfully with gonadotrophins or GnRH as described previously. Problems with intercourse may be amenable to sexual counselling. The problem of surgical treatment of obstructive azoospermia has already been discussed.

In some patients treatment is clearly of no benefit. Men with severe oligospermia, small testes and raised FSH levels are likely to remain infertile; androgen replacement may be necessary sooner or later in those with biochemical evidence of Leydig cell failure (for example patients with Klinefelter's syndrome). In the remaining patients, the 70–80% with oligospermia or poor sperm motility, the question of whether any treatment is likely to improve fertility is still unresolved. Ligation of a varicocoele has been reported to improve semen quality, but it is doubtful whether surgical treatment increases the pregnancy rate.

The medical treatment of idiopathic oligospermia includes a large number of drugs and hormones. Oral androgens, testosterone rebound, gonadotrophins and antioestrogens have been widely used but the very fact that no one treatment has been universally adopted in idiopathic oligospermia suggests that there are no studies which demonstrate the efficacy of therapy. Problems in interpretation of reports of 'successful treatment' include the absence of strict criteria for selection of patients, lack of suitable control groups and poor criteria for documentation of 'improvement' in semen quality. Such data as are available suggest that the pregnancy rate in the partners of men with oligospermia is unaffected by hormone treatment of the subfertile male.

Sexual differentiation

NORMAL SEXUAL DIFFERENTIATION

In normal development, gonadal and phenotypic sex follow an orderly process of development, which is initially determined by the genetic or chromosomal sex fixed at conception (Fig. 7.1).

The primitive gonad is bipotential, having an inner medulla capable of developing into a testis and an outer cortex which may become an ovary. The primitive germ cells migrate into the gonad from the endoderm of the primitive yolk sac at 4–6 weeks of gestation. Further development will depend on the sex chromosomal constitution, a Y chromosome or Y determined H-Y anitgen being essential for testis formation and subsequent male development. In the presence of a second X, or in the absence of a second sex chromosome (i.e.

45XO), development will follow the female pattern, although XX is required for normal ovary formation. At the end of the second month the genital organs are undifferentiated and comprise a paired duct system, a medial Müllerian and a laterally placed Wolffian duct, together with the primitive genital tubercle.

In the female, the Wolffian system regresses and the Müllerian ducts develop to form fallopian tubes, the uterus and upper third of the vagina. The external genitalia undergo relatively little change, the genital tubercle becomes the clitoris and the genital swellings and urethral folds form the labia. In the male, the Müllerian system regresses, and the Wolffian ducts develop to form the excretory ducts of the testis, the rete testis, epididymis and vas deferens. The posterior portion of these ducts also gives rise to the prostate and seminal vesicles.

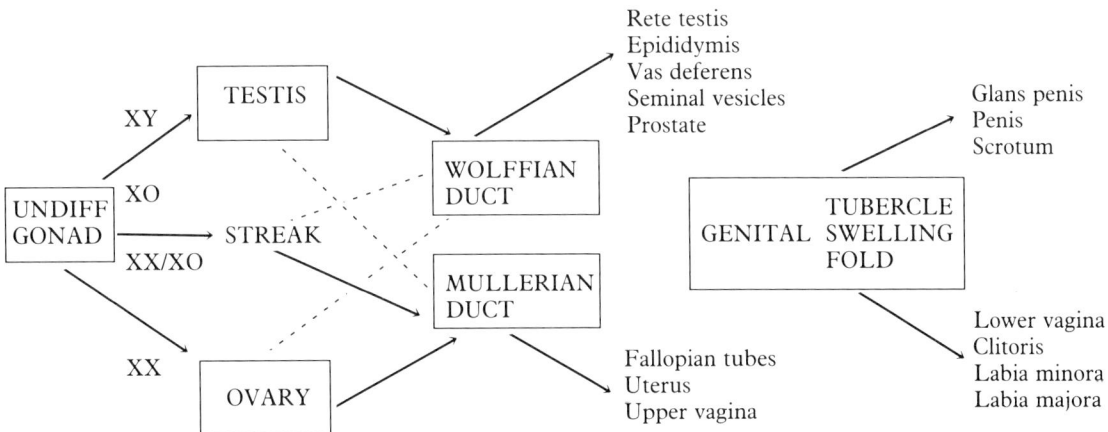

Fig. 7.1   Normal sexual differentiation

The genital tubercle becomes the glans penis, while the shaft is formed by simultaneous fusion and elongation of the urethral fold and groove. The genital swellings fuse to form the scrotum into which the testes descend, together with their Wolffian derivatives.

There is now good evidence to suggest that internal and external genital development in the male is hormone dependent. The secretion of chorionic gonadotrophin from the placenta, having an LH-like action, stimulates fetal Leydig cell production of testosterone. Testosterone inhibits regression of Wolffian duct derivatives and stimulates their differentiation into accessory sex structures. The external genital structures, however, are only fully responsive to dihydrotestesterone, which is formed from testosterone by the tissue enzyme 5α-reductase. The Sertoli cells of the fetal testis secrete a small polypeptide (Müllerian inhibiting factor, MIF), which produces local regression of the Müllerian duct system. The ovary, in contrast, appears to be hormonally inactive in utero.

ABNORMAL SEXUAL DIFFERENTIATION

Patients with abnormalities of sexual differentiation may present with abnormal external genitalia in the newborn period, growth disturbance in later childhood, or with inappropriate or absent secondary sexual development at adolescence. In this chapter the major emphasis will be given to abnormal genital development.

Abnormal gonadal development

True hermaphroditism is very rare; persistence of both cortical and medullary elements of the primitive gonad may lead to bilateral ovotestes, or lateralised sexual dimorphism may result in a testis and Wolffian duct derivatives on one side and an ovary and Müllerian structures on the other. The recognition of the H-Y antigen may explain the apparent absence of demonstrable Y chromosomes in some of these cases. In most instances however, abnormal gonadal development follows a primary abnormality in sex chromosomal constitution.

Chromosome abnormalities

Klinefelter's syndrome

This is the commonest sex chromosomal anomaly with an incidence of 1 in 400 males. The diagnosis is made only rarely in childhood. The classical appearance is shown in Figure 7.2 and the typical findings in Table 7.1. The usual karyotype is XXY, but XXXY and XY occur, when mental deficiency and gonadal failure are more pronounced. Mosaic forms XY/XXY may have normal appearances and sexual function.

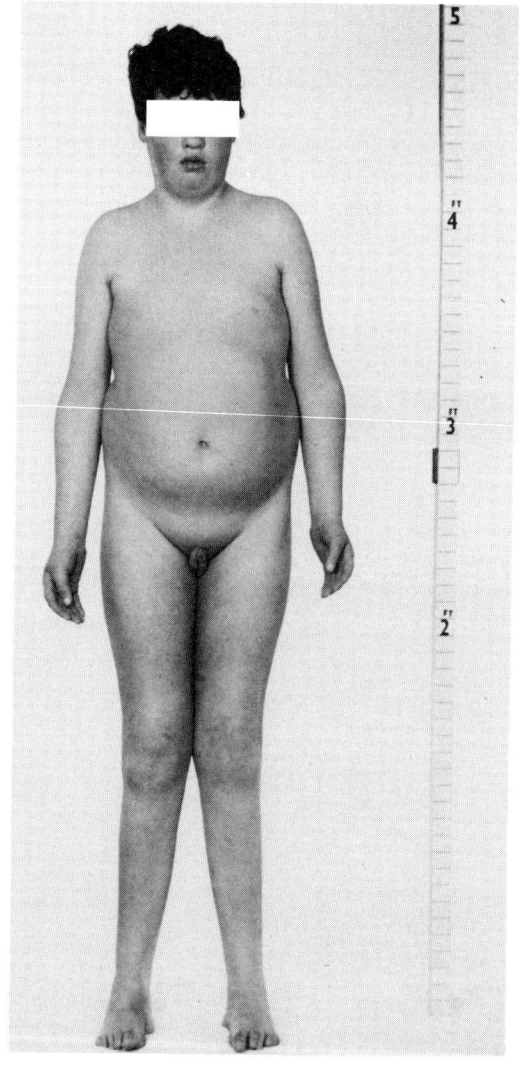

Fig.7.2 Klinefelter's syndrome. Typical appearance in childhood.

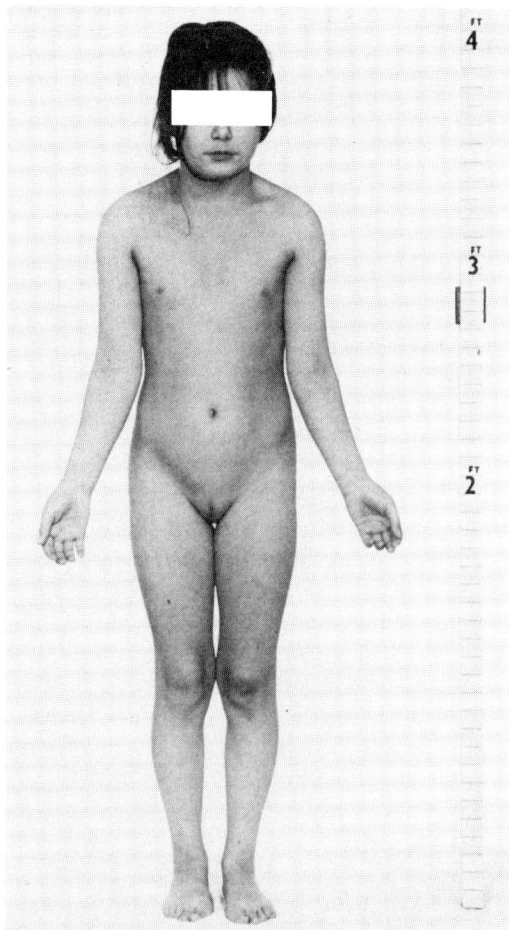

Fig. 7.3 Turner's syndrome. Typical appearance in a 14-year-old girl.

Table 7.1 Klinefelter's syndrome

Clinical features	Laboratory findings
In childhood	
Normal or tall stature	Sex chromatin positive
Eunuchoid proportions	Serum testosterone decreased
Truncal obesity	Serum gonadotrophins increased
Mild mental deficiency	Oligo- or azoospermia
In adolescence and later	
Small firm testes (6 ml volume)	
Gynaecomastia	
Reduced secondary sexual development, libido, musculature	

Turner's syndrome

Turner's syndrome has an incidence of 1 in 2500, although the incidence in aborted fetuses is much higher. About 70% of cases have the classical XO karyotype, the remainder having mosaic XO/XX forms or deletions of the short or long arm of an X chromosome. The physical appearances and clinical findings in XO cases are usually easily recognised (Figs. 7.3, 7.4, Table 7.2), but subjects may have near normal phenotypes. 'Streak' gonads are present in patients with an XO karyotype. Loss of either the long or short arm of one X chromosome appears to be associated with gonadal dysgenesis, whereas loss of genetic material from the short arm appears to be associated particularly with

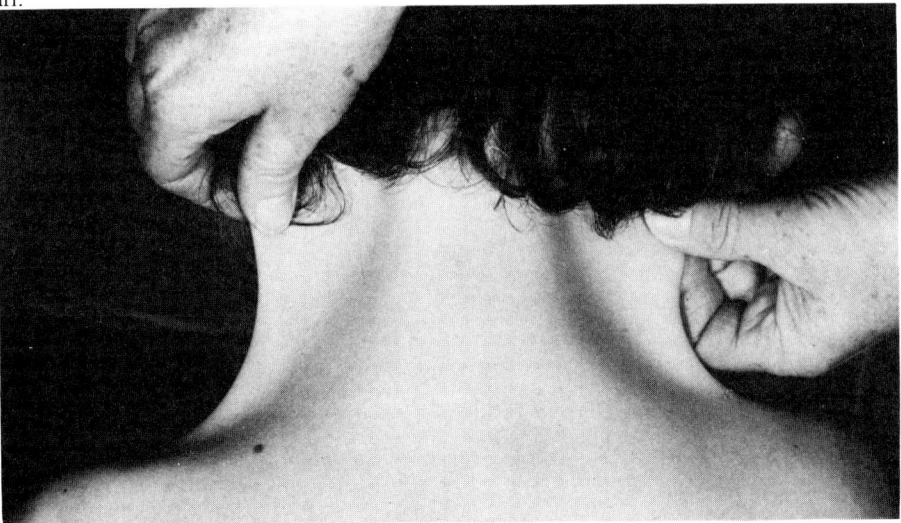

Fig. 7.4 Turner's syndrome. Neck webbing

Table 7.2 Turner's syndrome

Clinical features	Laboratory findings
In childhood	
Lymphoedema of hands and feet	Sex chromatin negative (70%)
Small, deeply-set nails	Vaginal smear oestrogen
Neck webbing, triple hairline	Serum gonadotrophins elevated
Low birth weight	
Pigmented cutaneous naevi	
At adolescence and later	
Retardation of growth and bone age	
Osteodystrophy, cubitus valgus	
Amenorrhoea, absent breast development	
Pubic and axillary hair present	

short stature. Spontaneous sexual development and menstruation may occur regularly in a few patients with XX/XO mosaicism. The Turner phenotype also occurs rarely in males with XY karyotypes (Noonan's syndrome).

Male pseudohermaphroditism

In male pseudohermaphroditism, development of external male genitalia is incomplete despite the presence of a normal male karyotype and well differentiated testes. The abnormality is due to a functional androgen deficiency, which may arise from defective testosterone synthesis or from defective target tissue response (Table 7.3). The

Table 7.3 Aetiology of male pseudohermaphroditism

Androgen synthesis defects
20,22-Desmolase deficiency
3β-Hydroxysteroid dehydrogenase deficiency
17-Hydroxylase deficiency
17,20-Desmolase deficiency
17-Reductase deficiency

Leydig cell hypoplasia
Idiopathic fetal gonadotrophin deficiency

Defective target tissue response to androgens
5α-Reductase deficiency
Complete androgen insensitivity (testicular feminisation syndrome)
Partial androgen insensitivity

Miscellaneous
Various dysmorphological syndromes
Persistent oviducts
Iatrogenic

genital anomaly may range from apparently normal female appearance to a male pattern with severe hypospadias. Accessory structures of Wolffian duct origin are usually deficient or absent. Secretion of MIF is unaffected so that Müllerian structures are absent. An isolated defect in Sertoli cell production of MIF may, however, occur in the presence of normal testicular androgenic activity resulting in the persistence of oviducts in an otherwise normal male.

Androgen synthesis defects

This recessively inherited group of disorders are the result of deficiency of the various enzymes involved in the synthesis of testosterone from cholesterol. They may result in defective virilisation of the fetal genitalia alone, or be combined with defects in the production of cortisol and aldosterone by the adrenal, since many of the enzyme pathways in early steroid synthesis are common to both glands. The steps involved in androgen synthesis have been described in Chapter 5. The proximal defects of 20,22-desmolase and 3β-hydroxysteroid dehydrogenase deficiencies result in deficiency of aldosterone and cortisol as well as testosterone synthesis, so that severe salt loss occurs in addition to poor genital virilisation (Fig. 7.5). Females with 3β-hydroxysteroid dehydrogenase deficiency have some virilisation of their external genitalia since the production of the weak androgen dehydroepiandrosterone is sufficient to produce androgenic effects in the female, but it does not induce full virilisation in the male. The enzyme 17-hydroxylase is not required for aldosterone production and stimulation of this pathway by ACTH results in potassium loss and hypertension. Deficiencies of the more distal enzymes in the testosterone pathway, 17,20-desmolase and 17-reductase, result in androgen deficiency without adrenal hormone disturbance.

Defective target tissue response to androgens

5α-reductase deficiency In androgen responsive tissues, testosterone, after entering the cell, is converted by the intracellular enzyme 5α-reductase to its biologically active form 5α-dihydrotestosterone (DHT). The steroid DHT

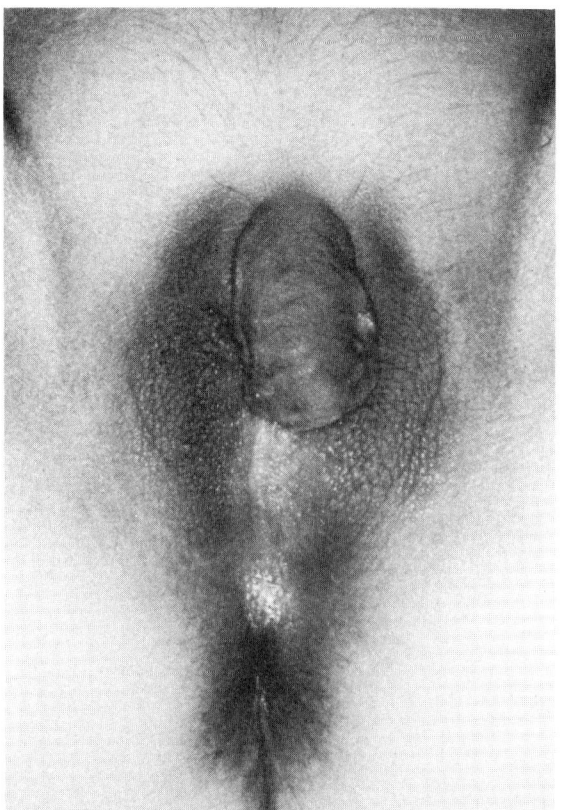

Fig. 7.5 Appearance of external genitalia in a male infant with a 3β-dehydrogenase deficiency.

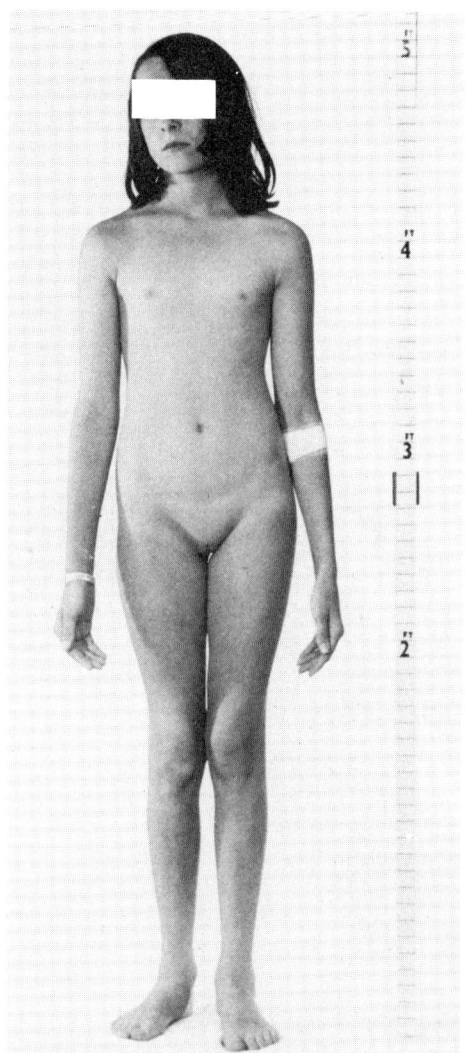

Fig. 7.6 Testicular feminisation syndrome. Typical appearance in childhood.

binds to a cytoplasmic receptor protein, initiating protein synthesis within the cell. Reported cases of 5α-reductase deficiency, a condition with autosomal recessive inheritance, have a selective impairment of the masculinisation of the external genitalia with normal Wolffian duct derivatives. Masculinisation occurs at puberty with normal spermatogenesis.

Complete androgen insensitivity – testicular feminisation syndrome. In this inherited condition, a female phenotype occurs paradoxically in XY males (Fig. 7.6). The external genitalia are of normal female appearance, but the vagina is short and blind. Normal testes are present, which may be cryptorchid or situated in the labia majora or inguinal herniae. Müllerian regression occurs normally, but Wolffian duct derivatives do not develop. Good breast development but no sexual hair growth occurs at puberty. There is an increased incidence of testicular gonadoblastoma after puberty. The exact aetiology of this defect remains to be established, but a defect in the cytoplasmic receptor for DHT, or in its subsequent action, appears most likely.

Incomplete androgen insensitivity. Some patients with XY karyotype and normal testicular testosterone production, appear to have an incomplete or partial insensitivity to androgens. A wide spectrum of defects has been described. The genitalia may be predominantly female in appearance, but with clitoral hypertrophy. Breast development occurs at puberty but with some virilisation. In other cases a male phenotype with hypospadias develops, but gynaecomastia may occur at puberty. The variety of defects probably represent as yet undefined abnormalities in the complex intracellular pathways of androgenic action.

Female pseudohermaphroditism

In female pseudohermaphroditism virilisation of the external genitalia occurs in the presence of an XX karyotype, normal ovaries and Müllerian duct derivatives, and usually potentially normal female puberty. The degree of virilisation may vary from clitoral enlargement with posterior labial fusion, to virtually male appearances with perineal hypospadias. The principal causes are listed in Table 7.4. Typical genital appearances are shown in Figure 7.7.

Table 7.4 Aetiology of female hermaphroditism

Variants of congenital adrenal hyperplasia
21α-Hydroxylase deficiency
11β-Hydroxylase deficiency
3βHydroxysteroid dehydrogenase deficiency

Maternal androgen administration

Maternal androgen secreting tumour

Miscellaneous
Dysmorphic syndromes
Associated renal and anal abnormalities

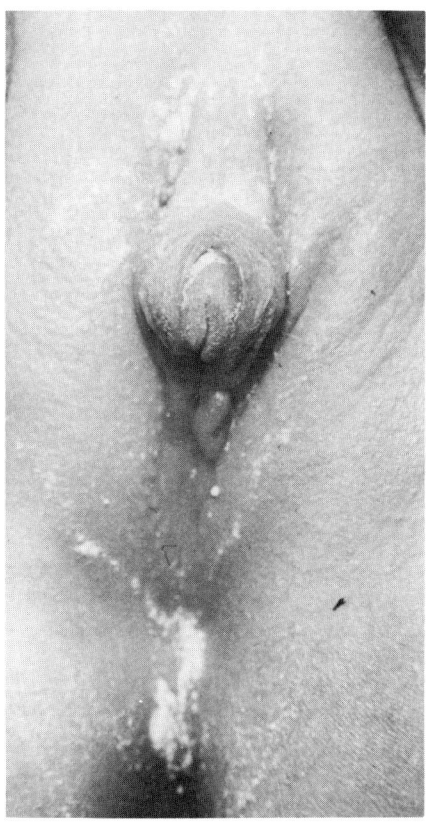

Fig. 7.7 Typical genital appearance of a virilised female infant with 21-hydroxylase deficiency.

Congenital adrenal hyperplasia

This group of disorders results in excess secretion of adrenal androgens in response to pituitary ACTH stimulation (Ch. 5). The normal pituitary-adrenal feedback mechanism is cortisol dependent, and all variants share a defect at some level in cortisol production. The commonest disorder, accounting for 95% of patients with congenital adrenal hyperplasia, is 21-hydroxylase deficiency. In about 50% of affected patients aldosterone production is also significantly impaired, and clinical features of salt loss also occur. There is a broad correlation between the degree of virilisation of the external genitalia and the severity of salt loss. The precursor steroid prior to the 21-hydroxylase block, 17-hydroxyprogesterone, is shunted into the androgen pathway, resulting in excess production of dehydroepiandrosterone, androstenedione, and ultimately testosterone. Deficiency of the enzyme 11β-hydroxylase, while leading to similar overproduction of adrenal androgens, also results in excess production of 11-deoxycortisol and 11-deoxycorticosterone in the aldosterone pathway. These steroids have weak sodium retaining effect, and when produced in excess may result in hypertension.

Paradoxically, as previously mentioned, deficiency of 3β-hydroxysteroid dehydrogenase results in excess production of the weak androgen dehydroepiandrosterone, leading to virilisation in female fetuses. Severe salt loss is present in both sexes.

Maternal androgen production or administration

The virilisation of female fetuses by androgens, secreted by maternal ovarian or adrenal tumours, although rare, is well documented. In some cases the diagnosis has been made in the mother retrospectively after birth of a virilised infant. Progesterone or its derivatives, may have sufficient androgenic action to produce some virilisation of female infants when given in the first trimester of pregnancy (Fig. 7.8). Their use for threatened abortion in early pregnancy has now been discontinued.

The investigation and management of ambiguous genitalia in the new born

Careful examination should be performed to determine the precise anatomical nature of the external genitalia and to identify vaginal and urethral orifices. The perineum and groins should be palpated carefully for gonadal swellings.

The most important initial investigation is the determination of the karyotype. Buccal smear examination for the presence of sex-chromatin (Barr) bodies, and Y fluorescent techniques are useful screening tests, but may be unreliable in the first few days of life. Full chromosomal analysis is essential for the determination of normal XX, XY or sex chromosome mosaicism. Further investigation may include studies of androgen synthesis and androgen binding or measurement of steroid metabolites in blood and urine appropriate for the diagnosis of congenital adrenal hyperplasia (Ch. 5).

Assignment of sex of rearing

This is a very important decision with far reaching consequences, and hasty decisions cannot easily be reversed without great psychological trauma. The concern expressed by the parents to have a rapid decision should be resisted until full information is available. In general, female pseudohermaphrodites should be reared as females, especially virilised female infants with congenital adrenal hyperplasia, who, with appropriate treatment, can lead normal reproductive lives. Sex assignment in male

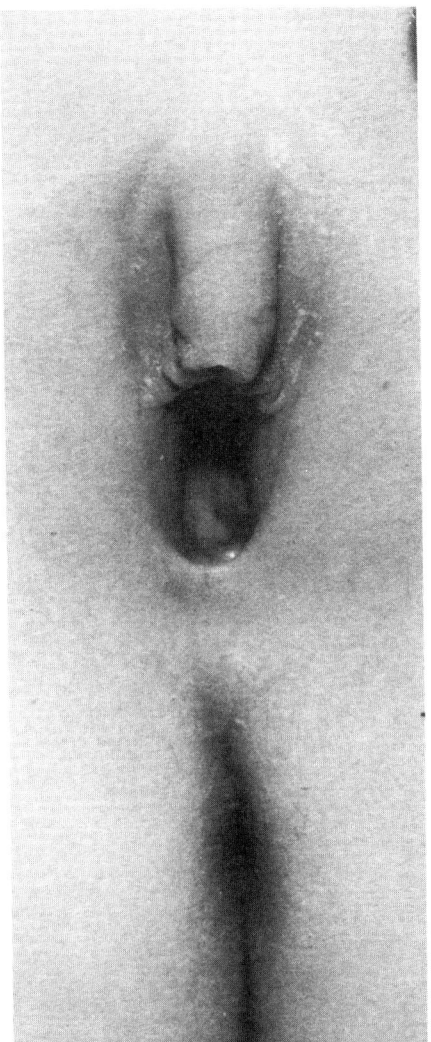

Fig. 7.8 Virilisation of genitalia in female infant due to maternal progesterone therapy.

pseudohermaphrodites is much more difficult, because a poorly developed phallus can rarely become a functioning penis, and a female role is often the most appropriate. Consideration should also be given to the nature and adequacy of further development at puberty.

Gut hormones

The gut hormones, often termed gastrointestinal regulatory peptides, play a major role in regulating the normal function of the gastrointestinal tract, gall bladder and pancreas. Clinically, however, their importance lies in their association with a variety of syndromes due to overproduction by tumours. A number of these peptides are used in gastrointestinal function tests, which utilise their physiological and pharmacological properties.

PHYSIOLOGY

A great number of peptides have now been isolated from the gastrointestinal mucosa and pancreas. Many of these peptides are also found in the central nervous system and in peripheral nerves. The major peptides with their primary localisation and postulated physiological actions are listed in Table 8.1. Insulin and glucagon are not usually considered as gut hormones, but syndromes of tumour overproduction of these two peptides are discussed below. A number of other peptides have been extracted from the gastrointestinal tract and pancreas including somatostatin, bombesin, thyrotrophin releasing hormone and the enkephalins but their role is less certain. Several other biologically active substances, for example prostaglandins and 5-hydroxytryptamine, are found within the gastrointestinal mucosa, but their role in the physiology of the bowel remains to be defined. In addition, abnormalities of hormone

Table 8.1 Principal gastrointestinal hormones

Peptide	Principal sources	Physiological actions
Gastrin	Gastric antrum and duodenum	Gastric acid and pepsin secretion
Cholecystokinin/pancreozymin	Upper small intestine	Gall bladder contraction Pancreatic enzyme secretion
Secretin	Upper small intestine	Pancreatic bicarbonate and water secretion
Gastric inhibitory polypeptide	Upper small intestine	Insulin release Inhibition of gastric secretion and motility
Motilin	Upper small intestine	Stimulates gut motility
Pancreatic polypeptide	Pancreas	Unknown, cholecystokinin antagonist
Vasoactive intestinal polypeptide	Throughout gut	Unknown, neural regulation of gastrointestinal motor tone, motility and secretion.
Neurotensin	Ileum	Unknown, regulates ileal absorption
Substance P	Throughout gut	Unknown, inhibits gastric and pancreatic secretion and stimulates intestinal motility
Enteroglucagon (Glicentin)	Ileum and colon	Unknown, slows intestinal transit and increases mucosal growth

Table 8.2 Tumour syndromes

Syndrome	Hormone	Usual presentation
Zollinger-Ellison	Gastrin	Multiple or recurrent peptic ulcers
VIPoma	Vasoactive intestinal polypeptide	Watery diarrhoea and hypokalaemia
Glucagonoma	Glucagon	Skin rash, wasting
Somatostatinoma	Somatostatin	Not defined
Carcinoid	5-Hydroxytryptamine + various peptides	Diarrhoea, flushing, asthma, cardiac lesions

release have been described in various diseases affecting the gastrointestinal tract. For example, in coeliac disease there is a failure of release of hormones predominantly secreted by the upper small bowel (cholecystokinin, secretin, gastric inhibitory polypeptide), while hormones predominantly secreted by the lower small bowel (enteroglucagon and neurotensin) are increased. These findings, while of physiological interest, have not yet proved to be of diagnostic value. Similarly, measurement of serum gastrin, despite profound effects on gastric acid secretion, has not proved helpful in the management of simple peptic ulcer disease.

Peptides in gastrointestinal function tests

A commercially available pentapeptide containing the C-terminal five peptides of gastrin (pentagastrin) is fully active in promoting gastric acid secretion and is used as a test of maximal secretory capacity of the stomach. This test is sometimes used in assessing new drugs for their efficiency in reducing gastric acid secretion and to confirm the diagnosis of achlorhydria. Secretin and pancreozymin are used to assess pancreatic exocrine function. Gastric and duodenal juices are aspirated after injection of secretin and pancreozymin; the volume of secretion and bicarbonate and enzyme (amylase or trypsin) output are determined. Diminished output of bicarbonate and enzymes is found in chronic pancreatitis and carcinoma of the head of the pancreas and thus differentiates these conditions from non-pancreatic steatorrhoea. Secretin and pancreozymin are also used to stimulate the flow of pancreatic juice to facilitate cytological detection of malignancy at endoscopic retrograde pancreatography (ERCP). Glucagon is

used for both its hyperglycaemic properties and to inhibit peristalsis during radiological and endoscopic procedures.

TUMOUR SYNDROMES

Several well defined syndromes have been described in association with overproduction of specific hormones by tumours of gastrointestinal hormone secreting cells. These tumours are most commonly located in the pancreas or within the gastrointestinal mucosa, but have been described in association with tumours elsewhere. The major syndromes are listed in Table 8.2.

Pathology

Tumours of the gastrointestinal endocrine cells have similar histological characteristics and are often referred to as 'carcinoids'. True carcinoid tumours originate from the enterochromaffin cells (cells which reduce silver salts), while the remaining gut hormone secreting tumours do not. The histological features of such tumours are sufficiently characteristic to enable easy diagnosis when the tumour is in the gastrointestinal mucosa or pancreas, but isolated liver secondaries may be mistaken for anaplastic carcinoma. It is often not possible to determine whether any particular tumour is malignant on histological criteria alone, but most are slow growing and metastasize late.

Zollinger-Ellison syndrome (ZES)

The coincidence of islet cell tumours of the pancreas and severe ulcer diathesis was recognised by Zollinger and Ellison in 1955. It was later shown that ZES has associated hypersecretion of gastrin and it is thus also known as the gastrinoma syndrome. Gastrinomas are usually located in the pancreas, upper duodenal mucosa or rarely in the gastric antrum. Sixty per cent are malignant and 50% recur after apparently successful surgery. Twenty per cent are associated with the multiple endocrine adenomatosis (MEA) type I syndrome; this association should be suspected in the presence of hypercalcaemia or hypoglycaemia (Ch. 9). In general gastrinomas are slow growing and it is possible to live for many years with multiple secondaries if gastric hypersecretion can be controlled.

Clinical features

The ZES can present at any age. Two thirds of patients have chronic symptoms and one third episodic symptoms. Although some patients present with fulminating ulcer disease with perforation, haemorrhage, oesophagitis and stricture formation, the majority of patients have a more benign course. Approximately one third of patients will have had surgery for apparently simple ulcer disease, with remissions lasting from 1 month to 20 years. Forty per cent of patients present with dyspepsia alone, 20% with diarrhoea alone and 40% with both. The syndrome should be suspected in any patient with duodenal ulceration which does not respond to treatment or rapidly recurs following surgery, patients with multiple duodenal or jejunal ulcers, patients with peptic ulcers associated with diarrhoea or steatorrhoea, or patients with excessive gastric secretion coexisting with peptic ulcer.

Diagnosis

The diagnosis is made by demonstrating hypersecretion of gastric acid and hypergastrinaemia. A spontaneous gastric acid secretion of 20 mmol/hour is almost diagnostic and levels of 10 mmol/hour are suspicious. The diagnosis is confirmed by demonstration of a fasting plasma gastrin level of more than 300 pmol/l. A number of other conditions are associated with elevated gastrin concentrations including retained gastric antrum,

antral G-cell hyperplasia, chronic renal failure and pernicious anaemia. Hypergastrinaemia may be present following vagotomy and in patients receiving H_2-antagonist drugs.

Treatment

The tumour. If appropriate, attempts should be made to localise the tumour. Techniques used include duodenoscopy and ERCP, ultrasound scanning with aspiration cytology, computerised tomography and laparoscopy; these are rarely successful and selective angiography is more useful, locating tumours of 6 mm diameter. Percutaneous transhepatic venous catheterisation may be required together with coeliac axis catheterisation – measurement of peptide concentration gradients will demonstrate the exact site or sites of the tumour. If the primary tumour can be located, metastasis excluded, and the patient is otherwise fit, then it should be resected. Blind resections do not often abolish the hypergastrinaemia because of multiple primary tumour sites; total pancreatectomy is not warranted. Depending on the localisation of the tumour or tumours, a Whipple's operation or local resection may be performed. If the condition coexists with a parathyroid adenoma this should be removed first. A reduction in serum calcium to normal levels often leads to a fall in serum gastrin and clinical remission of ulcer symptoms and diarrhoea. If there is evidence of metastatic disease, cytotoxic treatment with streptozotocin may induce remission in some patients; its use is limited by renal, haemotological and hepatic toxicity. Other approaches in patients with massive liver deposits include hepatic artery ligation and selective hepatic arterial embolisation.

Gastric hypersecretion. Management of ZES has been revolutionised by H_2-receptor antagonist drugs. Continuous therapy with cimetidine can produce prolonged clinical remissions. Some patients respond initially to conventional dosage but many require up to 3 g daily. Careful clinical surveillance with gastric acid measurement and periodic endoscopy will indicate the need to increase dosage. The large doses required frequently cause gynaecomastia in men. A few patients escape control despite large doses but can usually be controlled by changing to ranitidine or addition of pirenzepine. There have also been reports of prolonged remissions with a combination of vagotomy and H_2-antagonist therapy. Omeprazole, a proton-pump inhibitor which produces more complete suppression of gastric acid secretion, is currently under trial, and may become the medical treatment of choice in this condition. In patients with fulminant ulcer disease or those not controlled by conservative measures, total gastrectomy should be performed.

VIPoma

The syndrome of watery diarrhoea, hypokalaemia and achlorhydria (WDHA) associated with pancreatic tumours was described by Verner and Morrison in 1958. It was shown subsequently to be associated with hypersecretion of vasoactive intestinal polypeptide (VIP) and is now variously known as VIPoma, WDHA or Verner-Morrison syndrome. The disease is sometimes referred to as 'pancreatic cholera' but 20% of cases are due to extra pancreatic VIP secreting tumours of neural crest origin: ganglioneuromas and ganglioneuroblastomas. These patients are usually children. Fifty to sixty per cent of the pancreatic tumours are malignant, whereas most of the neural crest ones are benign. A few patients with apparently typical features of VIPoma have normal VIP levels. Some of these have other endocrine tumours, e.g. calcitonin-producing medullary carcinoma of the thyroid, carcinoid tumours and carcinoma of the lung. Some have no other obvious pathology and have been described as having 'pseudo-Verner-Morrison syndrome'. The pathogenesis of this syndrome is unknown, although some patients have generalised pancreatic endocrine cell hyperplasia and in others excess ingestion of laxatives and diuretics may be a factor.

Clinical features

Symptoms which have been described in the Verner-Morrison syndrome are:

1. Watery diarrhoea (up to 6 litres per day)
2. Hypokalaemia and metabolic acidosis
3. Achlorhydria or hypochlorhydria
4. Flushing of skin
5. Weight loss
6. Impaired glucose tolerance
7. Hypercalcaemia
8. Tetany (hypomagnesaemia)
9. Biliary disturbance (large gall-bladder with dilute bicarbonate-rich bile)

The most profound symptom is that of profuse water diarrhoea, often occurring in explosive bursts without much associated colic. The stool, which can average 6 l daily, contains little fat, much bicarbonate and has a high potassium concentration, so that patients rapidly become dehydrated, hypokalaemic and acidotic.

Diagnosis

The diagnosis in a patient with watery diarrhoea and hypokalaemia is supported by demonstration of achlorhydria, or by absence of gastric hypersecretion. The presence of hypercalcaemia and/or hyperglycaemia is suggestive. The diagnosis is confirmed by finding a high plasma VIP, always in excess of 60 pmol/l. The tumour is localised using similar techniques to those described for gastrinomas. CT scanning plays a more important role in the diagnosis of neural tumours as a source of VIP secretion.

The carcinoid syndrome

In comparison with the other gut and pancreatic tumours described in this chapter, carcinoid tumours are relatively common, comprising 0.5-1% of all gastrointestinal tumours; only a few (5%) are associated with the typical carcinoid syndrome consisting variously of flushing, diarrhoea, heart lesions and asthma. The majority of tumours associated with the carcinoid syndrome are derived from argentaffin cells of the mid-gut intestinal epithelium, giving rise to appendiceal and ileal tumours. Tumours of the hindgut (colon and rectum) are less common and rarely produce the carcinoid syndrome. Tumours of the foregut (bronchus, pancreas, stomach, duodenum and biliary tract) are rare and often associated with atypical syndromes. Carcinoid tumours produce a number of biologically active compounds, each of

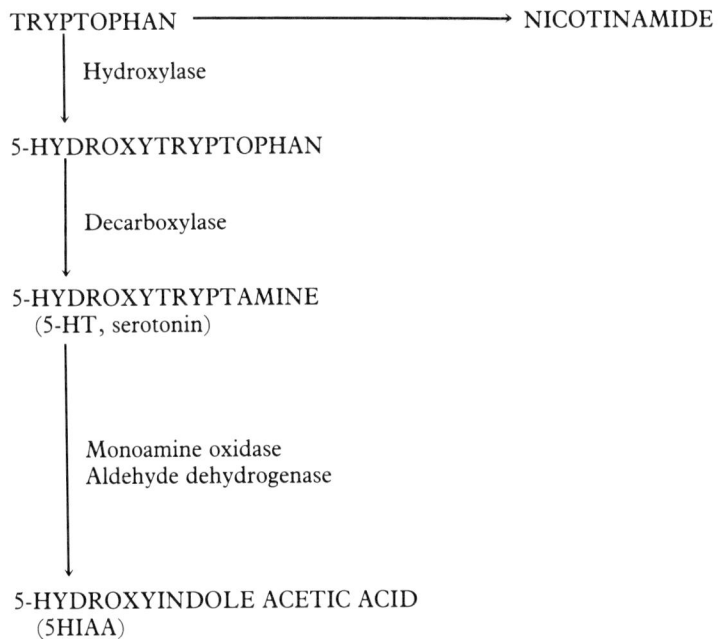

Fig. 8.1 Synthesis and metabolism of 5-hydroxytryptamine.

which may be responsible for specific features of the syndrome. 5-Hydroxytryptamine (5HT, serotonin) may contribute to both diarrhoea and cardiac lesions. The synthesis of large quantities of 5HT diverts dietary tryptophan from production of nicotinamide (Fig. 8.1) and may result in pellagra-like skin lesions. Prostaglandins may also contribute to diarrhoea and facial flushing. A variety of other peptides associated with the tumours have been identified. Bradykinin is liberated from a plasma kininogen by excess kallikrein and contributes to flushing, asthma and perhaps also diarrhoea. The role of motilin and substance P produced by carcinoid tumours is less certain.

Clinical features

The clinical features are:

1. Flushing
2. Diarrhoea
3. Heart lesions
   a. right sided (mid-gut)
   b. left sided (bronchial)
4. Asthma
5. Rare
   a. skin lesions
   b. peptic ulcer
   c. arthralgia.

Attacks of flushing are usually spontaneous but may be induced by alcohol, meals or emotion. The area affected is usually confined to the head and neck. Eventually, permanent telangiectasia are seen and pellagra-like or sclerodermatous skin lesions may develop. Diarrhoea is usually watery, although some patients have intermittent steatorrhoea. In classical carcinoid syndrome right sided heart lesions, either pulmonary stenosis or tricuspid incompetence occur in over half of affected patients. In the rare bronchial carcinoid, or if there is a right to left intracardiac shunt, left-sided heart lesions occur. Asthma is uncommon; peptic ulcer and arthralgia are rare, but definite, associations with carcinoid syndrome. Gastrointestinal carcinoids in the portal vein drainage territory produce carcinoid syndrome only after metastasis to the liver. Tumours may also present with local symptoms; ileal tumours may cause intussusception, obstruction or rarely bleeding. Appendiceal carcinoids may be found in patients with otherwise typical appendicitis.

Diagnosis

The diagnosis of carcinoid syndrome is confirmed by finding excess 5-hydroxyindole acetic acid (5HIAA) (Fig. 8.1) in a 24-hour urine collection. Since excretion of 5HIAA is variable the diagnosis can be excluded only after three urine collections. Chlorpromazine and its metabolites may produce false negative results while ingestion of bananas, pineapples and other fruits give false positive results. It is likely that estimation of specific plasma peptides may replace urinary 5HIAA estimation and allow detection of tumours before metastasis.

Treatment

The tumour. Resection of a bronchial carcinoid is often curative. In other carcinoids, presence of the syndrome implies metastasis, but nevertheless debulking procedures produce useful remission of symptoms. If the tumour is localised to one lobe of the liver, hemihepatectomy is performed. In other cases, enucleation of large metastases can be helpful. Where disease is more widespread, hepatic artery ligation or selective hepatic artery embolisation can produce prolonged remissions. Cytotoxic therapy is less useful than in other gastrointestinal endocrine tumours.

The syndrome. Various features of the syndrome may respond to drugs directed at the effects of one or other of the biologically active compounds. 5-hydroxytryptamine antagonists, including methysergide and cyproheptadine, are often effective in controlling diarrhoea. Likewise parachlorophenylalanine, which inhibits the hydroxylation of tryptophan to 5-hydroxytryptophan, a precursor of 5-HT (Fig. 8.1), may control diarrhoea. Flushing is more difficult to control. Short-term control has been reported with α-adrenergic blockade with phenoxybenzamine, probably because it prevents the release of kallikrein in response to circulating catecholamines. A combination of histamine H_1 and H_2 receptor antagonists may control severe flushing. Other drugs used to control flushing include chlorpromazine, prochlorperazine and steroids. Oral nicotinamide should be given to any patient with skin lesions.

Glucagonoma

A rare syndrome in which glucagon producing tumours of the pancreas are associated with a peculiar skin rash was recognised by Mallinson in 1974. Other clinical features of this syndrome are:

1. Skin rash – necrolytic, migratory erythema
2. Glossitis and angular stomatitis
3. Diabetes mellitus
4. Anaemia
5. Severe wasting
6. Psychiatric disturbances.

The skin rash (Fig. 8.2) is usually the diagnostic hallmark and consists of a bullous dermatosis affecting particularly the groin, perineum, buttocks, distal extremities and central face. Healing takes place with characteristic hyperpigmentation. The rash is often painful and characteristically the histology shows necrolysis of the upper epidermis. Since many of the clinical features are apparent only at a late stage, many patients also have symptoms due to the tumour itself.

Diagnosis depends on the demonstration of hyperglucagonaemia and hypoaminoacidaemia. The plasma glucagon is at least five times higher than the normal fasting concentration and therefore above the level seen in severely ill, metabolically stressed patients. The hypoaminoacidaemia is believed to reflect increased hepatic gluconeogenesis induced by glucagon. Diagnosis is almost always achieved at a late stage in the syndrome since early tumours do not produce specific clinical symptoms.

The rash of glucagonoma often responds to oral zinc therapy. Over half of glucagonomas have metastasised at the time of diagnosis, but since clinical features are related to elevated hormone concentrations, reduction of tumour bulk is advisable. Surgical resection, partial hepatic resection of secondaries, hepatic artery ligation or embolisation

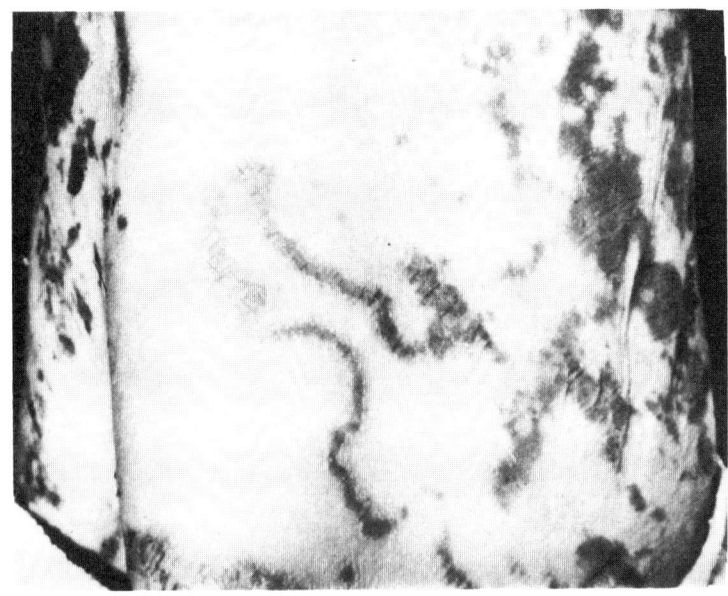

Fig. 8.2   Skin rash characteristic of glucagonoma (by courtesy of Professor S Bloom).

have all produced remissions. Cytotoxics are usually unhelpful but occasional responses to streptozotocin have been reported.

Somatostatinoma

Many pancreatic tumours have been shown to contain somatostatin-staining cells. Recently a number of patients have been described with high circulating levels of tumour-secreted somatostatin, but no typical clinical picture of excess hormone secretion has emerged. A common association is impaired glucose tolerance; other features include malabsorption, hypochlorhydria, flushing and gallstones. Many of the tumours are mixed or associated with pancreatic polypeptide cell hyperplasia and secretion of other peptides may affect the clinical picture. The diagnosis depends on finding elevated fasting somatostatin levels and resection of the tumour should be attempted.

Insulinoma and the investigation of hypoglycaemia

Insulinomas were the first pancreatic hormone secreting tumours to be recognised, largely because of the profound consequences of excess secretion of insulin. Most tumours are small, half being 1 cm or less in diameter. In 13% of cases they are multiple and multiple tumours may be associated with the multiple endocrine adenomatosis (MEA) type I syndrome. The diagnosis is suspected in patients with symptoms which may be due to hypoglycaemia. Symptoms may be neurological — bizarre behaviour, poor concentration, incoordination, diplopia, slurred speech, tingling around the mouth, transient loss of consciousness, fits or even coma, or adrenergic symptoms due to adrenaline release in response to hypoglycaemia may predominate — sweating, tremor, palpitations, tachycardia and pallor. If any of these symptoms coincide with demonstrated hypoglycaemia, then the diagnosis of insulinoma should be considered. Other causes of hypoglycaemia need to be excluded (Table 8.3). A scheme for the investigation of hypoglycaemia is outlined in Figure 8.3.

Diagnosis

The diagnosis of insulinoma is made by demonstrating a low plasma glucose concentration in association with an inappropriately high plasma insulin. The majority of insulinomas may be diag-

Table 8.3 Causes of hypoglycaemia

Reactive (post-prandial) hypoglycaemia	Fasting hypoglycaemia

Gastrointestinal causes:
   gastrectomy
   gastrojejunostomy
Early diabetes mellitus
Galactosaemia (childhood)
Fructose intolerance (childhood)
Idiopathic reactive hypoglyaemia
	Insulinoma
	Alcoholism
	Hypopituitarism
	Addison's disease
	Liver failure
	Factitious hypoglycaemia
	   self-administration of insulin
	   self-administration of sulphonylureas
	Extrapancreatic sarcomas
	Neonatal islet cell hyperplasia
	   (nesidioblastosis)

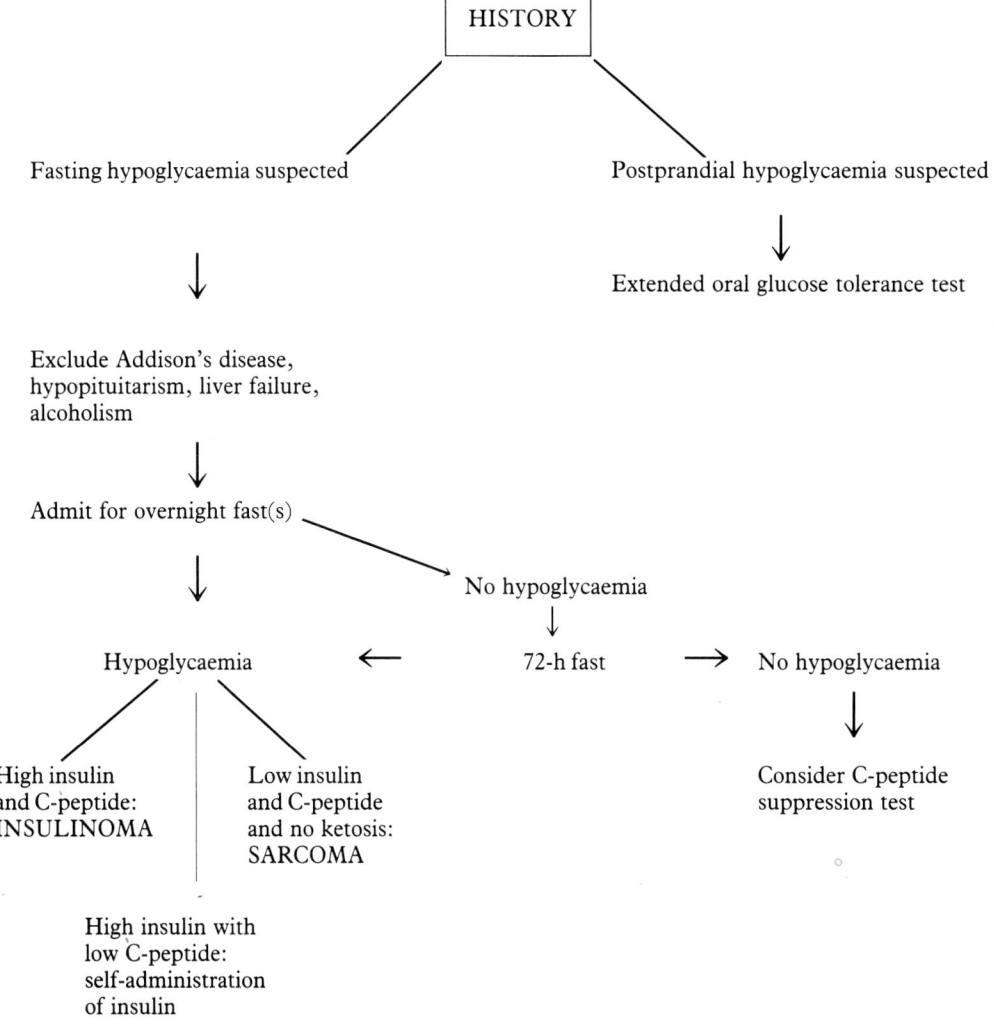

Fig. 8.3 Investigation of hypoglycaemia.

nosed by measurement of glucose and insulin levels after overnight fasts performed on three occasions. The diagnostic yield is increased by extending the fast to 72 hours. A glucose level should be checked at the end of the fast and whenever the patient has symptoms suggestive of hypoglycaemia; a simultaneous sample for measurement of plasma insulin should be taken and insulin concentration measured if the blood glucose level proves to be less than 2 mmol/l. In normal subjects a plasma glucose of less than 2 mmol/l is associated with suppression of insulin secretion and a plasma insulin level of 1.5 mu/l or less. In patients with insulinoma, insulin secretion is not suppressed by hypoglycaemia and plasma levels of 5-40 mu/l are found. In the diagnosis is not established by fasting or biochemical findings are equivocal, and clinical suspicion remains, then a C-peptide suppression test may be performed. Purified insulin is administered to induce hypoglycaemia and plasma C-peptide concentration measured by radioimmunoassay. In normal subjects, C-peptide secretion is suppressed by hypoglycaemia, but it remains elevated in insulinoma.

Tumour localisation

Since insulinomas are usually very small at pres-entation, most of the conventional investigations are valueless in locating the tumour. In expert hands selective pancreatic angiography will localise 60–80% of tumours. More consistent success is obtained by selective transhepatic venous blood sampling from the portal vein and its tributaries, the site of tumour being indicated by a sudden step-up in hormone concentration. In many cases localisation is achieved only at laparotomy.

Treatment

If the tumour is localised, surgical removal is successful in 90% of cases. If the tumour cannot be localised either preoperatively or at laparotomy some advocate blind distal pancreatectomy but this will miss two out of three of tumours. In these cases, or in patients with non-resectable tumours, medical treatment consistant of frequent high car-bohydrate meals and diazoxide (100–600 mg daily) should be tried. Malignant insulinomas are rare and difficult to treat. Streptozotocin will induce biochemical remission in 60–70%, allowing reduc-tion in diazoxide dosage. Long-acting analogues of somatostatin have been shown to suppress insulin release for 24 hours and may prove useful in some cases.

Ectopic hormones and multiple endocrine adenomatosis

INTRODUCTION

Endocrine syndromes may arise in association with neoplasms of organs or tissues that are not generally recognised as the normal site of production of that hormone. A tumour may produce a fully active hormone, a partially active or inactive precursor, or a hormone that is a stimulatory or inhibitory factor for the normal endocrine gland. Many more ectopic hormones are now recognised because specific assays can identify ectopic hormone production in the absence of clinical features.

Mechanisms of ectopic hormone production

There are several mechanisms whereby tumours may synthesise and secrete ectopic hormones. In some instances it may represent enhanced basal capacity already existing in that tissue. Another possibility is that many of the tumours producing ectopic hormone are derived from APUD (amine precursor uptake and decarboxylation) cells:

1. Hypothalamic endocrine cells
2. Pineal cells
3. Pituitary corticotrophic cells
4. Thyroid C cells
5. Argyrophil cells of lung, thymus, urogenital tract
6. Enterochromaffin cells
7. Adrenomedullary cells.

The capacity of apparently different tissues to produce the same peptide hormones may be due to derivation of the tissues from the same common embryological precursor. The APUD cells were thought to be derived from the neural crest but are now thought to be derived from neuroectoderm of epiblast. An alternative theory is that the APUD phenomenon does not mean that cells are of common ectodermal origin but that dedifferentiation has occurred; this may occur in tissue of any embryological origin. It is of interest that certain histological cell types appear to be related to specific endocrine function. This has been best documented in lung cancer, where abnormal adrenal function and inappropriate secretion of vasopressin are found in oat cell but rarely squamous tumours.

Humoral hypercalcaemia, on the other hand, occurs almost entirely in squamous tumours and is rarely, if ever, seen in small cell or large cell tumours or in adenocarcinomas. 'Big' adrenocorticotrophic hormone (ACTH) and beta-lipotrophin, calcitonin and beta-human chorionic gonadotrophin (HCG) are found in the plasma of a considerable proportion of patients with all histological types of lung cancer. Another interesting feature of tumours of APUD cell type is that several hormones are often produced.

Evidence for ectotopic hormone production

The presence of a clinical syndrome or abnormal circulating level of a hormone or metabolite in a patient with malignancy is suggestive of ectopic hormone production if one or more of the following

features can also be shown:

1. Disppearance or remission of syndrome following treatment of the tumour.
2. Recurrence when tumour recurs or metastases occur.
3. Higher concentration of hormone in tumour extracts in comparison with adjacent normal tissue.
4. Arterial-venous differences in hormone concentration across the tumour.
5. Biosynthesis of hormone either from tumour when cultured in vitro or from cell extracts

One of the pitfalls in the diagnosis of ectopic hormone production is recognising when a patient with a tumour has a coexisting endocrine disorder that is aetiologically quite separate.

Clinical importance

The initial diagnosis of a tumour may be made because of ectopic hormone secretion and indeed the hormonal effects may, on occasion, be a more immediate threat to the patient than the tumour itself. Another clinically important feature of ectopic hormone production is as a tumour marker in assessing the effects of therapy.

Individual hormones

ACTH-related peptides

Ectopic ACTH production is one of the more commonly recognised ectopic hormone syndromes. It has been associated with a wide range of tumours (Table 9.1).

Table 9.1 Ectopic ACTH-LPH producing tumours

Relatively common		Rare
Oat cell lung	(60%)	Carcinoid
Thymus	(15%)	Ovary
Pancreatic islets	(10%)	Phaeochromocytoma
		Prostate
		Parotid
		Medullary carcinoma thyroid
		Gastrointestinal tract

A few ACTH-producing tumours, such as squamous cell carcinoma or adenocarcinoma, are not APUD tumours. Many ACTH-producing tumours also secrete beta-lipotrophin, which is part of the common precursor molecule (Fig. 9.1).

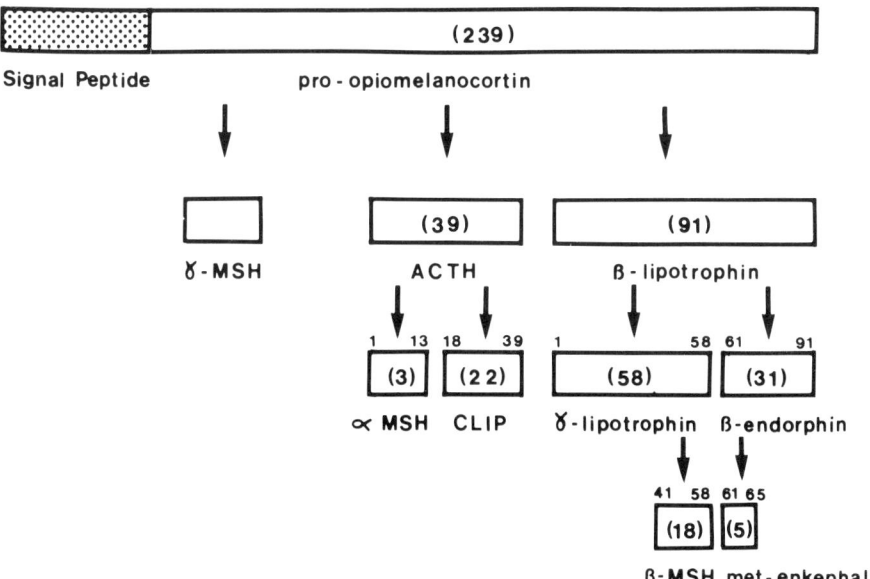

Fig. 9.1 Various peptides biosynthetically related to adrenocorticotrophic hormone (ACTH). CLIP is corticotrophin-like intermediate lobe peptide and MSH melanocyte stimulating hormone. The figures in parentheses refer to the number of amino acid residues in the peptides.

Beta-lipotrophin may be split further into gamma-lipotrophin and beta-endorphin. ACTH itself may be converted into alpha-MSH and corticotrophin-like intermediate lobe peptide (CLIP).

Clinical features.   The clinical features of Cushing's syndrome due to ectopic ACTH production often differ from the features of Cushing's disease (Ch. 5). Ectopic ACTH production from a clinically obvious tumour such as a bronchial carcinoma, results in weight loss, muscle weakness, hyperpigmentation, hypertension and peripheral oedema; weight gain and obesity are rare. The clinical features of ectopic ACTH production from a benign tumour such as a carcinoid tumour are often indistinguishable from Cushing's disease.

Investigations.   Profound hypokalaemic alkalosis may be present and plasma cortisol and ACTH levels are usually markedly elevated. However, the range of plasma ACTH levels overlaps with that found in pituitary dependent Cushing's disease. Within this overlap, ectopic ACTH production is usually from benign rather than malignant tumours. In theory, metyrapone and dexamethasone are without effect in ectopic ACTH secretion, but a partial response is found occasionally, perhaps because some tumours secrete corticotrophin releasing factor or have glucocorticoid receptors. These tests are, therefore, not reliable in the differentiation of ectopic ACTH production from pituitary-dependent Cushing's disease.

Treatment.   The tumour should be removed if possible. Medical treatment includes potassium replacement, and adrenocortical blocking drugs such as metyrapone and aminoglutethimide.

Arginine vasopressin (AVP)

Most of the ectopic AVP-producing tumours are thought to be derived from APUD cells and the vast majority are oat cell and small cell undifferentiated bronchial carcinomas. A few other tumours have been described in association with ectopic AVP secretion – other bronchial carcinomas and carcinoma of thymus, bladder, prostate and pancreas. In some tumours, ectopic production of AVP has been shown to be associated with production of neurophysin and oxytocin.

Clinical features.   Ectopic AVP produces a syndrome of nausea, vomiting, headaches, anorexia, confusion, fits and coma (Ch.3).

Investigations.   Hyponatraemia with increased urinary sodium excretion is found, resulting in urine osmolality being higher than serum. Renal function is normal.

It should be appreciated that there are no methods for differentiating ectopic AVP secretion from excessive AVP production by the hypothalamus and posterior pituitary and so the existence of an inappropriate antidiuresis syndrome in a patient with a tumour does not always indicate ectopic AVP production.

Treatment.   The tumour should be removed if possible. Medical treatment includes restriction of water intake to less than 1 litre per day and the use of demeclocycline for blocking the renal tubular effect of AVP (Ch. 3).

Gonadotrophins

The gonadotrophin produced by tumours is similar or identical to human chorionic gonadotrophin (HCG). Individual alpha and beta subunits may also be produced. Ectopic production of pituitary gonadotrophins does not occur. The term ectopic HCG-producing tumour should be reserved for those tumours derived from non-trophoblastic tissues (Table 9.2); this definition would exclude

Table 9.2   Ectopic HCG-producing tumours

Relatively common	Rare
Bronchial carcinoma	Carcinoma of: stomach,
Hepatoblastoma	kidney, oesophagus, ovary,
Renal cell carcinoma	bladder, pancreas, uterus,
Adrenal carcinoma	pancreatic islet
	Melanoma

trophoblastic tumours and teratomas containing trophoblastic cells, but would include tumours, such as primary adenocarcinomas, showing some differentiation into trophoblastic elements. It should be appreciated that HCG-like material has been found in normal liver and colon so that HCG-producing tumours arising from these organs may not be strictly ectopic HCG-producing tumours.

Clinical features.   HCG causes precocious puberty in boys and gynaecomastia in adult men. Excess HCG does not usually cause any symptoms

in women apart from irregular uterine bleeding in some patients.

Investigations. Elevated plasma levels of HCG may result in apparently elevated levels of LH because in some radioimmunoassay systems HCG will crossreact with anit-LH antisera. Plasma levels of FSH are low and, following injection of gonadotrophin-releasing hormone, there is usually no change in LH or FSH levels. Plasma oestradiol is usually elevated and plasma testosterone normal. Specific beta subunit measurements may be useful as a tumour marker, but alpha subunit measurements are less helpful because alpha subunits may be released by the normal pituitary gland.

Growth hormone

The association of acromegaly and bronchial carcinoid tumours may be due to the ectopic secretion of either growth hormone or growth hormone releasing factor by the tumour. A growth hormone releasing polypeptide and growth hormone have also been isolated from pancreatic tumours causing acromegaly.

Placental lactogen

Abnormal levels of placental lactogen have been found in patients with non-trophoblastic tumours including bronchial carcinomas, hepatoma, lymphoma, gastric and thyroid carcinomas and phaeochromocytoma. Gynaecomastia is rare unless oestrogen is also produced which may be due to coincident ectopic production of HCG.

Calcitonin

Ectopic calcitonin production is a common finding when looked for in APUD tumours and may also be found in other carcinomas of lung, breast and pancreas. Ectopic calcitonin production does not give rise to any clinical features.

Other hormones

Several hormones are rarely produced ectopically:

1. Insulin
2. Glucagon
3. Parathyroid hormone
4. Prolactin
5. Follicle-stimulating hormone
6. Luteinising hormone
7. Thyrotrophin.

MULTIPLE ENDOCRINE ADENOMATOSIS

In multiple endocrine adenomatosis benign or malignant tumours occur in various endocrine organs. The disorders are familial, being inherited as an autosomal dominant, and the clinical features in any one family tend to be similar. Some examples are new mutations. A basic classification is given in Table 9.3.

Table 9.3 Multiple endocrine adenomatosis

Basic classification	
Type I (Werner's syndrome)	Type II (Sipple's syndrome)
Tumours or hyperplasia of:	
Parathyroid	Thyroid C cells
Pancreatic endocrine cells	Adrenal medulla
Anterior pituitary	Parathyroid

Pathogenesis

Several hypotheses have been advanced to explain the association of these abnormalities. It could be that there is a genetic abnormality in all cells. Alternatively a tumorigenic factor could be incorporated into a cell population such as the APUD cells. This theory would not account for all tumours, some of which do not contain APUD cells. It is also possible that overproduction of hormone from one adenoma causes secondary changes in other endocrine glands. No linkage with genetic or chromosome markers has been discovered and no chromosomal abnormality reported apart from increase of chromosomal breakage in culture.

Pathologically there appears to be a continuous spectrum from hyperplasia to adenoma to carcinoma. Another characteristic pathological feature is that lesions are often multicentric.

MEA type I

A family history of tumour or hyperplasia of two or more of the endocrine glands noted in Table

Table 9.4 MEA type I

Tumour or hyperplasia	Hormones secreted
Parathyroid Pancreatic endocrine cells	Parathyroid hormone Gastrin Insulin Vasoactive intestinal polypeptide Glucagon Calcitonin Pancreatic polypeptide
Pituitary	Growth hormone Prolactin Adrenocorticotrophin Non-functioning

9.4 is found. A fifth of patients have tumours of three or more systems. The secretion of parathyroid hormone, gastrin, insulin and growth hormone are the most important from the clinical point of view.

Parathyroid glands

Chief cell hyperplasia is the most frequently encountered pathology, but single or multiple adenomas may be found. Tumours are usually benign though new adenomas may arise in normal glands left after the removal of an adenoma.

Pancreas

A proportion of these tumours may be malignant. Multiple tumours are characteristic.

Clinical features

Common presenting features are peptic ulceration, hypoglycaemia, hypercalcaemia and pituitary disease. Tumours may occur at any age but are rare in childhood and over 60 years of age. There may be no time interval, or months, or years between the discovery of one adenoma and the appearance of the next. The clinical features of the individual lesion of MEA I are not usually different from that observed in a sporadic non-familial case. The important point is to have a clinical awareness that a second or third gland may be involved if there is a typical family history of MEA I, or even in the absence of a family history if two or more adenomas have occurred. The proportion of individual tumours that belong to MEA I varies in different series but approximately 5% of patients with insulinomas, 15% of primary hyperparathyroidism and 25% of patients with gastrinomas belong to the MEA syndrome.

Management

Although hypercalcaemia in MEA I is commonly due to primary hyperparathyroidism, it is not necessarily so. The hypercalcaemia may be due to a pancreatic tumour, especially the VIP watery diarrhoea hypokalaemic achlorhydria syndrome (Ch. 8).

At parathyroid surgery it is recommended that all four parathyroid glands are identified. When multiple gland disease is found, as suggested by the combined weight of two glands in excess of 100 mg, three and a half glands should be excised and a marker left near to the remaining half gland. Alternatively all four glands should be removed and parathyroid tissue implanted at an easily accessible site.

It should be noted that peptic ulcer disease occurs in 10–30% of patients with isolated primary hyperparathyroidism and needs to be distinguished from Zollinger-Ellison syndrome. The management of gastrinoma is detailed in chapter 8 but includes total gastrectomy and H2-histamine receptor blockade. Streptozotocin may be considered for malignant tumours of the pancreas.

Once the diagnosis of MEA I is made both patients and first-degree relatives should be screened every 1–2 years by the following methods:
1. History
2. Serum calcium
3. Fasting blood glucose
4. Serum gastrin.

MEA type IIa

A family history or tumours or hyperplasia of two or more of the endocrine glands noted in Table 9.5 are found. The subtype MEA IIb (or type

Table 9.5 MEA type IIa

Hyperplasia or tumour	Hormones secreted
Thyroid C cells	Calcitonin (ACTH, serotonin, VIP occasionally)
Adrenal medulla	Catecholamines
Parathyroid	Parathyroid hormone

III in some classifications) is distinguished by the addition of a variety of neurological abnormalities, by the relative rarity of overt parathyroid disease and the poor prognosis.

Medullary thyroid carcinoma

Thyroid C-cell hyperplasia may precede the development of frank malignancy by many years. The hyperplasia is bilateral. Similarly tumours are characteristically multicentric, composed of pleomorphic cells surrounded by amyloid (Ch. 4). The tumour is part of MEA type II in 20% of all patients with medullary thyroid carcinoma. Putting it the other way round, it is true to say that the majority of medullary carcinoma of the thyroid occurs sporadically.

Familial medullary thyroid carcinoma should be suspected if the carcinoma is bilateral, if there are multiple sites of C-cell hyperplasia, or if there is coexisting phaeochromocytoma, hyperparathyroidism or mucosal neuromas.

Phaeochromocytoma

A spectrum of pathology is found ranging from diffuse or nodular hyperplasia of the adrenal medulla to large multicentric phaeochromocytoma. Accessory adrenal glands may be involved and extra-adrenal paraganglioma are not uncommon. Both benign and malignant phaeochromocytomas penetrate the capsule, invade adjacent veins and have a pleomorphic appearance with mitoses. Metastases usually occur within 10 years and should be determined by the evidence of distant spread or invasion of adjacent soft tissue, lymph nodes or other organs. The spectrum of pathology and the absence of symptoms in young people having early disease may explain the differences in the reported incidence of the phaeochromocytoma component of MEA type II which varies from 13–21% in populations detected through medullary thyroid cancer screening programmes, to 50% found clinically in older patients reported in the literature. Only 6% of reported phaeochromocytomas are part of the MEA type II.

Parathyroid

There is evidence of parathyroid disease, usually hyperplasia of the parathyroid glands, in up to half of patients with MEA type IIa but it is only a minority who have clinical symptoms.

Clinical features and investigations

Thyroid. Medullary carcinoma of the thyroid is often the earliest feature to be diagnosed. The most common presentation is an asymptomatic thyroid nodule or multinodular goitre. Cervical lymphadenopathy, hoarseness, or dysphagia may be the first symptom. Occasionally diarrhoea is a prominent symptom which may be due to serotonin, prostaglandins or other peptides produced by the tumour. Thyroid scans are not helpful in early diagnosis but calcification may be seen in the thyroid or in metastases on plain X-ray. Elevated plasma levels of immunoreactive calcitonin are a consistent biochemical marker for the detection of disease or its recurrence. The calcitonin secreted is immunologically heterogeneous; at least five distinct molecular sizes are secreted and decreased biological activity is common. When basal plasma levels of calcitonin are within the normal range stimulation with pentagastrin and calcium gluconate will result in an abnormally high response in patients or relatives with preclinical disease. The following precautions should apply when interpreting plasma calcitonin levels.

1. Elevated plasma levels of calcitonin may be due to ectopic secretion of calcitonin from a variety of neoplasms and is a common finding in APUD tumours.

2. Elevated plasma levels of calcitonin occur in pregnancy and chronic renal failure.

3. False negative stimulation tests may occur and it is suggested that more than one stimulus should be used.

Phaeochromocytomas. These tumours may be clinically silent, with no hypertension, or show all the usual features of catecholamine-secreting tumour. Tumours of the adrenal gland produce both adrenaline and noradrenaline, whereas extraadrenal tumours usually secrete noradrenaline only.

Management

Thyroid. It is important to exclude and treat coexisting phaeochromocytoma first. The treatment of medullary carcinoma is total thyroidectomy with or without a modified neck dissection. Replacement thyroxine is required long term and plasma calcitonin measurements are used for follow-up. The prevalence of residual cancer increases with increasing age; obvious residual tumour should be resected. Radioiodine therapy, external irradiation to the neck and chemotherapy are of no value; radiotherapy may be useful for bone metastases. The overall 10-year survival rate is about 50%.

Adrenal. Bilateral total adrenalectomy and excision of any extra-adrenal paragangliomas is advised followed by maintenance glucocorticoid and mineralocorticoid replacement therapy.

Screening. The screening tests useful for MEA type II are:

1. History and examination
2. Plasma calcitonin
3. Urinary metanephrine excretion.

MEA type IIb (type III). MEA type IIb refers to medullary carcinoma of the thyroid and phaeochromocytoma with characteristic coarse

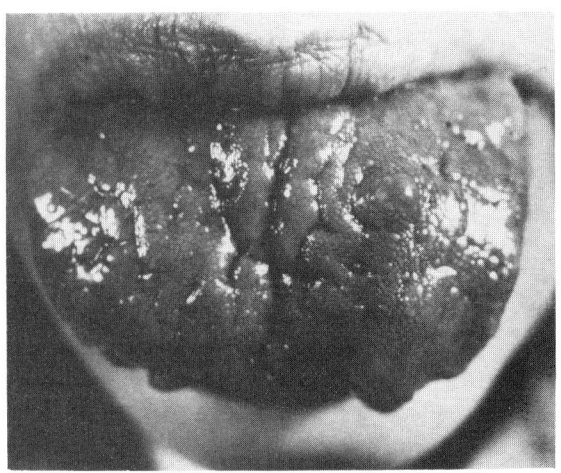

Fig. 9.2 Neuromas in multiple endocrine adenomatosis type IIb (III)

facial features (Fig. 9.2). The lips are patulous and multiple mucosal neuromas are found on the eyelids, lips, tongue and occasionally throughout the gastrointestinal tract. These tumours should be called ganglioneuromas because they contain ganglion cells in addition to tortuous nerve trunks. Though neurofibromatosis may be associated with phaeochromocytoma the cutaneous tumours are different histologially with predominantly fibrous strands. Patients may also have a marfanoid appearance, pectus excavatum, lax joints and kyphoscoliosis, and prominent corneal nerves on slit lamp examination. Hyperparathyroidism is not part of the MEA type IIb syndrome.

Patients with MEA type IIb tend to present with symptoms at an earlier age than MEA type IIa and have a poorer prognosis.

Calcium metabolism

CONTROL OF CALCIUM METABOLISM

During normal health the concentration of calcium in serum is controlled between a very narrow range. This is achieved by regulating the movement of calcium by the intestine, bone and kidney (Fig. 10.1). The bone acts as a large reservoir of calcium containing 97% of the total body calcium with a mere 10 mmol (400 mg) entering

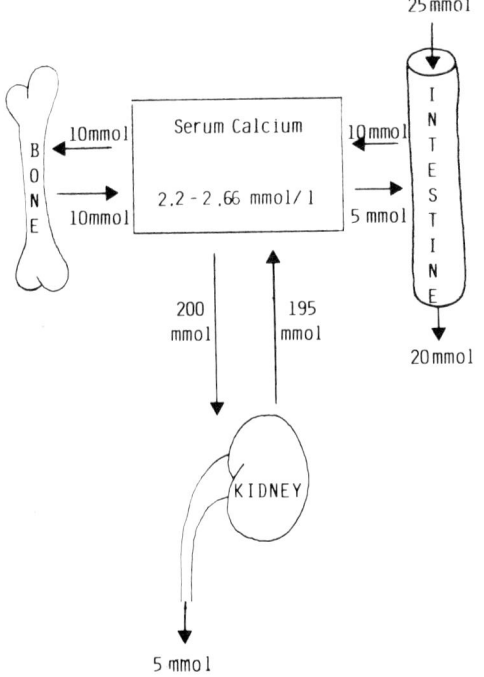

Fig. 10.1 Calcium balance. The largest daily fluxes of calcium occur in the kidney (1 mmol=40 mg).

and leaving the skeleton each day, whereas the kidney filters over 200 mmol (8000 mg) of calcium per day. The kidney is therefore well equipped to deal with minute-to-minute fluctuations in calcium, whereas the bones are likely to be involved in more chronic regulation. Net intestinal absorption amounts to 5 mmol (200 mg) of calcium daily and changes in this are unlikely to affect calcium homeostasis acutely. If, however, long-term calcium losses exceed net calcium absorption the deficit is resorbed from bone, leading eventually to demineralisation.

Two separate but inter-related hormones are involved in the control of calcium metabolism – parathyroid hormone (PTH) and the vitamin D system. Parathyroid hormone is secreted by the parathyroid glands and, like many peptide hormones, is formed first as a larger precursor molecule. Both a prepro-PTH and pro-PTH have been characterised and are cleaved within the parathyroid gland to produce the 84 amino-acid native PTH. This peptide is secreted intact in response to hypocalcaemia. The amino-terminal 34 amino acids contain all the biological activity of the intact molecule, whereas the carboxy-terminal portion is biologically inert. Once in the systemic circulation, PTH is cleaved into a number of fragments, most of which are devoid of biological activity and which have longer half-lives than the active molecule. For this reason, especially in the presence of renal failure, biologically inactive fragments may predominate in the peripheral blood.

PTH exerts its major effects on kidney and bone. Its renal effects are to increase calcium reabsorption and to decrease phosphate reabsorption. Its major

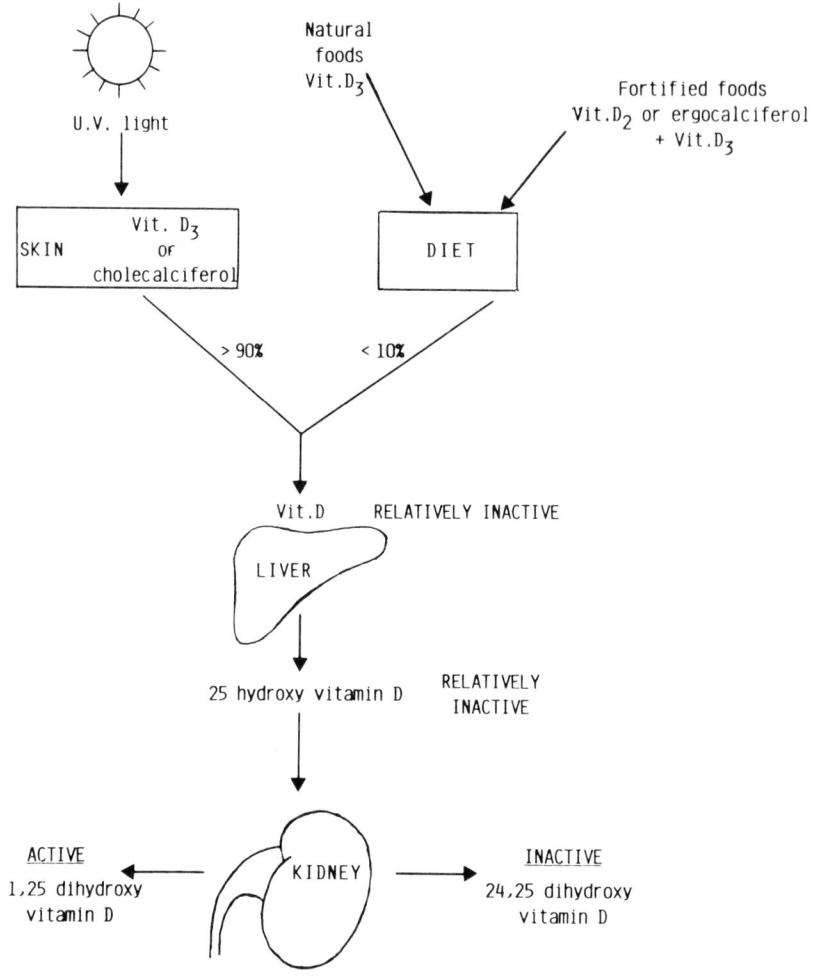

Fig. 10.2 Vitamin D metabolism. The major source of vitamin D is the action of sunlight on the skin.

action on bone is to increase calcium resorption by increasing osteoclastic activity, but it also appears to have anabolic effects and under certain circumstances may cause calcium deposition. The mechanism of PTH action appears to be mediated by a direct effect on osteoblasts, the bone-forming cells rich in alkaline phosphatase enzyme. The stimulated osteoblast results in increased activity of the osteoclast and hence increased bone resorption. In most situations there is a close link between the activity of osteoblasts and osteoclasts so that the change in activity of one cell leads to a similar change in activity of the other cell type. All these actions of PTH are produced by interaction

with PTH receptors in the target tissue leading to stimulation of adenylate cyclase activity.

Vitamin D metabolism is depicted in Figure 10.2. Vitamin D is formed in the skin by the action of ultraviolet light and is also present in the diet. The compound formed in the skin is cholecalciferol or vitamin D_3. The diet includes foods which naturally contain vitamin D_3, together with foods specifically fortified with vitamin D, usually a synthetic compound ergocalciferol [vitamin D_2]. Under normal circumstances, it appears that the skin is the major source of vitamin D with at least 90% being produced there. Both vitamin D_2 and D_3 are handled identically and the term vitamin D will be used for both. The relatively inert vitamin is first hydroxylated in the liver to produce 25-hydroxy vitamin D (25-OH vit D). This hydroxylation increases biological activity slightly but the subsequent renal hydroxylation to produce 1,25 dihydroxy vitamin D (1,25 diOH vit D) results in a very active metabolite. The kidney also has the ability to convert 25-OH vit D to 24,25 dihydroxy vitamin D (24,25 diOH vit D), a compound devoid of activity. Under situations of calcium lack, the kidney preferentially makes the active metabolite 1,25 diOH vit D, the production of which is also stimulated by PTH. When calcium supplies are adequate, 24,25 diOH vit D production is increased and 1,25 diOH vit D synthesis falls. 1,25 diOH vit D acts on the small intestine to increase calcium absorption, a process involving a calcium binding protein present within the intestinal cells. Vitamin D is essential for normal bone formation and its lack results in rickets or osteomalacia. When present in excess, both calciferol and its active metabolites cause increased bone resorption and this explains why hypercalcaemia occurs when these compounds are used in non-physiological doses.

Calcium is present in serum in three forms: ionised, protein-bound and complexed. The complexed form constitutes a very small fraction (1–2%), with calcium complexed to citrate and phosphate. About one half of serum calcium is protein bound, mainly to albumin and to a lesser degree to globulin. For this reason, changes in serum proteins can markedly alter total calcium measurements without any change in ionised calcium concentration, the physiologically important form of the element. During dehydration or prolonged venous stasis serum proteins increase and this may increase total calcium by up to 0.3 mmol/l. Low protein states are common in ill patients, especially hypoalbuminaemia, and this may have profound effects on total calcium concentration. Despite the presence of numerous correction formulae, none makes an accurate correction for protein levels and they are best avoided. Blood for calcium measurement should be taken in the non-fasting state using minimal venous stasis. An associated serum protein measurement is

Table 10.1 Causes of hypercalcaemia

Common
Malignancy
Primary hyperparathyroidism

Less common
Familial benign hypercalcaemia (FBH)
Sarcoidosis
Thyrotoxicosis
Vitamin D poisoning
Acute renal failure

Rare
Immobilisation
VIPomas
Tuberculosis
Milk-alkali syndrome
Addison's disease
Lithium
Thiazide diuretics
Parenteral feeding

---

always advisable.

HYPERCALCAEMIA

Hypercalcaemia has many causes as illustrated in Table 10.1. The vast majority of cases are due either to malignancy or to hyperparathyroidism; these two diagnoses account for approximately 97% of all cases of hypercalcaemia.

Symptoms of hypercalcaemia

The symptoms of hypercalcaemia are unrelated to the cause but are related directly to the severity. They are non-specific and may mimic disorders of many systems. The clinical features are:
1. Tiredness and lethargy
2. Proximal muscle weakness
3. Polyuria, nocturia and thirst
4. Nausea, vomiting and constipation
5. Depression, psychosis and impaired consciousness.

Hypercalcaemia can only be diagnosed biochemically.

Signs of hypercalcaemia

Apart from muscle weakness, usually of a proximal type, signs of hypercalcaemia are infrequent. Band keratopathy is rare except in severe, prolonged hypercalcaemia especially if associated with renal impairment.

Hypercalcaemia of malignancy

Hypercalcaemia is a common complication of malignancy. The incidence varies considerably depending at which stage of the disease hypercalcaemia is looked for. In hospital, carcinoma of the breast and lung account for nearly half of the cases seen, with approximately 5% of cases being complicated by hypercalcaemia. The incidence of hypercalcaemia varies with tumour type; in lung cancer it is more common in squamous cell tumours than in oat cell tumours, unlike ectopic ACTH and inappropriate ADH secretion. Many other tumours can be complicated by hypercalcaemia. Myeloma has the highest prevalence of hypercalcaemia with approximately one-third of cases being hypercalcaemic. When hypercalcaemia complicates malignancy, the malignant process is usually very obvious and almost invariably disseminated. It is unusual for hypercalcaemia to be detected before the diagnosis of malignancy is made. Most patients with malignancy have low serum albumin concentrations, making the severity of the hypercalcaemia more marked than may first appear.

Diagnosis

Diagnosis is usually easy because the malignant process is obvious. No single biochemical test differentiates hypercalcaemia of malignancy from hyperparathyroidism. Measurement of serum albumin is often low in malignancy, but rarely so in hyperparathyroidism. Measurements of serum chloride, bicarbonate, phosphate or urinary indices of phosphate handling are of no value in the individual case because of marked overlap between the two conditions. Serum PTH is rarely increased in malignancy and if clearly so should suggest the simultaneous presence of primary hyperparathyroidism. Ectopic PTH secretion by malignant tumours is thought to be rare and, although many cases of hypercalcaemia probably have a humoral

basis, the humoral agent has not yet been identified.

Treatment

Not all patients with hypercalcaemia of malignancy should be treated, but therapy should be considered if specific treatment is being offered for the malignant state, or if relief of hypercalcaemic symptoms would improve the quality of the patient's life. When severe, hypercalcaemia should be treated initially with intravenous fluids; 6–8 l of fluids are given daily, usually as N-saline and 5% dextrose. Potassium supplements are nearly always necessary as hypokalaemia commonly develops. Careful fluid balance charts need to be kept and diuretics given if any evidence of heart failure develops. Such treatment alone will usually improve the state of the patient, although the serum calcium rarely returns to normal. Alternative parenteral therapies include the use of calcitonin, which does not appear to offer much advantage over fluids alone, or steroids in high dose. Overall, less than 50% of patients with hypercalcaemia of malignancy respond to steroids although higher response rates can be expected in myeloma, Hodgkin's disease and leukaemia. Another effective agent is mithramycin, given in a dose of 20 μg/kg intravenously as a single bolus injection. Recent studies suggest that a variety of intravenous bisphosphonate drugs may also be useful and possibly safer.

Once hypercalcaemia is under control oral therapy is instituted. Oral phosphates are effective in about 80% of cases when given in a dose of 500 mg 6-hourly, but their clinical usefulness is reduced by the high incidence of gastrointestinal disturbances, especially diarrhoea. Oral steroids, starting with prednisolone 20–40 mg daily, are well tolerated and are effective in about 50% of cases. Steroids are probably the treatment of choice, with the dose being reduced in responsive patients to the minimum required for the maintenance of normocalcaemia.

Hyperparathyroidism

The term hyperparathyroidism means overproduction of PTH. Primary hyperparathyroidism is

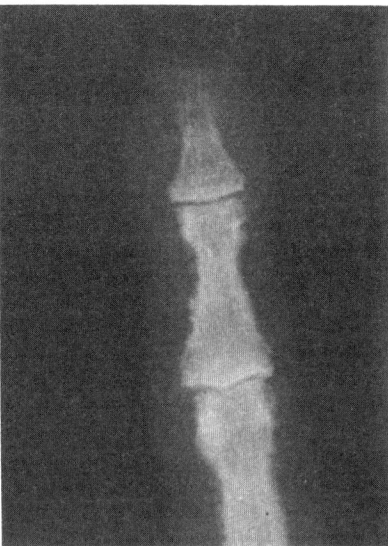

Fig. 10.3 Subperiosteal bone resorption affecting phalanges.

autonomous overproduction, leading to hypercalcaemia. A secondary increase in PTH secretion occurs in hypocalcaemic states, especially in vitamin D deficiency, renal failure and malabsorptive diseases. If hypocalcaemia is persistent, this leads to a secondary hyperparathyroid state. It should be stressed that this is initially a normal physiological response to hypocalcaemia. Occasionally the secondary hyperparathyroid state progresses to an autonomous hyperparathyroid state causing hypercalcaemia – tertiary hyperparathyroidism – seen most frequently in patients with chronic renal failure.

Primary hyperparathyroidism

This condition has been recognised with increasing frequency during the past 20 years, due mainly to the introduction of biochemical screening. As a consequence, the mode of presentation has altered considerably.

Incidence

Surveys in both the UK and USA show 400–500 cases of hyperparathyroidism per million population. The disorder is three times more common in females and increases with age, 90% of cases being aged over 50 years.

Presentation

In the past, presentation with renal stones or bone disease was common. With the advent of biochemical screening cases usually now have only mild, non-specific symptoms, or are asymptomatic.

Diagnosis

The diagnosis of hyperparathyroidism depends upon the demonstration of persistent hypercalcaemia and a high normal or elevated PTH concentration in the blood. Few, if any, other tests are necessary. Measurements of serum phosphate, chloride, bicarbonate and urinary phosphate are of no value. The finding of a low haemoglobin, high ESR, low albumin or high globulin is uncommon in primary hyperparathyroidism and should raise the possibility of another cause of hypercalcaemia. Steroid suppression tests are indicated rarely and should be reserved for cases with unusual features (see below). Failure to suppress on steroids does not prove hyperparathyroidism but complete suppression of the hypercalcaemia makes the diagnosis extremely unlikely. Although X-rays are rarely abnormal in hyperparathyroidism in the absence of chronic renal disease, the presence of subperiosteal resorption on hand X-ray (Fig. 10.3) is diagnostic of hyperparathyroidism. The absence of these changes does not help in diagnosis.

Hyperparathyroidism may be associated with pancreatic islet cell and pituitary tumours (multiple endocrine adenomatosis, type I), or with thyroid medullary carcinoma and phaeochromocytomas (multiple endocrine adenomatosis, type II) (Ch. 9). Although within these syndromes hyperparathyroidism is common, they are so rare that the routine search for other endocrine tumours in cases presenting with apparently uncomplicated hyperparathyroidism is not justified. In familial cases the hyperparathyroidism is usually due to four gland hyperplasia.

Management

The only effective treatment of hyperparathyroidism is surgical removal of the abnormal parathyroid tissue. At present there is no effective medical treatment. The options are therefore long-term conservative management or parathyroidectomy. Many clinicians now offer surgery to all young patients (i.e. below 50 years), irrespective of symptoms, while in older patients surgery is reserved for those with significant complications or symptoms of the disease. Such a policy results in conservative treatment of most elderly patients.

Surgery should be performed only by experienced parathyroid surgeons. Preoperative localisation of the abnormal parathyroid by radioisotope scanning is probably not indicated in patients who have not had previous neck surgery. Experienced surgeons will find the affected gland or glands in over 95% of cases. A single parathyroid adenoma is found in 90% of patients with primary hyperparathyroidism with only 10% of cases having hyperplasia of all four parathyroid glands. The single adenoma (very rarely two adenomas) should be removed and histology confirmed by frozen section. At least one normal parathyroid gland should be identified. When hyperplasia of four parathyroid glands is present, most surgeons remove all four, transplanting fragments of one of the glands to the forearm. Here the gland functions well and, should it become hyperactive in the future, it can

be dealt with simply without recourse to further neck surgery.

Following operation the serum calcium will have fallen to normal values usually within 24 hours. Mild hypocalcaemia may then follow for several days but it is generally asymptomatic. Occasionally, especially when the preoperative calcium is very high or bone disease is present, there may be a phase of more severe postoperative hypocalcaemia and rarely permanent hypoparathyroidism may result.

Familial benign hypercalcaemia (FBH) or familial hypocalciuric hypercalcaemia (FHH)

This familial condition with dominant inheritance has been well documented only recently. It mimics primary hyperparathyroidism biochemically, but parathyroidectomy virtually never results in normocalcaemia even though the parathyroid glands may appear enlarged.

Presentation. Most cases so far diagnosed have come to light after a failed parathyroidectomy for presumed primary hyperparathyroidism. The finding of affected family members has led to the diagnosis. Affected patients have few if any symptoms and the hypercalcaemia is usually an incidental finding.

Diagnosis. Up to one third of cases have elevated PTH concentrations in serum and there is very considerable overlap between urinary calcium measurements in FBH and hyperparathyroidism. The serum magnesium tends to be high normal whereas in hyperparathyroidism it is usually low normal. Although familial hyperparathyroidism may occur, it is extremely unusual for children to be hypercalcaemic, whereas in FBH affected individuals are hypercalcaemic from birth. A logical policy is to consider family screening in all asymptomatic hypercalcaemic patients below the age of 40 who would be referred for parathyroidectomy should a diagnosis of hyperparathyroidism be made.

Management. The purpose of making the diagnosis of FBH is to avoid parathyroidectomy. To date it appears that the condition is benign. Rarely, however, affected neonates may suffer from severe, life-threatening hypercalcaemia which may require a total parathyroidectomy to control the disorder. Fortunately, such cases are extremely uncommon.

Vitamin D poisoning

Large doses of calciferol (i.e. 100 000 units/day or more), or more potent vitamin D metabolites will cause hypercalcaemia if given for long enough. Therefore the use of these compounds requires constant monitoring.

Sarcoidosis

Although hypercalciuria is common in sarcoidosis, hypercalcaemia is rare and often intermittent. It is likely that less than 1–2% of cases of sarcoidosis are complicated by hypercalcaemia.

Presentation. Usually the presentation is that of clinical features of sarcoidosis with routine investigations revealing hypercalcaemia. Occasionally symptoms of hypercalcaemia will be the first presentation of the disease. Hypercalcaemia may be more common after prolonged exposure to sun.

Aetiology. Studies have shown that 1,25 diOH vit D levels are higher than expected during the hypercalcaemia phase, reverting to normal when the patient becomes normocalcaemic. Recent evidence suggests that alveolar macrophages in sarcoidosis have the capacity to produce this active metabolite. As expected, PTH concentrations are not increased.

Diagnosis. Hypercalcaemia due to sarcoidosis is corrected by steroid administration. The failure to respond to steroids or a high PTH concentration suggests concomitant hyperparathyroidism. The patient in whom hypercalcaemia occurs before there is clinical evidence of sarcoidosis is more difficult to diagnose, as there are no specific biochemical changes which differentiate it from other causes of hypercalcaemia. The finding of a persistently low PTH measurement in a hypercalcaemic patient without malignancy should lead to a steroid suppression test. Correction of the hypercalcaemia should raise the possibility of sarcoidosis, providing there be no evidence of vitamin D ingestion. A positive Kveim test or the finding of non-caseating granulomata on liver biopsy may then clinch the diagnosis.

Treatment. Hypercalcaemia complicating sarcoidosis is best treated with corticosteroids, the lowest dose of prednisolone being used to correct the biochemical abnormality. Once control has been achieved the steroids should be withdrawn slowly to see if the hypercalcaemia has remitted.

Thyrotoxicosis

Hypercalcaemia is a rare, but well-recognised, complication of thyrotoxicosis. The thyrotoxicosis is always clinically severe and not readily overlooked. The hypercalcaemia is probably due to increased calcium release from bone and PTH levels are low. The hypercalcaemia may take 4–6 weeks to resolve with antithyroid treatment. Persistent hypercalcaemia usually means concomitant hyperparathyroidism.

Other causes of hypercalcaemia

Many other causes of hypercalcaemia have been reported. They are rare and include the milk-alkali syndrome, VIPomas, phaeochromocytomas, Addison's disease, the recovery phase of acute renal failure and immobilisation. Clinically the associated condition is usually apparent.

An approach to the investigation of a patient with hypercalcaemia

With the knowledge of the causes of hypercalcaemia and their presentation it is possible to put forward a logical method of investigation.

It must be remembered that in 97% of cases either hyperparathyroidism or malignancy will be the cause and that malignancy, if present, will usually be obvious. The initial history and investigations should be directed at looking for evidence of a malignancy and clinical evidence of the rarer forms of hypercalcaemia. Screening procedures that raise the likelihood of malignancy are anaemia, high ESR, low albumin, high globulins and abnormal liver function tests. If malignancy, thyrotoxicosis or vitamin D treatment are not found, the serum PTH concentration should be measured. If elevated or in the high normal range the diagnosis of hyperparathyroidism can be made and no further investigations are required, except in young asymptomatic patients where the possibility of familial benign hypercalcaemia exists. In the few patients who remain undiagnosed, the possibility of an occult neoplasm, or one of the rarer causes of hypercalcaemia becomes more likely. A steroid suppression test is now indicated. Suppression of the calcium into the normal range would favour certain malignancies, sarcoidosis or vitamin D toxicity.

HYPOCALCAEMIA

Hypocalcaemia is a less common biochemical abnormality than hypercalcaemia. Perhaps the commonest cause of low total calcium measurement is a reduction in serum proteins. Unfortunately, no correction formula corrects adequately for protein changes and the errors are particularly marked when the proteins are moderately or severely reduced. The symptoms and signs of hypocalcaemia are illustrated in Table 10.2.

Table 10.2 Clinical features of hypocalcaemia

Symptoms	Signs
Paraesthesiae, especially circumoral and in the peripheries	Chvostek's sign
Tetany	Trousseau's sign
Tiredness	Cataracts
Convulsions	Papilloedema

Renal failure

Both acute and chronic renal failure can cause hypocalcaemia, due in part to phosphate retention and formation of insoluble complexes, and to the inability to produce 1,25 diOH vit D in the kidney. When chronic renal failure develops, the inability to produce adequate amounts of this potent metabolite leads to the development of osteomalacia. Coupled with this, however, is

Table 10.3 Signs and symptoms of renal osteodystrophy

Symptoms	Signs
Tiredness and lethargy	Muscle weakness, especially proximal
Bone pain	
Itching	Bone tenderness and deformity
Muscle weakness and walking difficulties	Soft tissue calcification e.g. corneal
	Bone fracture
	Loss of height due to vertebral compression

hyperparathyroid bone disease due to the secondary hyperparathyroid state that develops in an attempt to correct hypocalcaemia. Both diseases are usually present in chronic renal failure although in any one case, one or other may predominate. The renal osteodystrophy of chronic renal failure causes a variety of symptoms, signs and complications as shown in Table 10.3.

Biochemical changes include a moderately reduced serum calcium, a raised phosphate, a raised alkaline phosphatase, and an increase in serum PTH. Radiological changes include the changes of osteomalacia, with Looser's zones, subperiosteal resorption and bone cysts. The bone may appear more dense than normal and the vertebrae may show dense bands at their upper and lower margins with a translucent mid-zone giving rise to the so called rugger-jersey spine (Fig. 10.4).

Prevention

Assuming that the renal failure is irreversible, attempts to minimise bone disease depend on reducing the high serum phosphorus and giving vitamin D metabolites. By reducing serum phosphorus the incidence of metastatic calcification can be reduced and it is hoped that the degree of hypocalcaemia is also lessened. In the past, the mainstay of such treatment has been the use of drugs to bind phosphate in the gut, especially oral aluminium hydroxide. Recently it has been realised that some aluminium is absorbed and that aluminium toxicity can develop, in turn leading to a severe form of osteomalacia. For

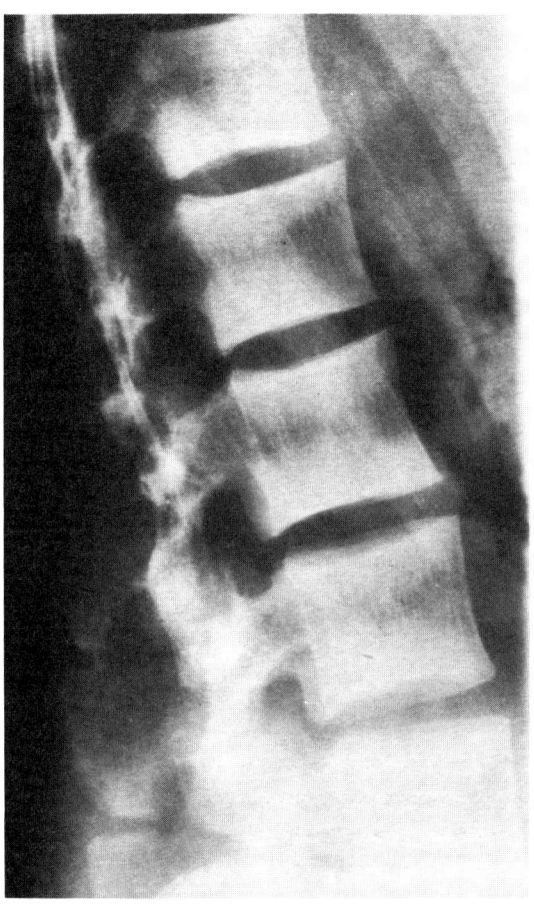

Fig. 10.4 Rugger-jersey spine. (Reproduced with kind permission of Gower Medical Publishing.)

this reason alternative phosphate binders are being sought and calcium carbonate is being evaluated. As the kidney cannot produce 1,25 diOH vit D in chronic renal failure, the bone disease is resistant to calciferol. The use of 1,25 dihydroxy vitamin D (calcitriol), or 1α hydroxycholecalciferol (One-alpha), which is converted in vivo to 1,25 diOH vitamin D, is therefore more appropriate, although it is not yet known whether such therapy will prevent the development of bone disease.

Treatment of established disease

Established bone disease may respond very well to the active vitamin D metabolites and this is especially true when osteitis fibrosa predominates. Failing this, and especially when hypercalcaemia is present, parathyroidectomy may be required.

The presence of severe osteomalacia should raise the possibility of aluminium toxicity which can be diagnosed on bone biopsy.

Vitamin D deficiency

Vitamin D deficiency in children causes rickets and in adults it results in osteomalacia.

Causes

Vitamin D deficiency is most commonly encountered in Britain in the Asian patient at times of increased vitamin D requirement, e.g. childhood, adolescence and the child-bearing years. The explanation of the disorder in Asians is unclear: it cannot be due to simple dietary vitamin D deficiency, as the vast majority of vitamin D in the body results from production in the skin. The disease is seen particularly in vegetarians with a high chapatti intake. The elderly, especially if housebound, frequently have subclinical vitamin D deficiency, but clinical disease appears to be uncommon. Other causes include malabsorptive disorders and chronic cholestatic liver disease.

Symptoms

In children the disease particularly affects the long bones causing pains especially in the knees, which are worse on exercise. Bone deformity may lead to knock knees (genu valgum) or less commonly to bow legs (genu varum). Growth retardation is common. In the adult diffuse bone pain predominates especially affecting the ribs, spine, pelvis and thighs. Difficulty with walking is common. Signs of hypocalcaemia, tetany and convulsions occur rarely in both age groups.

Signs

Bone tenderness and deformity may be present. Chvostek's sign may be positive. Muscle strength is reduced, especially proximally, and the combination of muscle weakness and pelvic pain produces a characteristic waddling gait.

Diagnosis

The biochemical changes of vitamin D deficiency are hypocalcaemia, which is usually mild but occasionally severe, a slightly reduced serum

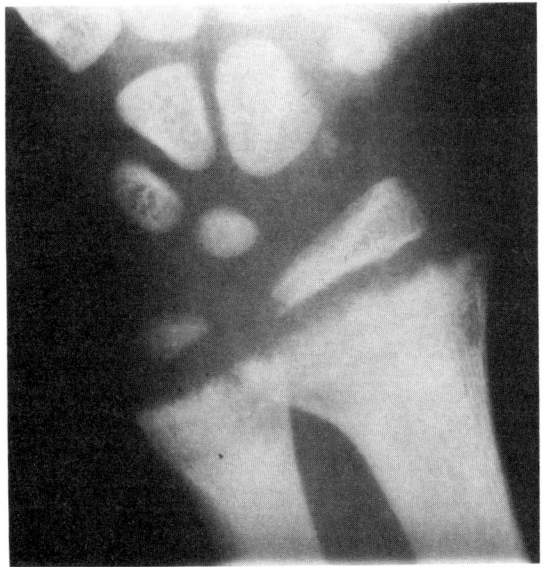

Fig. 10.5 Metaphyseal widening in rickets. (Reproduced with kind permission of Gower Medical Publishing.)

phosphate concentration and an elevated alkaline phosphatase. The serum PTH level is increased but usually need not be measured, while measurements of the vitamin D metabolites are rarely required.

Radiological changes when present are characteristic. In children the ends of the long bones show major changes with metaphyseal widening and irregularity (Fig. 10.5). In adults, Looser's zones or pseudofractures are found, especially in the pelvic rami, femoral necks, ribs and scapulae (Fig. 10.6). Bone biopsy is indicate rarely, but if performed shows marked widening of the osteoid seams and increased osteoclastic bone resorption.

Treatment

Treatment is usually simple and comprises small doses of cholecalciferol (1000–2000 units/day). This is best given as calcium with vitamin D tablets which each contain 500 units of vitamin D. Larger doses are virtually never required, except in the presence of severe gut or liver disease, or in the very rare anticonvulsant osteomalacias. There is no indication for the use of more potent vitamin D metabolites. Treatment is usually continued for the period of increased vitamin D requirement,

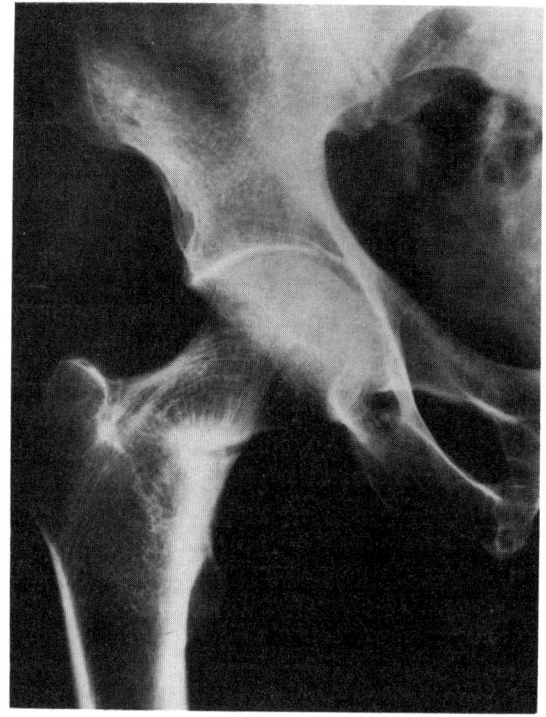

Fig. 10.6 Looser's zone of femoral neck. (Reproduced with kind permission of Gower Medical Publishing.)

e.g. throughout pregnancy or the adolescent growth spurt.

Vitamin D resistant rickets

Apart from renal failure there is a group of conditions causing rickets or osteomalacia which is characterised by a marked resistance to vitamin D therapy.

Vitamin D dependent rickets. This condition, inherited in an autosomal recessive manner, produces a biochemical disorder identical to vitamin D deficiency rickets. It heals only, however, with doses of vitamin D of around 50,000–75,000 units per day; healing is then complete. It probably represents deficiency of the renal 1-hydroxylase enzyme.

Hypophosphataemic rickets. These disorders are resistant to vitamin D even in massive doses. The biochemistry is different from vitamin D deficiency with a normal serum calcium but a very low phosphate concentration. PTH concentration is normal. Multiple renal tubular defects may be present, resulting in glycosuria, phosphaturia and

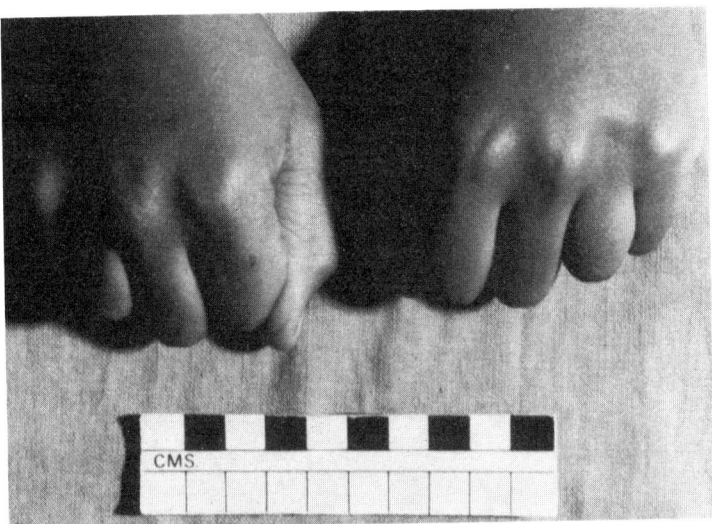

Fig. 10.7 Short fourth metacarpals of pseudohypoparathyroidism.

aminoaciduria. Occasionally, unusual tumours of the skin, muscle or connective tissue may be present, removal of which leads to complete healing of the disease. Various forms of inheritance may be found and treatment is with phosphate supplements combined with moderate doses of vitamin D or vitamin D metabolites.

Hypoparathyroidism

Hypoparathyroidism most commonly occurs as a consequence of neck surgery – parathyroidectomy, thyroidectomy or laryngectomy. Rarely it is an idiopathic disorder associated with other autoimmune diseases. When due to surgery it usually presents within days of the operation, though occasionally its presentation may be delayed for a number of years.

Symptoms

The symptoms are those of hypocalcaemia (see Table 10.3). When the onset is very gradual, few symptoms may be present until profound hypocalcaemia occurs.

Signs

Generalised twitchiness of muscle may be present, together with tetany in which the hands become flexed at the metacarpophalangeal joints and extended at the interphalangeal joints, described as the 'main d'accoucheur'. Chvostek's sign may be positive, that is facial contraction produced by tapping over the facial nerve in front of the ear, as may Trousseau's sign, which is the development of 'main d'accoucheur' following the application of an inflated sphygmomanometer cuff to the arm for several minutes.

Diagnosis

The biochemical changes are characteristic with a low calcium and high phosphate concentration associated with normal alkaline phosphatase and normal indices of renal function. Serum PTH concentration is low. Pseudohypoparathyroidism is a condition producing identical biochemical changes but in association with an elevated serum PTH. The defect is a resistance to PTH action and it may be associated with short stature, round facies, short metacarpals and mental retardation (Fig. 10.7).

Treatment

Acute treatment of hypoparathyroidism, required if symptoms are severe, is with intravenous infusion of calcium. Long-term treatment is with oral vitamin D. This can be either in the form of calciferol 50 000–100 000 units daily or

One-alpha or calcitriol (1–2 μg per day). Frequent measurements of serum calcium are required to detect the development of hypercalcaemia.

Hypomagnesaemic hypocalcaemia

Magnesium deficiency induces a secondary hypocalcaemia which is very resistant to conventional treatment. In severe hypomagnesaemia, both PTH secretion fails and PTH resistance develops. The commoner causes of hypomagnesaemia are alcoholism, severe gastrointestinal disease and drug therapy, especially prolonged aminoglycoside or cis-platinum therapy. Treatment is with magnesium supplements. This treatment alone corrects hypocalcaemia completely.

COMMON BONE DISEASES

Osteoporosis

Osteoporosis is a condition in which diminished amounts of normal bone are present. It occurs when bone resorption exceeds bone formation for a prolonged period of time.

Bone mass increases during childhood and then remains roughly constant during early adult life, to begin falling around the 5th decade. This loss is progressive and is more obvious in females than males in whom it appears to be temporally related to the menopause. Osteoporosis alone is asymptomatic, symptoms arising only when complications, particularly fractures, occur. Bone consists of compact and trabecular bone and it is the latter which is most affected by osteoporosis, therefore the vertebral column is affected commonly by the disorder. Osteoporosis may be localised or generalised. Table 10.4 lists the causes of osteoporosis. The most common forms of generalised osteoporosis are seen in elderly women and in patients on long term high dose corticosteroid therapy.

Diagnosis

The diagnosis of osteoporosis is fraught with difficulty. The most widely applied technique is bone radiography, but in excess of 25% of the bone mineral has to be lost for the diagnosis to be clear. The most accurate of the more readily

Table 10.4 Causes of osteoporosis

Localised	Generalised
Immobilisation, e.g. fracture	Oestrogen deficiency,
Local disease, e.g. rheumatoid	e.g. post-menopausal
arthritis	women, Turner's syndrome
Sudeck's atrophy	Testosterone deficiency
	Cushing's syndrome
	Thyrotoxicosis
	Alcoholism
	Chronic liver disease
	Immobilisation
	Idiopathic
	Prolonged heparin therapy

available techniques is absorption densitometry in which a loss of around 5% in bone mineral can be detected.

Presentation

The major complication of osteoporosis is bone fracture which affects three areas predominantly, the wrist, hip and vertebral column. Fractures of the wrist and hip are normally traumatic, occurring after falls. Vertebral fractures are frequently spontaneous and not infrequently painless. The consequent wedging of the vertebrae causes progressive loss of height and the development of thoracic kyphosis, so common in the elderly. When symptomatic, vertebral fractures cause a sudden, severe localised back pain which settles usually after 3–4 weeks. Chronic back pain is a difficult symptom to assess in osteoporosis, particularly in elderly patients as similar radiological changes are found frequently in asymptomatic subjects. Despite the frequency of vertebral collapse in osteoporosis, nerve compression syndromes are extremely rare.

Management

Hip and wrist fractures are treated conventionally and unite in a normal fashion. Vertebral fractures when painful are treated with bed rest and analgesics followed by mobilisation as soon as possible. Treatment of the osteoporosis itself can be considered under prevention and management of the established disease.

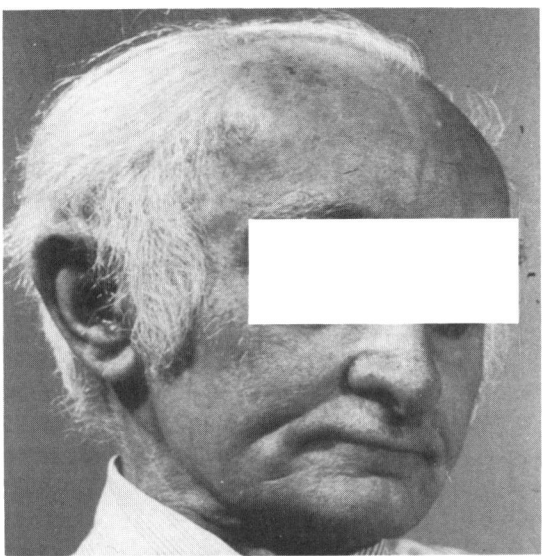

Fig. 10.8 Appearance of head in Paget's disease. A hearing aid is being used. (Reproduced with kind permission of Gower Medical Publishing.)

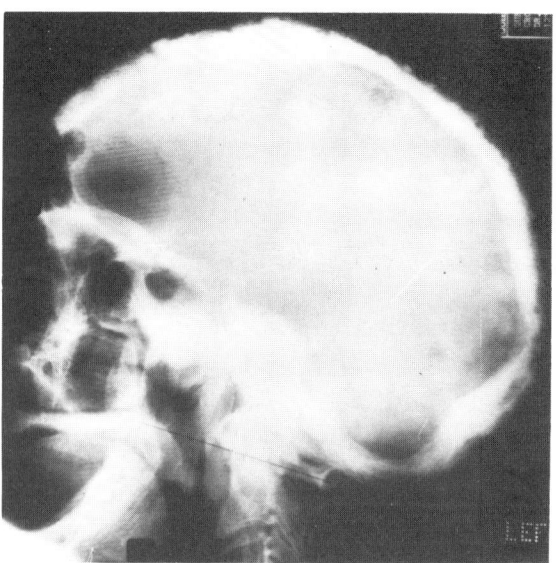

Fig. 10.9 Skull X-ray appearance in Paget's disease. (Reproduced with kind permission of Gower Medical Publishing.)

Prevention

The development of postmenopausal osteoporosis has been shown clearly to be delayed or even prevented by the administration of oestrogen replacement therapy. At present it is not possible to identify those patients at greatest risk of developing symptomatic osteoporosis in the future, who would most obviously benefit from treatment. Because the risks of prolonged oestrogen therapy are not understood fully, long term oestrogen replacement has not achieved widespread use in the UK.

Epidemiological studies have shown that osteoporosis is less common in groups who are more physically active and who have a higher dietary calcium intake.

Treatment of established osteoporosis

The management of established osteoporosis is controversial. Many therapies have been advocated but few, if any, have been shown clearly to improve bone density or to reduce the incidence of the most dangerous complication – hip fracture.

Most clinicians agree that vitamin D levels may be reduced in the elderly, especially if housebound. Some studies have suggested that osteomalacia is an important factor in the aetiology of hip fracture,

but the value of vitamin D therapy in this situation is not established. Calcium supplementation and/or cyclical oestrogen therapy are the two most common therapeutic regimes used in practice and have the advantage of being well tolerated and relatively free of serious side effects. Anabolic steroids, fluoride and calcitonin are also used but have greater side effects or are very costly.

Paget's Disease

Paget's disease is a condition in which abnormal bone is produced. There are areas of both increased and decreased bone formation, with new bone being laid down in a disorganised manner. The bone involved usually becomes expanded, showing areas of both increased and decreased density, with the former usually predominating. In Britain it is a common disorder with over 5% of people over the age of 50 having radiological evidence of the condition. Within the UK the prevalence varies, being highest in north-east England.

Presentation

In the majority of patients Paget's disease is an asymptomatic condition found by chance during radiological investigation of other conditions.

Table 10.5   Paget's disease — bones affected

Common	Pelvis, sacrum, skull, tibia, vertebrae
Less common	Scapula, humerus, clavicle, patella, radius, ulna, os calcis
Uncommon	Ribs
Rare	Fibula, mandible
Very rare	Metatarsals, metacarpals, phalanges

When causing symptoms it most frequently presents with either bone pain or deformity (Fig. 10.8, Fig.10.9). Bone pain is usually a chronic, burning pain. The bones most likely to be involved are shown in Table 10.5. Other complications are:

1. Pain
2. Fracture
3. Nerve entrapment e.g. auditory nerve, spinal cord
4. Sarcoma < 1% of affected patients

Although often described, hypercalcaemia and cardiac failure due to Paget's disease are very rare. Many patients with Paget's disease have osteo-arthritis of the joints adjacent to the Pagetic bone, which may itself be the cause of the pain experienced by the patient.

Differential diagnosis

The most frequent condition mistaken for Paget's disease is metastatic malignancy, especially the sclerotic secondaries of carcinoma of the prostate. Of particular importance in differentiating between the two is whether or not the bone is expanded; enlargement of bone strongly supports a diagnosis of Paget's disease (Fig. 10.10). It should be remembered that both conditions cause increased uptake of radioisotope on bone scans and that the serum acid phosphatase concentration may be elevated in Paget's disease, although the alkaline phosphatase in such cases is usually disproportionately higher.

Diagnosis

The diagnosis is usually made on the radiological appearance alone. The serum alkaline phosphatase

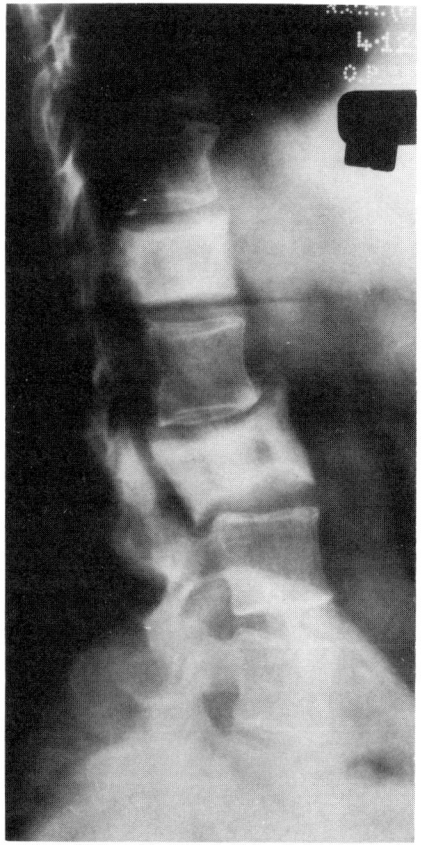

Fig. 10.10   Paget's disease of the spine. Note expansion of vertebral bodies.

is elevated, especially in extensive disease. The urinary hydroxyproline excretion, a measure of bone resorption, is usually increased in Paget's disease but such measurements are not required routinely.

Treatment

Asymptomatic patients do not require treatment. Pain due to Paget's disease should be treated initially with analgesics and only those patients resistant to such treatment considered for more specific therapy. Currently two treatments are generally available – calcitonin and the bisphosphonate, sodium etidronate. Calcitonin is injected subcutaneously and causes transient flushing and nausea at the time of injections. The response rate is variable (30–80% in different series) with one third of patients who respond subsequently relapsing biochemically and occasionally clinically. Sodium etidronate is an oral agent, the use of which is restricted initially to a 6-month course as prolonged treatment may be associated occasionally with the development of osteomalacia. Pain is relieved in about 60% of patients.

Diabetes mellitus

DEFINITION

Diabetes mellitus is characterised by an elevated blood glucose concentration. Acutely, this results in the classical symptoms of thirst and polyuria while chronic hyperglycaemia may play a role in the development of specific complications of the disease. An elevated blood glucose concentration may be the hallmark of diabetes but it is by no means the sole biochemical abnormality which is found. Weight loss, ketonuria and acidosis are common presenting features of insulin-dependent diabetes, while the chronic effects of inadequate treatment of insulin-dependent diabetes upon growth during adolescence are well recognised. In non-insulin-dependent diabetes abnormalities of circulating lipoproteins commonly accompany the raised blood glucose concentration. The link between these many facets of carbohydrate, protein and fat metabolism lies in the major hormonal regulator, insulin.

Biochemically, diabetes must be considered as a disorder of insulin effect. In insulin-dependent diabetes, the underlying reason is readily apparent – there is grossly diminished or absent secretion of the hormone from the β cells of the islets of Langerhans. In non-insulin-dependent diabetes the basic defect is less clear. Insulin secretion may be diminished such that, while circulating concentrations lie within the normal range, they are inappropriately low for the prevailing blood glucose concentration. Alternatively, insulin may be unable to exert a full effect upon target tissues due to either reduced sites of action on the cells or to an impairment of intracellular effect.

Thus, the biochemical definition of diabetes mellitus is a lack of insulin effect upon tissues, resulting in abnormalities of carbohydrate, protein and fat metabolism. Superimposed upon the biochemical abnormality of diabetes is the clinical syndrome resulting from long-term disordered metabolism. The main features of the syndrome are a specific microangiopathy, neuropathy and more frequent and accelerated macrovascular disease.

Diagnosis

In the past few years attempts have been made to obtain greater uniformity in the diagnosis of diabetes. Recommendations for this have come from the Diabetes Data Group of the National Institutes of Health in the USA and the World Health Organisation (WHO). The guidelines of the WHO, which in turn are similar to those suggested by the Diabetes Epidemiology Study Group of the European Association for the Study of Diabetes, have been adopted by the British Diabetic Association.

In the presence of symptoms of diabetes or specific long term complications such as microangiopathy, a single raised blood glucose concentration confirms the diagnosis. A fasting venous whole blood glucose of >7.0 mmol/l or a random venous whole blood glucose concentration >10.0 mmol/l is abnormal and will lead to the diagnosis of diabetes in more than 60% of patients. A fasting venous whole blood glucose concentration <7.0 mmol/l excludes diabetes. Fasting whole blood glucose concentrations between 5.5 and

6.9 mmol/l and random whole blood glucose concentrations between 7.0 and 9.9 mmol/l are considered equivocal.

It should be noted that differences exist in glucose concentration between venous and capillary blood and between whole blood and plasma. When blood is drawn from a fasting patient venous and capillary blood are similar, but, postprandially, capillary whole blood is approximately 10% higher than venous whole blood. Thus, to diagnose diabetes on a random capillary whole blood glucose measurement, the concentration would have to be 11.0 mmol/l or more. Similarly, since red blood cells contain little intracellular glucose due to rapid metabolism, the presence of these cells in a blood sample serves to dilute the plasma glucose. Plasma glucose measurement is therefore approximately 10% higher than whole blood glucose measurement and diagnostic values must be adjusted accordingly.

When fasting or random glucose measurements are equivocal it is appropriate to proceed to an oral glucose tolerance test. The WHO recommendations set down a standardised procedure and interpretation of the test (Table 11.1). Traditionally it has been stressed that the diet preceding the test should contain a minimum amount of carbohydrate. In practice, this is rarely of importance, although diets containing less than 150 g carbohydrate may lead to an abnormal glucose tolerance test – a phenomenon labelled 'starvation diabetes'. Of more importance is that the test should commence with the patient

fasted for a minimum of 10 hours. After blood and urine specimens are taken, a 75 g glucose load is drunk. The glucose is dissolved in flavoured water, the flavouring reducing the incidence of nausea, and the total volume should be approximately 300 ml. Too viscous solutions of glucose have an osmotic effect upon the gut and may result in a flat glucose tolerance test. The posture of the patient during the test makes some difference to the result and the patient should sit quietly. The WHO bans smoking during the test, although there is considerable evidence that it does not affect the result.

It is customary to take blood at 30-minute intervals from the time the patient completes ingestion and to take urine at hourly intervals. Urinary glucose is of no consequence in diagnosing diabetes, but is useful if renal glycosuria is suspected and may give an approximate indication of the renal threshold for glucose if diabetes is confirmed.

The criteria for interpretation of blood glucose concentrations are shown in Table 11.1. A word is necessary about the category called 'impaired glucose tolerance': only a few patients with impaired glucose tolerance show worsening to diabetes and many show spontaneous reversion to normal blood glucose levels. Patients falling into this category cannot, however, be assumed to be normal; the prevalence of macrovascular disease in this group is greater than in a control population. The unique status of diagnosis during pregnancy is not clarified in the WHO recommendations. The significance

Table 11.1 Diagnostic values during an oral glucose tolerance test in adults (1 mmol/l = 18 mg/100 ml)

| | Glucose concentration (mmol/l) | | |
	Venous whole blood	Capillary whole blood	Venous plasma
Normal			
Fasting	< 5.5	< 5.5	< 6.0
2 h	< 7.0	< 8.0	< 8.0
Diabetes mellitus			
Fasting	> 7.0	> 8.0	> 8.0
2 h	>10.0	>11.0	>11.0
Impaired glucose tolerance			
Fasting	5.5–6.9	5.5–6.9	6–7.9
2 h	7.0–9.9	8.0–10.9	8–10.9

of the diagnosis of impaired glucose tolerance in pregnancy and the relationship to gestational diabetes is not yet apparent. Interpretation of results obtained from glucose tolerance testing must always be considered in the light of the clinical situation. A deterioration in glucose tolerance occurs with age; the catabolic response to illness may alter diagnostic significance as, for example, after myocardial infarction; drugs, particularly thiazide diuretics, corticosteroids, and the contraceptive pill may have dramatic effects.

Types of diabetes

Currently two classifications coexist. An aetiological classification divides the two major types of diabetes into type 1 and type 2, while a clinical classification divides patients into insulin-dependent and non-insulin-dependent diabetes mellitus (Table 11.2). The terms type 1 and insulin-dependent and type 2 and non-insulin-dependent are not always synonymous. It is true that type 1 diabetic patients are, or will be, insulin-dependent and that the majority of type 2 diabetic patients are not dependent upon insulin, yet there are considerable numbers of patients who aetiologically are type 2, but clinically show an inadequate response to diet or tablets. Traditionally, insulin-dependent means that the patient is dependent upon insulin for the avoidance of ketoacidosis.

Table 11.2 Classification of diabetes and glucose intolerance

Clinical	Aetiological
Insulin-dependent	Type 1
Non-insulin dependent	Type 2
a. obese	
b. non-obese	
Associated with other diseases	—
Gestational diabetes	—
Impaired glucose tolerance	—

The aetiology and pathogenesis of type 1 diabetes mellitus (Table 11.3)

Inheritance

Considerable attention in recent years has been focussed upon human leukocyte antigens (HLA)

Table 11.3 Aetiological classification of diabetes

	Type 1	Type 2
Genetic susceptibility	HLA-linked	Not identified
Environmental factors	Viruses	Obesity
	Toxins	
Immunity	Islet cell antibodies	Absent

in type 1 diabetes. By comparing the frequency of these antigens in patients with type 1 diabetes and in non-diabetic populations it has been shown that certain HLA occur more frequently in diabetic patients. The strongest association of type 1 diabetes is with DR3 and DR4. Genetic studies have shown that a combination of DR3 and DR4 occurs more commonly than homozygous DR3 or homozygous DR4 in type 1 diabetic patients. This finding suggests genetic heterogeneity within type 1 diabetes. There is further support for this concept in that, although DR3 and DR4 are associated with a similar type of diabetes, there appear to be minor differences in the response to the disease between patients in whom the association is with DR3 and those in whom the association is with DR4. Patients with DR3 tend to show persistence of islet cell antibodies and occurrence of other organ specific autoimmune diseases. In patients with DR4 there is no tendency to autoimmunity but an increase in production of antibodies to viruses and heterologous insulin administration. There is also an increased risk of developing the disease before the age of 16 years.

In identical twins, concordance for diabetes (i.e. both twins have diabetes) is approximately 50% when the age of presentation is below 45 years. In both concordant and discordant pairs there is a high prevalance of DR3 and DR4 with a low prevalence of DR5, DR7 and DR2.

Environment

With only half of pairs of identical twins concordant for type 1 diabetes it is safe to conclude that inheritance is not the only factor determining the development of the disease. Current evidence suggests that viruses are the most likely environmental stimuli, although chemical toxins and other unidentified agents cannot be excluded and may be important in certain subgroups of patients.

Much of the evidence implicating viruses is circumstantial but when added together it provides considerable weight in favour of the viral theory. A disease resembling type 1 diabetes can be produced in laboratory rodents by inoculation with certain viruses. These include reovirus, encephalomyocarditis virus, and Venezuelan equine encephalitis virus. Perhaps more importantly in view of the findings in humans, the virus Coxsackie B4 will also produce diabetes in animals. Indirect evidence implicating viruses in the development of type 1 diabetes in humans comes from studies in children. A greater number of cases present in autumn, winter and spring with a marked reduction in incidence during the summer. This pattern can be linked with seasonal variation in incidence of viral infection. If viral antibodies are sought in the blood of children developing type 1 diabetes, Coxsackie B4 virus antibodies are found more commonly than in control groups. A history of influenza or influenza-like illness is also found more commonly, as is a history of mumps infection, although a large UK survey of children developing diabetes indicates that the excess of mumps is only of the order of 1%. More direct evidence of viral aetiology comes from studies of children born with congenital rubella of whom 20% develop diabetes.

Other possible environmental agents in type 1 diabetes are chemical toxins. Alloxan and streptozotocin have been widely used to destroy β cells in experimental animals. Further suggestive (if obscure) evidence of chemical toxins comes from Iceland where type 1 diabetes in young males appears to increase in relation to the eating of smoked cured mutton by the parents around the time of conception.

Immunological factors

As with both genetic and environmental factors, the precise role of the immune response in determining the development of type 1 diabetes is unclear. It is well established that at diagnosis the majority of patients have antibodies to islet cells present in their serum. There are a variety of antibodies in this family, including complement-fixing antibodies. Between 60% and 90% of newly diagnosed type 1

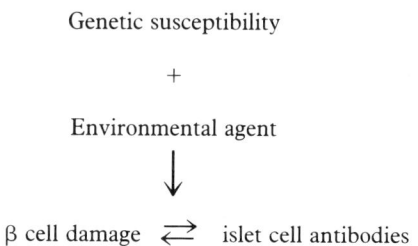

Genetic susceptibility

+

Environmental agent

↓

β cell damage ⇌ islet cell antibodies

Fig. 11.1 Possible mechanism of the development of type 1 diabetes.

diabetic children have islet cell antibodies present but, in contrast to other organ specific immune diseases, the antibody tends to disappear as the time from diagnosis increases. Only 10–15% of patients show persistence of islet cell antibodies and these tend to be female patients with a later age of onset and a high prevalence of other endocrine autoantibodies. Islet cell antibodies occur in a small number of normal people and in relatives of type 1 diabetic patients, situations in which their significance is unknown.

Pathogenesis

Piecing together the evidence from the foregoing sections, the most attractive hypothesis for the pathogenesis of type 1 diabetes is that, given a particular genetic susceptibility, an environmental agent such as a virus or chemical initiates β cell damage. The immune response to this is the production of islet cell antibodies which may continue β cell destruction (Fig. 11.1). Eventually sufficient damage results to cause insulinopenia and hence diabetes.

As was discussed in the section on definition of diabetes, the hormone insulin has effects upon carbohydrate, protein and fat metabolism (Table 11.4). It has both stimulatory effects upon storage and inhibitory effects upon breakdown and is the major anabolic hormone opposing the catabolic effects of catecholamines, glucagon and cortisol. The most potent stimulator of insulin secretion in everyday life is food and it is pertinent to consider the effects of insulin in the fed and the fasted state.

Following a meal, the rise in circulating nutrients is checked by insulin secretion. While

Table 11.4 Actions of insulin

Carbohydrate metabolism
    Enhanced glycogen storage
    Inhibition of glycogenolysis
    Inhibition of gluconeogenesis
    Enhanced peripheral glucose uptake

Protein metabolism
    Enhanced protein synthesis
    Inhibition of proteolysis

Fat metabolism
    Enhanced triglyceride storage
    Inhibition of triglyceride breakdown

certain tissues such as brain, peripheral nerves, retina, renal medulla and erythrocytes can take up glucose from the circulation independent of insulin, the major metabolic tissues such as muscle and fat have a requirement for insulin to stimulate glucose uptake. Once inside these cells glucose metabolism via glycolysis and the tricarboxylic acid cycle is rapid such that there is little intracellular free glucose. The effect of insulin upon protein synthesis is less well characterised. Circulating amino acid concentrations are reduced by insulin and effects of insulin upon protein synthesis have been attributed to increasing intracellular availability of amino acids. This is probably incorrect and the explanation may be very much more complex. In man de novo synthesis of fatty acids occurs in the liver. The liver does not require insulin for glucose uptake and following glycolysis, acetyl CoA is available for fatty acid synthesis. Fatty acids are esterified and endogenous triglyceride is released from the liver as very low density lipoprotein (VLDL). The uptake of triglyceride by peripheral tissues is insulin dependent. Stepwise breakdown of triglyceride allows uptake of fatty acids by adipocytes and this is dependent upon lipoprotein lipase. Both this breakdown and subsequent re-esterification of the fatty acids with α-glycerophosphate derived from glucose are regulatory sites for insulin.

In the postabsorptive period, low concentrations of insulin allow maintenance of blood glucose concentration by hepatic glucose production. Both glycogenolysis and gluconeogenesis are involved and both are sensitive to inhibition by a rise in insulin concentration. Proteolytic rates can be reduced by insulin, suggesting a permissive effect upon

protein breakdown of low insulin concentrations. Breakdown of stored triglyceride is influenced by the enzyme hormone-sensitive lipase, which is also inhibited by insulin.

To this skeleton of insulin effects upon metabolism should be added the process of ketone body synthesis. The ketone bodies, 3-hydroxybutyrate, acetoacetate and acetone, are synthesised in the liver from non-esterified fatty acids. The uptake of fatty acids by the liver is directly proportional to the circulating concentration and, since this is raised in insulin deficiency, there is enhanced ketogenesis. It is probable that in insulin deficiency, glucagon directs fatty acids into ketone body formation rather than into triglyceride synthesis. This, and other consequences of insulin deficiency are outlined in Table 11.5

Table 11.5 Consequences of insulin deficiency

1. Increased hepatic glucose production
   Impaired peripheral glucose uptake

2. Increased protein breakdown
   Impaired protein synthesis

3. Increased triglyceride breakdown
   Impaired triglyceride storage

4. Enhanced ketogenesis
   Impaired peripheral utilisation of ketone bodies

Type 2 diabetes mellitus

The aetiology and pathogenesis of type 2 diabetes are defined even less clearly than those of type 1 diabetes.

Inheritance

In type 2 diabetes, population studies show no association with HLA phenotypes. This should not be taken to mean that inheritance plays no part in aetiology, since in identical twins, when one twin develops diabetes over the age of 45 the concordance rate approaches 100%. The interval between the two twins becoming concordant for diabetes may be up to 5 years, so that in any cross-sectional study there will always be a few discordant pairs. Since the twins do not develop diabetes until after 45 years of life this must arouse suspicion of an environmental stimulus or 'trigger' leading to overt diabetes.

Environment

The most frequently encountered environmental factor contributing to the development of type 2 diabetes is obesity. Surveys show that up to 75% of patients developing type 2 diabetes are overweight and the fall in incidence during World War II, when intake of refined sugar and total calories fell, is well documented.

Other major environmental factors which may precipitate type 2 diabetes include trauma, major illness and drug therapy. The association of corticosteroid treatment and diabetes is not unexpected since corticosteroids are potent catabolic hormones with actions opposed to those of insulin. Thiazide diuretics also play a role in the development of diabetes acting through an impairment of insulin secretion. Oral contraceptive drugs produce minor disturbance of the glucose tolerance test but, at times, frank diabetes may occur; the development of diabetes during pregnancy (gestational diabetes) is also well recognised.

Immunological

Islet cell antibodies are absent from the sera of type 2 diabetic patients and indeed their presence would lead to a strong suspicion that the patient had type 1 diabetes. Similarly, any association of other endocrine autoimmunity is with type 1 and not type 2 diabetes.

Pathogenesis of type 2 diabetes

If non-obese, non-diabetic patients are compared with obese patients the latter have hyperglycaemia and hyperinsulinaemia. This is true for fasting insulin, insulin measured during an oral glucose tolerance test, or insulin measured throughout a normal day. Since blood glucose concentration is raised despite high circulating insulin concentration, the implication is that insulin resistance is present.

Insulin exerts its metabolic effects by binding to specific areas on the target cell membrane (insulin receptors). Binding activates a second messenger system which amplifies and translates into specific metabolic actions. Thus, insulin action may be impaired in any one of three ways. Firstly, by

secretion of an abnormal β cell product; secondly, through changes in binding to the receptor and, thirdly, by defects in postreceptor metabolic actions (Table 11.6). Receptor and postreceptor defects are believed to play an important role in the pathogenesis of type 2 diabetes. Mild insulin resistance in obesity or in patients with impaired glucose tolerance is characterised by a decrease in insulin receptor number. In more severe forms of obesity and diabetes, changes in receptor number coexist with impaired postreceptor events.

The major group of circulating insulin antagonists are the catabolic hormones. Diabetes is well recognised as a feature of excessive corticosteroid secretion in Cushing's syndrome, excessive growth hormone secretion in acromegaly and in phaeochromocytoma (Table 11.7). Following myocardial infarction glucose intolerance or precipitation of frank diabetes is common. The catabolic response to myocardial infarction includes massive catecholamine secretion, which both inhibits insulin secretion and results in peripheral insulin antagonism. Excessive secretion of one or more catabolic hormones in response to concurrent illness is a major factor in the development of ketoacidosis.

Table 11.6 Causes of insulin resistance

1. Abnormal β cell secretion
2. Circulating insulin antagonists
3. Changes in insulin receptor binding
4. Postreceptor impairment

Table 11.7 Circulating antagonists to insulin

Hormonal:
catecholamines, glucagon, cortisol, growth hormone, thyroxine, oestrogens, prolactin, AVP

Metabolites:
non-esterified fatty acids
ketone bodies

Immunological:
anti-insulin antibodies
anti-insulin receptor antibodies

Other types of diabetes

There are a number of diseases which are associated with diabetes and do not fit into the categories type 1 and type 2 in the aetiological classification. These are:

1. Pancreatic disease
2. Hormonal disorders
3. Drug induced
4. Receptor abnormalities
5. Genetic syndromes
6. Miscellaneous.

The two best recognised categories are pancreatic disease and hormonal disorders.

Diabetes occurs as a consequence of pancreatic damage in chronic pancreatitis, carcinoma of the pancreas, following surgical resection and in haemochromatosis. It may also be a feature of acute pancreatitis, remitting with recovery. The relationship between carcinoma of the pancreas and diabetes is of interest and must be considered when obstructive jaundice develops in a patient with a recent history of onset of diabetes. Whether carcinoma of the pancreas develops more often in patients with long-standing diabetes is less clear, but actuarial studies suggest that this is the case. Diabetes associated with haemochromatosis is attributed traditionally to iron deposition in the pancreas, but impairment in liver function should not be ignored in its effect upon carbohydrate metabolism.

Hormonal disorders associated with diabetes include acromegaly, Cushing's syndrome, Conn's syndrome, phaeochromocytoma, glucagonoma and somatostatinoma. Drugs which may induce diabetes include corticosteroids, contraceptive preparations and thiazide diuretics, as already discussed. Genetic syndromes associated with insulin receptor defects include Leprechaunism, lipoatrophic diabetes, and the syndrome of insulin resistance and acanthosis nigricans. The last of these is described in young females with hirsutism and decreased insulin receptors. A second syndrome of insulin resistance and acanthosis nigricans, which may be acquired rather than genetic occurs mainly in non-Caucasian females, often with evidence of other autoimmune endocrine disease. Circulating antibodies to the insulin receptor can be identified in these patients and massive insulin resistance may be present. Paradoxically, the patient may experience hypoglycaemia since the antibody appears to have some insulin-like effects.

In addition to these syndromes, over 40 other genetic syndromes are associated with diabetes but most of these are rare. Maturity-onset diabetes of young people (MODY) is sometimes referred to as Mason-type diabetes after a family with the syndrome. The disturbance in glucose tolerance is mild and often responds to simple dietary treatment even in teenagers. Where patients have been followed for 30 or 40 years, they develop few diabetic complications. Recognition of the syndrome is important in saving a teenager from a life-time of unnecessary insulin therapy. The DIDMOAD syndrome comprises diabetes insipidus (DI), diabetes mellitus (DM), optic atrophy (OA) and deafness(D). More than one member of the family may have the syndrome and diabetes is insulin-dependent. Diabetes insipidus developing in a patient with diabetes mellitus is often difficult to recognise. Optic atrophy is said to occur more commonly in diabetes mellitus than in the general population and may reflect partial manifestation of this syndrome.

TREATMENT OF DIABETES

Deciding upon insulin treatment for a 10-year-old child with a short history of severe symptoms, appreciable weight loss and heavy ketonuria is straightforward. Similarly presentation of an obese 55-year old without symptoms, weight loss or ketonuria, will point to diet as first choice for therapy. Between these two ends of the spectrum, lie many patients with widely varying histories and presentations and choice of therapy becomes empirical. A number of factors influence the decision:

1. Age
2. Acute or chronic onset
3. Weight loss
4. Wasting
5. Ketonuria
6. Family history
7. Medical problems.

Age remains an important factor in choosing therapy despite the abandonment of the terms juvenile-onset and maturity-onset diabetes. Young people (i.e. less than 30 years old) are likely to be type 1 diabetic patients; insulinopenia is the pathogenic mechanism for this type of diabetes, demanding insulin treatment. Also of importance is a family history of diabetes. A parent or sibling with insulin-dependent diabetes suggests insulin-dependence in the newly-diagnosed patient.

In patients who are not young, then the length of history is of importance. A short (less than three month) history of acute symptoms accompanied by weight loss suggests a loss of the anabolic effect of insulin, in turn implying insulin deficiency. Since lipolysis is sensitive to inhibition by insulin, the presence of ketonuria may be considered to represent severe insulinopenia. If immediate insulin treatment is unwarranted then the choice of therapy lies between diet, and diet plus oral hypoglycaemic agents. Symptoms play less part in influencing the choice since both approaches readily relieve symptoms. The degree of obesity is a major consideration and it is good practice to document the percentage ideal body weight from comparative tables at diagnosis. In obese patients who are either symptomatic or asymptomatic then calorie restriction may be the only treatment necessary. Rather more difficult to manage is the underweight patient whose diet allows little manipulation.

Except in ketoacidosis, hyperosmolar coma, or with very high (greater than 30 mmol/l) blood glucose concentration, the degree of hyperglycaemia does not dictate therapy. Documentation is important for diagnosis, but not in indicating the type of diabetes, since blood glucose is influenced profoundly by preceding dietary intake and particularly the attempted relief of thirst by drinking large volumes of carbohydrate containing drinks.

Diet

Diet is the cornerstone of treatment of diabetes used either alone, or in combination with oral hypoglycaemic agents or insulin. Dissatisfaction with the traditional low-carbohydrate diet has resulted from both an appreciation that carbohydrate restriction implies an increase in fat intake for most patients, and doubts regarding this approach in the pathogenesis of arterial disease. The accent in prescribing diets in the treatment of diabetes now falls firmly upon total calorie intake

and the proportion of this to be eaten as carbohydrate.

Insulin-treated patients

The traditional way of assessing carbohydrate intake is by a 10 g system, when 10 g is referred to by the patient as a portion, line, or exchange. The benefits of this system are that the total amount of carbohydrate eaten per day may be constant, but by utilising different carbohydrates, 10 g portions of rice or potato, for example, can be exchanged from day to day to allow variety in the diet.

Assessing total calorie intake follows the same principles which are used in constructing a diet for anyone. Three questions need to be considered. Firstly, is the patient underweight or overweight? Secondly, how many calories are being eaten to maintain the present weight? And thirdly, does work involve heavy calorie expenditure, are there periods of intense recreational exercise and is there a major variation from day to day in energy expenditure? Consideration of these factors allows estimation of an appropriate total calorie intake.

Having ascertained a desirable daily calorie intake, the amount of calories to be eaten as carbohydrate is calculated. The optimal carbohydrate content of the diabetic diet is unknown, but there is abundant evidence that control of blood glucose is not made worse by high (50–75%) carbohydrate diets. It is reasonable to aim for 40–65% of total calories to be eaten as carbohydrate. It is suggested that carbohydrate should not be eaten in a highly refined form, since this results in large increments in blood glucose concentration, but rather that it be consumed in the form of complex carbohydrates, where digestion time plays a part in moderating the blood glucose rise which follows absorption. In addition, the gelatinous fibres pectin and guar have been shown to delay absorption of carbohydrate eaten simultaneously.

The amount of protein eaten in a Western diet tends to remain constant, despite alterations in other aspects of diet; usually 10–20% of total calories are eaten as protein. The remaining calories are eaten as fat and consequently the higher the percentage carbohydrate intake, the lower the percentage fat intake.

Non-insulin-dependent diabetic patients

The principles involved in prescribing a diet for non-insulin-dependent diabetic patients are similar to those described above. How many calories are to be allowed and what percentage should be eaten as carbohydrate. Energy expenditure and percentage ideal body weight of the patient lead to a rational approach to total calorie intake. Of total calories, 40–65% should be consumed as carbohydrate. Some feedback control of blood glucose concentration by insulin secretion persists in these patients, allowing less rigidity in the amount eaten per meal.

Oral hypoglycaemic agents

Certain considerations apply in the choice of patient suitable for oral hypoglycaemic agents. Firstly, the patient should have sufficient endogenous insulin secretion to inhibit fat breakdown and ketosis. This is equivalent to saying that they must not be insulin-dependent. Secondly, having ascertained this fact from the clinical presentation there is a theoretical choice of treatment by diet, or by diet plus oral agents. When diet alone is used in treatment, sufficient time must be allowed for the production of a beneficial effect. Reassessment should be undertaken after one month. Patients who show no response may then be considered for treatment by oral agents. It should be stressed that the commonest reason for non-response to diet, particularly in obese patients, is non-compliance with diet. Non-obese patients may, however, fail to respond despite following a prescribed diet. Secondary failure occurs when a patient is treated adequately by diet for some time before showing a loss of diabetic control. The majority of oral hypoglycaemic usage is in secondary failure of dietary treatment despite compliance.

There are two families of oral hypoglycaemic agents, sulphonylureas and biguanides; metformin is the only biguanide currently available in the UK.

Sulphonylureas

Despite prolonged use, the mechanism of action of these drugs remains unclear. In the short-term (less than six months), sulphonylureas lower blood glucose by stimulating insulin secretion. In the long-term, the improvement in blood glucose concentration persists but circulating insulin levels tend to revert to pretreatment values. This has led to the suggestion that the lowering of blood glucose is due, in addition, to an extrapancreatic mechanism of action.

Since sulphonylureas act initially by increasing insulin secretion, there is a tendency for their use to be accompanied by weight gain. They are, therefore, most suitable for use in non-obese patients and whether they should be used in obese patients, with high blood glucose concentrations despite diet, is problematical. The use of insulin in such patients produces the same dilemma and the use of metformin is an alternative to consider (see below).

There are a large number of different sulphonylureas available, and they are classified in two ways. The 'first generation' sulphonylureas include chlorpropamide and tolbutamide, while the remainder are termed 'second generation', the only real difference being that the latter are more potent on a weight-for-weight basis. Of more value is the classification into short- and long-acting sulphonylureas. Short-acting sulphonylureas are given more than once daily, while long-acting need only be given once per day.

Side-effects of sulphonylureas are uncommon. Occasionally a widespread skin rash may occur and there is little point in changing to another sulphonylurea. Hypoglycaemia during sulphonylurea therapy is particularly likely to occur with the use of long-acting preparations and is commoner in elderly patients with impaired renal function. Chlorpropamide, because of its long half life (approximately 36 hours), and glibenclamide, because of its potency, may produce severe, prolonged hypoglycaemia. The incidence is reduced by using short-acting sulphonylureas. Occasionally chlorpropamide therapy results in water retention, hyponatraemia and confusion. This side effect is utilised in the treatment of diabetes insipidus. The majority of other side-effects occurring with sulphonylureas are extremely uncommon, with the exception of facial flushing after alcohol in patients taking chlorpropamide. It has been suggested that chlorpropamide-alcohol flushing was associated with less microvascular and macrovascular disease than occurred in non-insulin-dependent patients who did not flush, but this view has been challenged.

Biguanides

Phenformin and metformin have been used extensively in the UK but the former has been withdrawn because of an association with the development of lactic acidosis. Both biguanides produce a hypoglycaemic effect through the same mechanism of action, but the accumulation, metabolism and excretion of the drugs result in metformin being safer.

Metformin produces a lowering of blood glucose concentrations through three actions:

1. Impairs glucose absorption
2. Inhibits gluconeogenesis
3. Increases peripheral glucose utilisation.

Glucose absorption from the gut is impaired, as is absorption of other sugars, amino acids and certain vitamins. Glucose production by the liver is inhibited through an effect upon gluconeogenesis, and there is evidence that peripheral utilisation of glucose is enhanced.

Metformin is of use in obese hyperglycaemic patients when dietary treatment is inadequate. The side effects of metformin are:

1. Anorexia
2. Nausea
3. Metallic taste in mouth
4. Diarrhoea
5. Macrocytosis
6. Lactic acidosis.

Anorexia and nausea may reduce calorie intake. Diarrhoea is more common with large doses and may lead to an erroneous diagnosis of 'diabetic diarrhoea' due to autonomic neuropathy with unnecessary investigation of the patient. Vitamin B_{12} absorption is reduced by metformin and leads occasionally to macrocytosis and rarely to macrocytic anaemia. Occasional cases of lactic acidosis occurring during metformin therapy have been reported but these are rare. Because of its renal excretion it is not suitable for patients with renal impairment. Inhibition of gluconeogenesis and

increased utilisation of glucose increase blood lactate concentration and metformin should not be used if associated disease, which further raises blood lactate, is present. Thus, respiratory disease and cardiovascular disease which produce peripheral hypoxia are contraindications to the use of metformin. Similarly liver disease, which reduces lactate extraction from the circulation, is a contraindication to metformin therapy.

Combined oral agent therapy

Since the reduction in blood glucose concentration by sulphonylureas and by metformin is produced by different mechanisms, the two types of oral agent may be used in combination when either on its own is only partially effective. Their use in this way may delay instigation of insulin therapy.

Principles of insulin therapy

In normal man insulin secretion is linked closely to blood glucose concentration. Insulin is secreted in response to a rise in blood glucose concentration, while a fall in blood glucose reduces secretion. A number of other secretagogues affect the β cell, of which amino acids are the most important. A second important factor in normal man is delivery of insulin into the portal circulation. This allows high concentrations to reach the liver where approximately 50% is removed; portal insulin concentration is thus twice the level in peripheral blood. Hepatic glucose production, which is vital for maintenance of blood glucose concentration during fasting, is quickly inhibited by small rises in portal insulin concentration. Initially, as food is absorbed, inhibition of glucose production helps to prevent an excessive rise in blood glucose and then, as peripheral insulin levels rise, utilisation of glucose is increased.

There are two major discrepancies between this arrangement in normal man and current methods of insulin administration to insulin-dependent diabetic patients. Firstly, delivery to the tissues is governed by the amount of insulin injected and the physicochemical properties of the type of insulin. Secondly, delivery of injected insulin is into the peripheral circulation rather than the portal circulation and the normal ratio of insulin between the two circulations is lost.

Normoglycaemia remains the major aim of treatment and probably the best approach is to define the pattern of insulin secretion throughout the day in normal people and try to imitate it. In normal people there is a continuous secretion of insulin throughout 24 hours supplemented by peaks of circulating insulin following meals and snacks (Fig. 11.2). Attempting to mimic this pattern, a very long-acting insulin can be given once daily with further injections of short-acting insulin before meals. This involves three injections per day and its theoretical advantages are limited by patient acceptance. A compromise is to give two injections per day of a mixture of short- and intermediate-acting insulin. The intermediate-acting insulin provides a basal level of insulin and gives some protection against massive blood glucose rises with the mid-day meal, while breakfast and the evening meal are covered by the short-acting insulin. This insulin regimen is the treatment of choice in insulin-dependent patients in whom the aim is good diabetic control.

It is quite clear that a single daily injection of long acting insulin can in no way imitate the insulin pattern of normal man. This type of regimen is used when good control is not the primary aim of treatment such as in elderly patients when relief of symptoms is all that is required.

Choice of insulin

Bovine, porcine and human insulin are available in short-acting and in longer-acting preparations. The

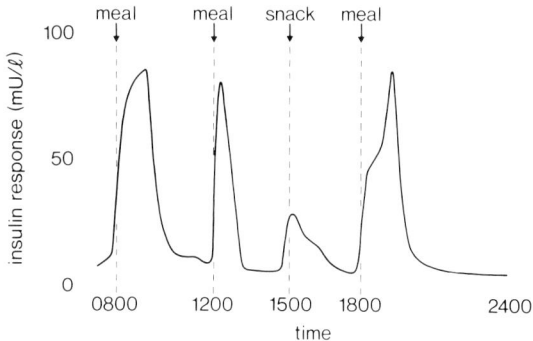

Fig. 11.2 Insulin concentrations during 24 hours in a normal person. (Reprinted from Kinson J, Nattrass M 1984 Caring for the diabetic patient. Churchill Livingstone, Edinburgh, by kind permission.)

basic 2 chain (A and B) structure linked by disulphide bonds is the same throughout these species and there is no difference in the biological potency. Duration of action of insulin is lengthened by additives to the insulin which slow absorption from the injection site and these are commonly zinc and protamine. Porcine insulin is chemically different to human insulin by one amino acid, where alanine replaces threonine at the B30 position. Beef insulin shows an additional two substitutions compared to human insulin, with valine replacing isoleucine at A10 and alanine for threonine at A8. All species can be prepared to a high standard of purity and individual insulins are designated monocomponent to denote highly purified insulin. All species of insulin, including human, are antigenic, although with highly purified insulins IgG antibody titres are low. Older types of insulin were considerably more antigenic. The presence of significant titres of antibodies may increase the dose of insulin required by a patient but it is uncertain whether their presence has other deleterious effects. There is no convincing evidence that they are harmful but highly purified insulins have become the first choice for insulin therapy.

Human insulin is prepared by modification of porcine insulin (semisynthetic or enzymatically modified porcine) or by bacterial synthesis (biosynthetic or recombinant). Bacterial plasmids can be modified to include the DNA sequence coding for insulin and under appropriate conditions they will then synthesise large quantities of human insulin which can be extracted. Current evidence suggests that while there is no difference in biological potency between porcine and human insulin there are small differences in absorption characteristics of the insulins and hence the duration of action.

Continuous subcutaneous insulin infusion

Continuous subcutaneous insulin infusion (CSII) is achieved by a small pump which drives a syringe to infuse insulin through a cannula positioned subcutaneously. Many different types of pump are available and most allow either changes in infusion rate or manual acceleration of infusion to increase insulin delivery with meals. Numerous studies show that good diabetic control can be obtained with this system by adjustment of the basal and bolus rates of insulin infusion by the patient or physician according to blood glucose measurements.

Aims of therapy

The aim of diabetic treatment is twofold. The relief of symptoms due to the biochemical disturbance is the first priority and can usually be achieved without too much effort. Diabetes is a life-long disorder, however, and the reduction of morbidity or the avoidance of complications is the long-term goal. This will include the treatment of complications as they arise and avoidance of their development by long-term correction of the biochemical disturbance. As yet, however, the important question of whether good diabetic control does indeed prevent the development of complications has not been answered. The majority of retrospective studies have suggested that patients with good diabetic control do develop fewer complications. However, it is possible that patients who do not develop complications have a type of diabetes which is inherently easier to control. Recent studies have attempted to obtain good control by intensive treatment, and then quantify change over a short time period. There is some evidence that the progression of capillary basement membrane thickening and development of microaneurysms is reduced with good control.

Monitoring therapy

At home patients may monitor symptoms, the amount of glucose in the urine and blood glucose. In diabetic clinics, treatment is assessed by blood and urine glucose measurement with due attention to symptoms and changes in weight. Measurement of glycosylated haemoglobin is being used more extensively to assess diabetic control. HbA normally comprises 90% of circulating haemoglobin. The remaining 10% is made up by A2, F, and the products of post-translational non-enzymatic reactions – HbA_{1a}, HbA_{1b}, and HbA_{2c}. HbA_{1c} is synthesised over the life of the red cell in proportion to the degree of glycaemia prevailing, and thus gives an integrated picture of diabetic control over the preceding six weeks.

The normal range of glycosylated haemoglobin is 5.5–8.5% of total haemoglobin. Levels within or close to this range can be obtained in patients treated by diet or diet and oral agents. Normal levels are more difficult to obtain in insulin-dependent diabetic patients. Even with rigorous control, the average in a group of patients can rarely be improved below 10%, whereas with poor control of diabetes it is difficult to glycosylate more than 22% of total haemoglobin. Low levels of glycosylated haemoglobin are obtained in patients with haemolytic anaemias since older erythrocytes contain more glycosylated haemoglobin.

Special problems with insulin therapy

Children and adolescents with insulin-dependent diabetes pose particular problems in the management of insulin therapy. The major aims in young patients are to avoid stunting of growth through inadequate diabetic control and reduction of the risk of diabetic complications in the future. Against the rigours of strict diabetic control must be weighed emotional and psychological factors. It is common for children and adolescents to react against their diabetes at some time. Virtually the converse situation occurs during pregnancy in the diabetic woman. Here the patient is usually aware of the increased risk to the fetus and, as a result, is highly motivated. There is no doubt that unexplained stillbirth has been reduced dramatically by the combination of improved diabetic control and advances in obstetric management. Pregnancy is one of the few times during life when normoglycaemia can be obtained and maintained for a finite period. There remains an excess mortality and morbidity in diabetic pregnancy due to congenital malformation. This occurs approximately twice as commonly in diabetic pregnancy, with an incidence of fetal malformation of 4.5%. A wide range of malformations is found, although sacral agenesis is more common than in a normal population. The majority of malformations involve organogenesis before the seventh week of pregnancy; it is postulated that poor control during organogenesis plays a part in the development of malformations and many groups now advocate prepregnancy diabetic clinics, attempting to improve control before and after conception.

COMPLICATIONS OF DIABETES

These fall into three groups: microvascular, neuropathy and macrovascular. All are generalised processes occurring throughout the tissues of the body. The pathogenesis of complications remains obscure and varies with different complications. The underlying histological change which occurs in microvascular disease is basement membrane thickening. This not only occurs in long-standing human diabetes, but can be reproduced in animal models exposed to chronic hyperglycaemia. In diabetic neuropathy there is considerable debate whether basement membrane thickening with subsequent capillary closure results in demyelination and axonal degeneration, or whether there is a more direct effect of chronic hyperglycaemia. The macrovascular disease which accompanies diabetes may not be a specific complication of the disorder since it has an identical histological picture to that which occurs in non-diabetic patients. In the diabetic patient it tends to occur at a younger age and be more extensively distributed.

Raised blood glucose concentrations may be harmful directly or through an alteration in tissue biochemistry or protein function. Excessive conversion of glucose to sorbitol by lens or nerve tissue may lead to tissue damage. Post-translational non-enzymatic glycosylation of proteins may alter the function of proteins such as albumin, lens protein or collagen. Glycosylation of haemoglobin at the binding site for 2,3-diphosphoglycerate may alter the oxyhaemoglobin dissociation curve sufficiently to impair oxygen delivery to tissues and cause tissue hypoxia.

Diabetic retinopathy

Diabetic retinopathy is the cause of blindness in between 5% and 20% of cases in the UK. Two major types of diabetic retinopathy are recognised, proliferative and background (Table 11.8). The latter is subdivided into two appearances, which may be identical in pathogenesis. In terms of treatment, it is important to detect diabetic maculopathy with its sight-threatening implication, while background retinopathy apparently sparing the macula may not need treatment, but does need careful follow-up.

Table 11.8 Diabetic retinopathy

Background retinopathy
1. Maculopathy
2. Without macular involvement

Proliferative retinopathy
1. Disc new vessels
2. Peripheral new vessels
3. Retinitis proliferans

Background retinopathy

The identification of background retinopathy depends upon the presence of microaneurysms, haemorrhages and exudates (Fig.11.3).

The following features are associated with background retinopathy:

1. Capillary dilatation
2. Capillary closure
3. Microaneurysms
4. Haemorrhages
5. Hard exudates
6. Soft exudates.

Microaneurysms.   These appear as small red dots on the retina. The presence of these with haemor-

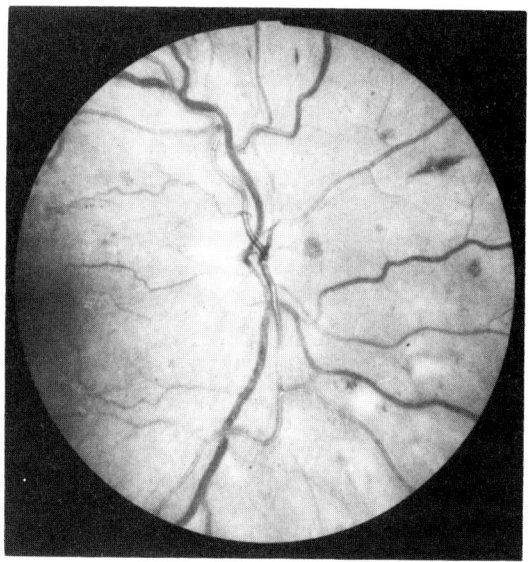

Fig. 11.3 Background retinopathy with haemorrhages and cottonwool spots.

rhages has led to the descriptive term 'dot and blot haemorrhages'. Microaneurysms are not haemorrhages, although their distinction from small haemorrhages may be difficult. Dilatation and capillary closure also occurs. Temporally, dilatation is the earliest lesion, followed by capillary closure which leads to areas of non-perfusion. Both of these lesions are difficult to recognise with an ophthalmoscope, although occasional large dilated capillaries may be observed. Microaneurysms are the earliest clinical sign consisting of fusiform dilatations of capillaries. Normal retinal capillaries are 5–12 μm wide and microaneurysms may have a diameter of 100 μm. Only those greater than 30 μm can be seen on ophthalmoscopy. A long natural history is well documented as is spontaneous disappearance.

Haemorrhages. The major part of the capillary bed of the retina is distributed in two layers – superficially in the nerve fibre and ganglion layer, and deep in the inner nuclear layer. The extracellular space of the deep layer is greater allowing a haemorrhage to assume a 'blot' shape. The majority of haemorrhages occurring with diabetic retinopathy are of this shape. Occasionally a flame-shaped haemorrhage in the superficial layer may occur but this should arouse suspicion of hypertensive retinopathy or coexisting hypertension.

Large haemorrhages may break through the inner limiting membrane to become preretinal. The appearance of a preretinal haemorrhage is of a large haemorrhage with a slightly curved or horizontal superior border. It may be difficult to identify the origin of such a haemorrhage which may also arise from bleeding from preretinal new vessels.

Haemorrhages may arise from leaking microaneurysms and may last from 1 to 6 months. A large preretinal haemorrhage may last longer and heal with fibrosis.

Hard exudates. Irregular creamy-white hard exudates of varying size are a feature of background retinopathy. They may occur at any site but are predominantly located between the superior and inferior temporal vessels, thus threatening the macula.

Histologically they consist of hyaline with fibrin deposition surrounded by fat. Macrophages can be seen in the deposit. The most likely origin is from capillary leakage although neuronal degeneration may contribute.

Soft exudates. Large soft exudates (cottonwool spots) may occur in background retinopathy. They are usually located within the region of the optic disc. Coexisting hypertension should be considered when exudates occur predominantly on the temporal side of the disc, but only about one-third of diabetic patients with soft exudates have hypertension. Soft exudates are located adjacent to ischaemic areas and result from interruption of normal axonal flow. The ischaemic lesion may be considerably larger than the exudate.

Many cottonwool spots herald a poor prognosis. The appearance is of exudative retinopathy and there is likelihood of new vessel growth. This appearance merits frequent review and treatment when appropriate.

Diabetic maculopathy (Fig. 11.4)

The significance of background retinopathy involving the macula lies in the threat to sight, which in turn determines treatment. Visual loss may occur from macular oedema or from a large plaque overlying the fovea. Microaneurysms, haemorrhages and exudates in the periphery of the retina do not require treatment but do indicate that a good view of the macula through a dilated pupil is

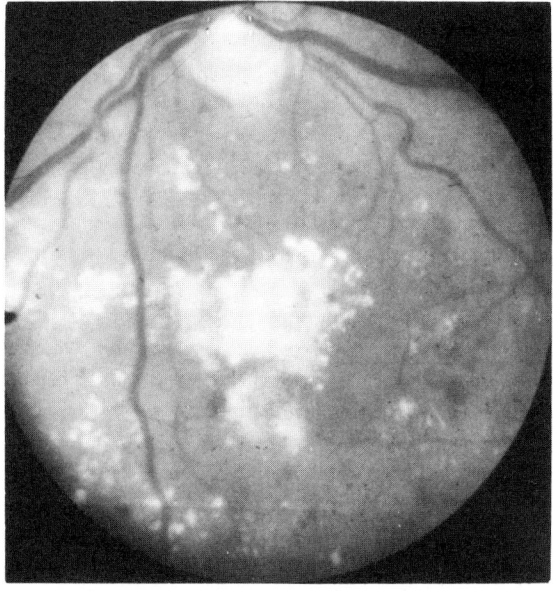

Fig. 11.4 Diabetic maculopathy.

mandatory as is careful follow-up with visualisation of the macula.

In general terms, maculopathy may be considered present when hard exudates lie in the immediate vicinity of, or involve the macula. They may lie lateral or superior to the macula or form a circinate pattern embracing the macula. Within the ring of exudates may lie microaneurysms and haemorrhages.

Focal maculopathy. Microaneurysms, haemorrhages, and circinate rings of exudates or plaques are obvious on ophthalmoscopy. Clinically the patient is typically aged 55, with diabetes for 15 years and a visual acuity of 6/6–6/24.

Cystoid maculopathy. A feature of cystoid maculopathy is that few exudates are present. Ophthalmoscopy is relatively unhelpful and detection is through maintaining a high degree of suspicion. This is aroused by poor vision and a rather featureless fundus. Fluorescein angiography reveals loculated (cystic) spaces which fill with fluorescein.

Ischaemic maculopathy. Rather like the cystoid type, the appearance is of few exudates but fluorescein angiography reveals areas of non-perfusion. These patients have a 30% chance of developing disc new vessels within 3 years.

The natural history of diabetic maculopathy which is untreated is of gradual visual loss. This may arise from macular oedema which, if left untreated, leads to permanent visual loss. Alternatively visual loss may arise from exudates encroaching on the macula; occasionally sudden visual loss is due to the appearance of a large plaque of exudate obliterating the macula.

Proliferative retinopathy (Fig. 11.5)

Proliferative retinopathy includes preretinal and intraretinal new vessel growth either over or around the disc, or in the peripheral retina. Left untreated there is progression to irreversible retinitis proliferans.

Disc new vessels. Disc new vessels arise from either the choroidal or retinal circulations. Fine tufts of new vessels can be observed on the surface of the disc and extend laterally or forwards. Sometimes arcades of new vessels may be seen. Generally the vessels are without connective tissue support,

although, if longstanding, fibrous tissue may grow along the vessel gradually leading to fibrous bands which can obliterate the vessels.

Unsupported vessels are at risk of rupture with preretinal or vitreous haemorrhage. This risk is reduced when supported by fibrous tissue but is replaced by a risk of fibrous traction which may lead to retinal detachment.

Peripheral new vessels. Peripheral new vessels are usually found in areas of poor perfusion. Progression is rapid from an intraretinal origin and they quickly become preretinal, piercing the inner limiting membrane. The origin may also be from large veins and rarely from retinal arteries.

The risk is of sudden and catastrophic haemorrhage. It is normal for the vitreous gel to collapse away from the retina with age and this process is accelerated in a patient with new vessel growth by previous haemorrhage and fibrous traction. New vessels may rupture during this process and, depending upon where the vessel bleeds, will lead to preretinal or vitreous haemorrhage. Further traction from fibrous healing leads to further retinal detachment.

New vessel growth occurs predominantly in long-standing insulin-dependent diabetic patients although not exclusively. The response of retinal neovascularisation may be an attempt at revascularisation. It has been suggested that chronically ischaemic areas of retina may release

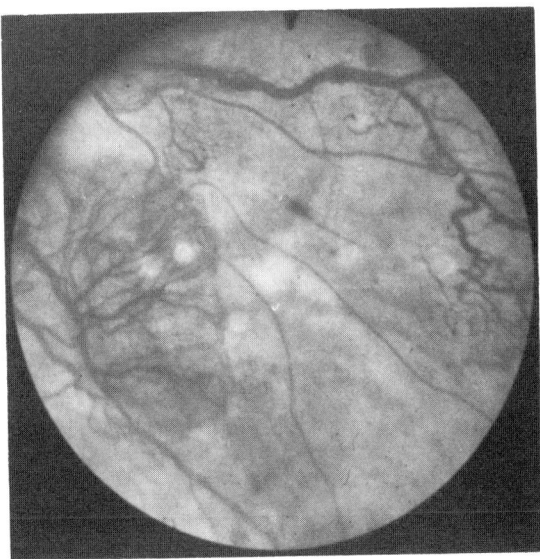

Fig. 11.5 Peripheral new vessel formation.

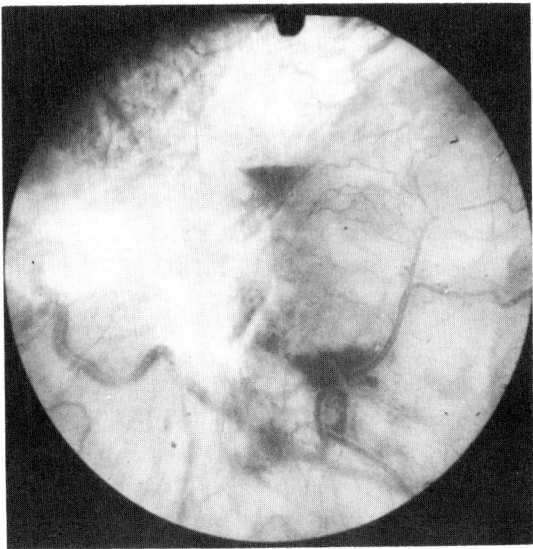

Fig. 11.6   End-stage diabetic retinopathy with haemorrhage, fibrosis and obliteration of disc.

a vasoproliferative substance which stimulates new vessel growth towards the area.

After bleeding, slow resolution of haemorrhage takes place, but replacement by fibrous tissue is likely. With repeated bleeding the end-point of retinitis proliferans is reached with retinal disorganisation by fibrous tissue (Fig. 11.6).

Investigation

Direct ophthalmoscopy is the means of detecting diabetic retinopathy, but is not without disadvantages. The periphery of the retina is difficult to visualise and the uniocular nature of the instrument makes an appreciation of depth difficult. This is particularly important in the recognition of macular oedema.

Colour photography of the retina is invaluable in providing a record of previous findings and thus following progression. Diabetic retinopathy is not graded from direct ophthalmoscopy, but this can be done from a composite picture of the retina derived from retinal photography. The patient's picture may then be compared with standard photographs.

Fluorescein angiography is an established technique for determining the extent of diabetic retinopathy. The passage of intravenously injected fluorescein through the retinal circulation is recorded by fundus photography. Invariably it reveals marked retinal abnormalities in patients with few changes apparent on ophthalmoscopy. New vessels, microaneurysms and leakage of dye are readily observed. The technique of fluorescein angiography is vital for prospective studies of diabetic retinopathy but there has been a re-evaluation of its role in routine clinical practice. It is not necessary to perform fluorescein angiography routinely before treatment of diabetic retinopathy but it is particularly valuable in investigating and monitoring the following, particularly the first three:

1.   Early retinopathy
2.   Evaluation of ischaemic areas
3.   Small new vessel growth
4.   Type of maculopathy
5.   Monitoring and management of photocoagulation.

In the normal retina there is a blood-retinal barrier which does not allow leakage. It has been shown that this barrier may break down in diabetic patients before retinopathy develops. Breakdown of the barrier can be detected by vitreous fluorophotometry when, following intravenous fluorescein, small quantities can be detected in the vitreous.

In some patients observation of the retina is precluded by cataract or vitreous haemorrhage. Ultrasound may be used to detect the presence and extent of haemorrhage, fibrosis, and retinal detachment.

Treatment

Background retinopathy without maculopathy rarely requires treatment. Gradual visual deterioration may result with maculopathy and intervention is warranted before permanent visual loss occurs. Hard exudates and macular oedema arise from microvascular abnormalities. Often dilated capillaries and microaneurysms are obvious in the area and destruction of these lesions is the treatment of choice.

New vessels may also be directly destroyed. This may be achieved safely for peripheral new vessels but is more difficult for new vessels in the region of the optic disc. Since it is believed that the latter arise in response to peripheral ischaemia an alternative approach is to destroy these peripheral areas. Fluorescein angiography may be used to locate the ischaemic areas but when these are profuse a systematic destruction of large areas of peripheral retina may be employed (pattern bombing).

Photocoagulation. Photocoagulation is the production of heat by absorption of light energy. Two light sources are in use. The xenon arc produces white light which is absorbed mainly by pigment epithelium. When applied to an area it destroys surface vessels, surface retina and intraretinal vessels. A surface burn on the retina may be seen on direct ophthalmoscopy. It is unsuitable for use on lesions lying near the fovea because of the size of the burn produced.

The argon laser produces green light which is absorbed by haemoglobin pigment. It has a small beam size and results in smaller burns. This allows the macula and optic disc to be approached, although close to the fovea the energy may be taken up by macular pigment with unwanted destruction. Vessels which are growing well forward into the vitreous can be picked-off with the argon laser.

Results of treatment. In the treatment of maculopathy there is adequate evidence that visual deterioration is arrested. Eyes with a visual acuity of better than 6/36 respond to treatment but improvement is not observed if visual acuity has deteriorated to 6/60 or worse.

Photocoagulation is also of benefit in the treatment of new vessels which arise from the disc. Visual deterioration to blindness is prevented and it is particularly beneficial in those eyes which fare worst if untreated, for example those which have already had a vitreous haemorrhage. Only in the treatment of peripheral new vessels is photocoagulation unproven. Side-effects of treatment include field defects, blurring, and loss of night vision. Complications may occur including foveal burns, haemorrhage and traction of the retina with detachment.

Other treatments. At various times other forms of treatment have been tried, including clofibrate, anticoagulants and fibrinolytic therapy. Clofibrate reduces exudates but does not improve vision and no benefit from anticoagulants or fibrinolytic agents has been demonstrated.

Pituitary ablation for neovascularisation is based upon the rationale that growth hormone may play some part in the genesis of proliferative retinopathy. Controlled studies of pituitary ablation are few but most authors report some beneficial effect. At best it may arrest progression of new vessels and may be necessary on the odd occasion when proliferative retinopathy is 'malignant' in its progression.

Vitreous shrinkage and detachment may result in haemorrhage from new vessels either into or behind the vitreous. Isolated haemorrhage will clear but when recurrent inevitably leads to fibrosis. Photocoagulation of the retina is prevented by vitreous haemorrhage and loss of sight may ensue. Vitrectomy involves piecemeal removal of the vitreous with replacement by clear fluid, such as saline. In competent, experienced hands more than 60% of patients who reach this stage benefit from vitrectomy.

Diabetic nephropathy

The hallmark of the clinical presentation is proteinuria, which is present in 5–15% of all diabetic patients. In insulin-dependent diabetic patients proteinuria is not present at diagnosis (or rather, if it is present it is not due to diabetic nephropathy), after 10 years of diabetes 1–2% have proteinuria, after 20 years the figure is 10–30%, and after 30 years almost 60% will have proteinuria. In non-insulin-dependent diabetic patients the relationship to time since diagnosis is less apparent, as would be expected from the discrepancy between duration of disease and time of diagnosis in this group. In these patients diabetic nephropathy may be present at diagnosis.

Initially proteinuria is intermittent, but it gradually becomes constant and heavier. A deterioration in renal function follows. The timing of these changes varies considerably from patient to patient. Many years may elapse before proteinuria becomes constant and even after this stage a patient may have 15 years before there is a decline in renal function. Peripheral oedema occurs at an early stage and may precede a fall in circulating albumin concentration. In contrast, hypertension tends to occur later in the disease and may be absent until the stage of advanced renal failure is reached.

Before the stage of advanced renal failure, progression is unpredictable and may occur in step-wise fashion. The onset of renal failure is

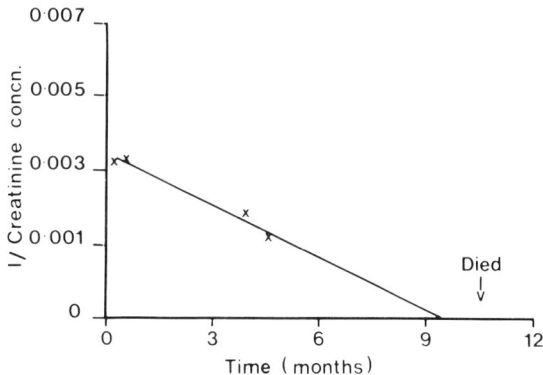

Fig. 11.7 Deteriorating renal function assessed by a plot of 1/creatinine concentration against time.

marked by a more predictable decline in renal function. When serum creatinine begins to rise steadily, it is possible to construct a graph of the reciprocal of the creatinine concentration against time (Fig. 11.7), which can be extrapolated to predict the number of months before the results are incompatible with life.

The prognosis is worse for patients who develop heavy proteinuria and for the few with nephrotic syndrome. Similarly, hypertension may accelerate progression of disease and adequate treatment of hypertension may influence the rate of deterioration.

Treatment

Transplantation and dialysis provide the only hope for diabetic patients with advanced renal failure. Treatment needs to be considered when the serum creatinine reaches 500 μmol/l and by this stage sufficient data for a reciprocal creatinine plot should have been collected. This indicates the time available for arrangements to be made.

A decision on whether to treat must be taken first. Arterial disease and calcification are commonly present in these patients, of whom 50% may be blind. Haemodialysis is the least successful treatment schedule, probably because of coexisting arterial disease. Better results are obtained with peritoneal dialysis and chronic ambulatory peritoneal dialysis is increasing in use. A number of centres report good results with this method although sepsis can be a major problem.

Considerable experience has been gained with

transplantation in a few centres. In diabetic patients the percentage surviving at three years is 80–90% of those given a live related donor kidney and 60% using a cadaver donor.

Histology

Basement membrane thickening is a fundamental lesion in diabetic nephropathy. This affects the glomerular capillaries leading to capillary obliteration. On light microscopy glomerular lesions are observed. Here lesions are gathered under the heading of diabetic glomerulosclerosis, although different histological types are recognised. Diffuse glomerular lesions and exudative glomerular lesions occur, but perhaps the best characterised is the nodular glomerular lesion of Kimmelstiel and Wilson (Fig. 11.8). In a normal-sized or enlarged glomerulus, single or multiple nodules can be seen. These nodules are acellular and confined to the periphery of the glomerulus. The chemical composition is unknown, but they are virtually pathognomonic of diabetes. The end point of the glomerular lesions is glomerular hyalinization.

Proteinuria

Standard reagent stick tests for protein in urine detect only concentrations of 10 mg/100 ml or greater. With more sensitive assay methods smaller quantities can be detected and the term microalbuminuria has been used for this finding. Increases in microalbuminuria are observed in diabetic patients within a short time of diagnosis and this is particularly true for excretion after exercise. The relevance of this finding to diabetic nephropathy is unclear, although it has been implied that these abnormalities may predict the development of diabetic nephropathy.

Diabetic neuropathy

There are many classifications of diabetic neuropathy but none is universally accepted. The majority of patients will have a type of neuropathy which fits into the following classification and described below.

1. Peripheral sensory polyneuropathy
2. Proximal painful neuropathy

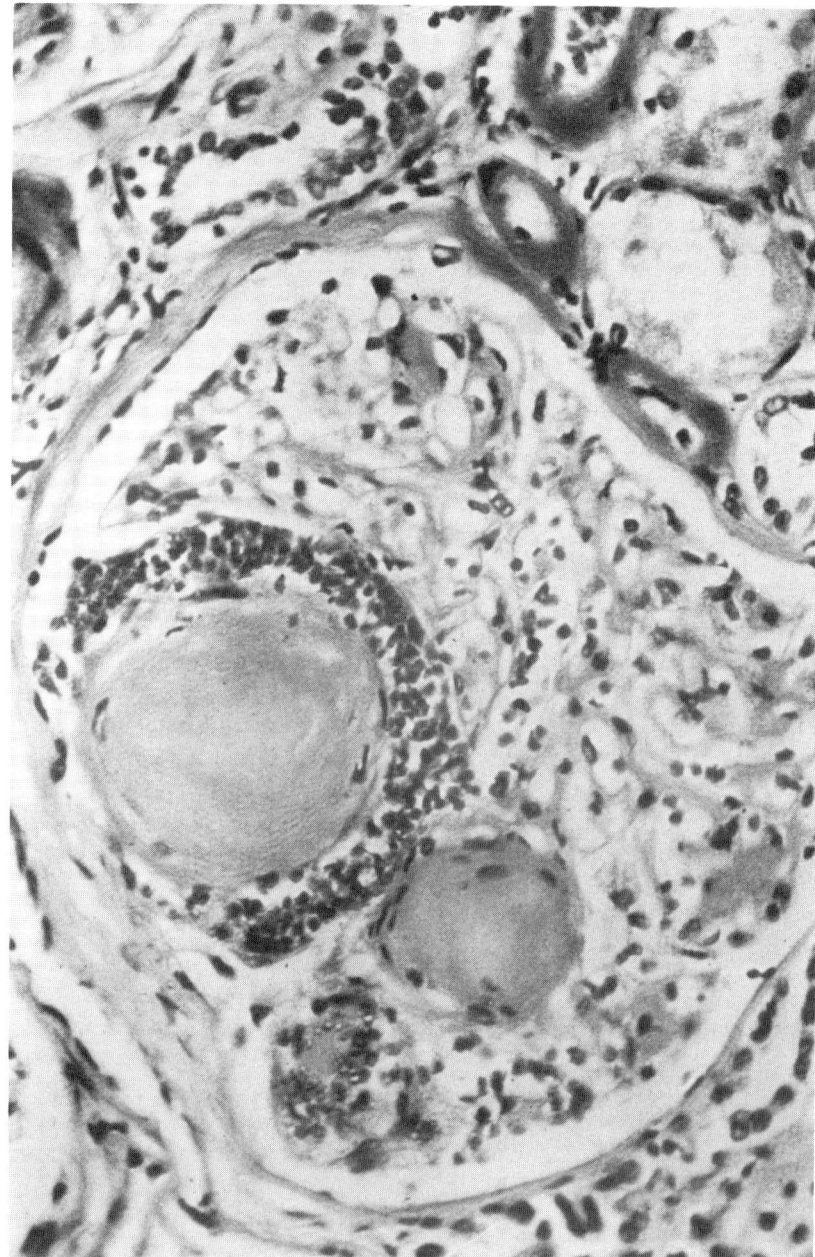

Fig. 11.8 Kimmelsteil-Wilson nodules in glomerulus.

3. Mononeuritis (multiplex)
4. Autonomic neuropathy.

Peripheral sensory polyneuropathy

This is the commonest type of diabetic neuropathy. It may be asymptomatic, recognised only on examination by diminished sensation distally and loss of reflexes, or at the other extreme it may be associated with perforating, infected foot ulcers.

When symptoms are present, they are usually due to altered sensory perception. Tingling and paraesthesiae occurring in the feet and lower legs are usually worse at night. Occasionally pain is a feature. Symptoms are usually symmetrical and confined to the feet and lower leg, but may also occur in the hands and arms. Symptoms may be present without obvious signs but glove and stocking sensory loss and diminished or absent knee and ankle reflexes can usually be detected. Wasting of the small muscles of the foot leads to arching and clawing of the foot. It is this change in shape which may alter pressure distribution through the sole of the foot with loss of spread and considerable pressure applied to localised areas. Calluses may form at these pressure areas and inattention to this finding can lead to ulceration. In contrast to ischaemic lesions, the foot is commonly warm with distended veins on the dorsum of the foot and readily detectable arterial pulsation.

Sensory loss may be so marked as to lead to severe traumatic lesions. Classically, the patient fails to realise the degree of sensory impairment and may sustain injuries unnoticed. Such lesions readily become infected, ulcerate and show resistance to healing. Typically the lesion is described as 'punched-out', surrounded by necrotic tissue and with variable degrees of infection. Infection may penetrate to bone. Large ulcerated areas may occur in the absence of pain, but small lesions may be excruciatingly painful.

Although proximal symptoms are not usually present, there may be marked proximal muscle wasting. This may result from the generalised nature of the neuropathy, through restriction of use, or through poorly controlled diabetes.

Sensory ataxia may be present and impairment of pain sensation may be of sufficient magnitude to result in painless joint destruction and disorganisation. In contrast to tabes dorsalis these 'Charcot joints' of diabetes usually involve the ankle and foot.

Proximal neuropathy

The predominant feature of this type of diabetic neuropathy is pain. Commonly this is confined to the thighs although occurrence in other sites is well documented. Pain is severe and debilitating and is rarely unilateral, although one side may be affected more than the other. The majority of patients are middle-aged or older and it can occur within a short time of diagnosis. The predominant finding is of marked weakness and wasting of the quadriceps and ilio-psoas muscles. Sensation is usually normal but reflexes may be diminished or absent. Wasting may be exacerbated by disuse, since movement may be painful. When affecting the thighs, the term diabetic amyotrophy has been used. Other sites may include the antero-lateral muscles of the lower leg and radiculopathy may well be a variant of this type of diabetic neuropathy. It has been suggested that there may be involvement of the spinal cord, since extensor plantar responses are found in some patients and the c.s.f. protein content is usually elevated. It should be emphasised that there is a tendency to show recovery. Pain may be severe and may necessitate opiate administration. There is a poorly defined overlap between this type of neuropathy affecting several muscle groups and mononeuritis multiplex.

Mononeuropathies

Isolated nerve lesions occur commonly in long-standing diabetes. The cranial nerves are most often affected, particularly the VIth cranial nerve with paralysis of the lateral rectus muscle. The IIIrd, IVth and VIIth nerves may also be affected. Involvement of the IVth nerve usually accompanies other nerve involvement while if the IIIrd nerve is affected the pupillary responses are spared. Onset is sudden without pain, or occasionally accompanied by headache. Recovery is usual, although the lesion may recur on the same or opposite side.

Isolated peripheral nerve lesions may occur and be either sensory or motor. Loss of sensation due to a lesion of the lateral cutaneous branch of the femoral nerve is well described as is the lateral peroneal nerve lesion leading to foot-drop. Other nerves which may be affected include the ulnar, median, radial and sciatic. Recovery may occur although this is less predictable for peripheral than for cranial nerve lesions.

The role of diabetes in the development of these lesions is circumstantial and it is unclear whether they are commoner than in the non-diabetic population. The distribution of isolated nerve lesions has led to the suggestion that the diabetic nerve is more vulnerable to damage at pressure points than the nerves of non-diabetic people.

Severe generalised neuritic pain is a feature of a small number of patients with long-standing diabetes. This occurs more commonly in young to middle-aged female patients with insulin-dependent diabetes and a history of excessive manipulation of their diabetes. Rather than this being a painful sensory polyneuropathy, careful examination shows it to be a mononeuritis multiplex.

Pathogenesis

Histological examination of nerve fibre preparations reveal segmental demyelination (Fig. 11.9). The myelin sheath is an integral part of the Schwann cell and damage may result from either a primary effect upon function of the Schwann cell or from primary axonal damage.

It has been postulated that sorbitol accumulation is important in the pathogenesis of neuropathy. Enzymes such as aldose reductase, which convert glucose to sorbitol, occur in a number of tissues including peripheral nerve, but in non-diabetic subjects only small amounts of sorbitol are formed. Metabolism of sorbitol is by conversion to fructose and this may be handled less well by the diabetic nerve.

Experimental drugs are available which inhibit aldose reductase activity and reduce conversion of glucose to sorbitol. These improve nerve conduction times in diabetic animals.

A second polyol, the cyclic hexitol, myo-inositol has been implicated in diabetic neuropathy. In contrast to sorbitol there is a fall in nerve myo-inositol following induction of diabetes in small animals.

An alternative to the sorbitol theory for damage to the diabetic nerve is that segmental demyelination and axonal loss may arise from disturbance in the blood supply to nerve. Electron microscopy of nerve from patients with long-standing diabetes reveals thickened basement membrane of capillaries supplying the nerve. Arteriolar lesions can be identified histologically with thickened hyalinised walls reducing vessel calibre.

Autonomic neuropathy

Autonomic neuropathy, as a feature of diabetic neuropathy, has received considerable attention in recent years. As with other complications of diabetes the process producing autonomic neuropathy is generalised, but the diversity of the autonomic nervous system leads to many different manifestations of damage:

1. Postural hypotension
2. Diarrhoea
3. Impotence
4. Atonic bladder
5. Pupillary abnormalities
6. Sweating abnormalities
7. Loss of hypoglycaemic awareness.

Disordered cardiovascular reflexes result in postural hypotension. Dizziness, faintness and even loss of consciousness may occur on moving from the recumbent to the standing position and symptoms may be worse in the morning. Other features of abnormal cardiovascular responses include a resting tachycardia, loss of sinus arrhythmia, an abnormal response to the Valsalva manoeuvre, and loss of the rise in blood pressure which occurs with sustained handgrip.

Disturbance of gastrointestinal motility can produce disabling symptoms. Diabetic diarrhoea is well recognised and is explosive and often worse at night. Rather less well recognised are disturbances of upper gastrointestinal motility. Impaired gastric emptying may result in a large distended stomach with considerable overnight residue and nausea may be a prominent symptom.

Impotence in male patients is common, occurring 2–5 times more frequently than in age-

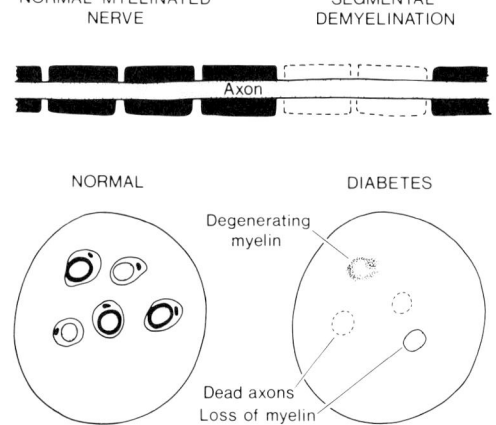

Fig. 11.9 Diagrammatic representation of histological lesion of peripheral nerve. (Reprinted from Kinson J, Nattrass M 1984 Caring for the diabetic patient. Churchill Livingstone, Edinburgh, by kind permission.)

matched, non-diabetic patients. This is usually erectile impotence and it is not clear whether loss of libido can be attributed to diabetic autonomic neuropathy. Fertility may be reduced in diabetic men by a number of causes. Impotence, reduced sperm counts, effects upon other endocrine systems and retrograde ejaculation may all play a part. Retrograde ejaculation is associated with the large atonic bladder of autonomic neuropathy. It has been suggested that autonomic neuropathy in female diabetic patients impairs orgasm.

Denervation of the bladder results in a large distended bladder, which may contain more than one litre of urine. The risk of ascending renal tract infection is increased when the bladder is atonic.

Pupillary abnormalities are common, particularly small pupils which dilate sluggishly. Argyll-Robertson pupils occur occasionally in diabetic autonomic neuropathy.

Other disturbances include loss of thermally induced sweating, particularly affecting the lower limbs, and gustatory sweating. The latter usually affects the head, neck and upper trunk and is precipitated by food. Certain foods may be potent stimuli, including cheese, chocolate and milk.

Loss of hypoglycaemic awareness can occur. Patients who previously experienced symptoms of impending hypoglycaemia may suddenly lose these and become unconscious without warning. The situation is compounded if symptoms of postural hypotension coexist. Counter-regulatory responses to hypoglycaemia are impaired in patients with autonomic neuropathy and a similar effect upon hypoglycaemic awareness can occur in patients treated with beta blockers.

Sudden death in diabetic patients has been attributed to autonomic neuropathy. Disordered cardiovascular reflexes and changes in respiratory reflexes may make death during sleep more likely and pose a hazard during general anaesthesia.

Diagnosis of autonomic neuropathy

The presence of a resting tachycardia implies loss of vagal inhibition upon heart rate but is insufficient

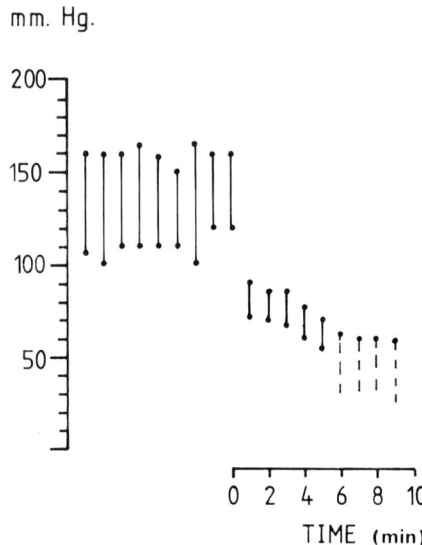

Fig. 11.10 Continuous blood pressure recording following standing (time 0) in a patient with autonomic neuropathy.

to diagnose autonomic neuropathy conclusively. A more useful feature of partial or complete denervation of the heart is loss of sinus arrhythmia or beat-to-beat variation in rate. In patients with autonomic neuropathy the increase in heart rate which accompanies standing is also lost. The Valsalva manoeuvre of forced expiration against a closed glottis produces an abnormal response in the presence of autonomic neuropathy. This can be performed by asking the patient to blow a column of mercury to a height of 60 mm for 15 s. The normal acceleration of heart rate during expiration which is followed by a rebound slowing is lost.

In practice, two findings should be taken as pointers for a further search for autonomic neuropathy. Peripheral neuropathy indicates that autonomic neuropathy should be carefully sought in both history and examination. Autonomic neuropathy does not always accompany peripheral neuropathy, but it is doubtful whether it ever occurs in the absence of peripheral neuropathy. Secondly, measurement of the blood pressure during lying and standing remains a most useful screening test (Fig. 11.10). A fall in systolic pressure > 30 mmHg on standing strongly favours the presence of autonomic neuropathy, which can then be confirmed by assessment of beat-to-beat variation.

Treatment

In the majority of patients with severe autonomic neuropathy there is little which can produce dramatic improvement. Postural hypotension may respond to fludrocortisone in high doses (0.6–1.2 mg/day), which increases plasma volume. Oedema is a side-effect limiting use. Tetracycline in small dosage (250 mg/day) may dramatically alleviate diabetic diarrhoea. While there is evidence of bacterial overgrowth in the gut of patients with diabetic diarrhoea, the response to such a small dose suggests that it is unlikely that the antibacterial action is important. Testosterone enhances libido, but is without effect upon erectile impotence and is thus inappropriate. Penile implants may be used in appropriate patients.

Macrovascular disease

In contrast to microangiopathy, which is a specific complication of diabetes, the basic arterial lesion of macrovascular disease is the same in diabetic as in non-diabetic patients. In addition, there is little evidence to suggest that the development or progression of arterial lesions in the diabetic patient can be influenced by attention to control of blood glucose concentration. What cannot be doubted, however, is that the prevalence of macrovascular disease amongst diabetic patients is in excess of that among non-diabetic patients. It also occurs at an earlier age in diabetic patients, tends towards a different distribution in the arterial tree and is increased in severity. Risk factors are similar to those in non-diabetic subjects.

1. Hypertension
2. Obesity
3. Lipid abnormalities
4. Cigarette smoking
5. Haemostatic abnormalities
6. Diabetes.

Cerebrovascular disease. The excess mortality among the diabetic population for cerebrovascular disease is between 1 and 2-fold. Mortality is increased with age and duration of diabetes. In general these figures are for cerebrovascular accident, but other results of cerebrovascular disease are seen in diabetic patients, particularly atherosclerotic dementia. In all respects the process appears

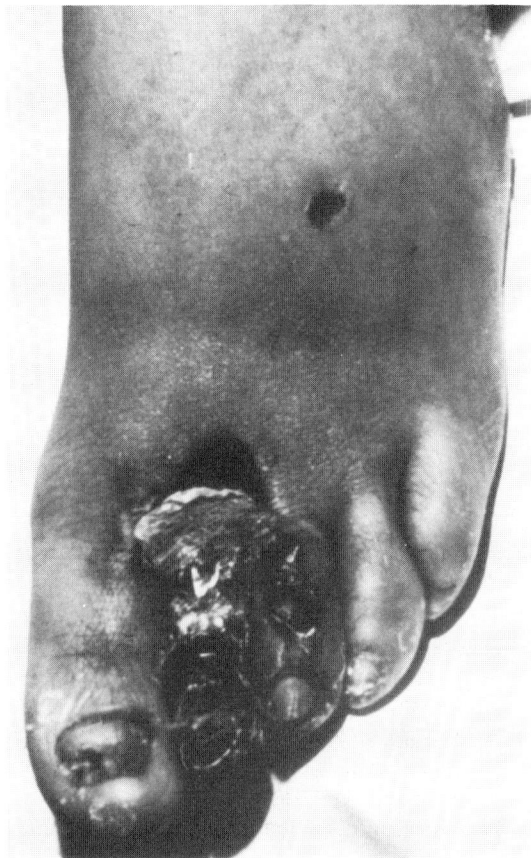

Fig. 11.11 Frank gangrene affecting second and third toes.

identical in diabetic patients to that of non-diabetic patients.

Coronary artery disease. Population studies such as that at Framingham have provided ample evidence that coronary artery disease has a higher prevalence in the diabetic population. This is true for both non-fatal disease and for fatal myocardial infarction. The excess mortality is most marked in diabetic women and in patients who die before the age of 40.

Peripheral vascular disease. Intermittent claudication is two to three times commoner in diabetic patients. Figures for peripheral gangrene are less well documented, but few would deny that it is a frequent accompaniment of diabetes, even allowing for a contribution from neuropathic sepsis (Fig. 11.11). Comparison of the distribution of the lesions reveals more widespread involvement of the tibial and peroneal arteries in diabetic patients than in non-diabetic patients, where lesions are more proximal. Radiological studies show intimal calcification to be similar in the two groups, while medial arterial calcification is twice as common in diabetic patients.

The diabetic foot

Both ischaemic and neuropathic ulceration occur in the feet of diabetic patients. An ischaemic ulcer may be accompanied by gangrene, occurring in a cold, pale, pulseless foot. In neuropathic ulceration the lesion is typically punched out, surrounded by necrosis of skin and occurs primarily over pressure points (Fig. 11.12). The ball of the foot and sites of trauma due to ill-fitting shoes are commonly affected. The foot may be clawed, is often warm with distended veins on the dorsum, and pulses may not only be present but have a bounding character. If infection is present, this may lie in the deep tissues and bony involvemnt can occur. Obvious cellulitis may be observed.

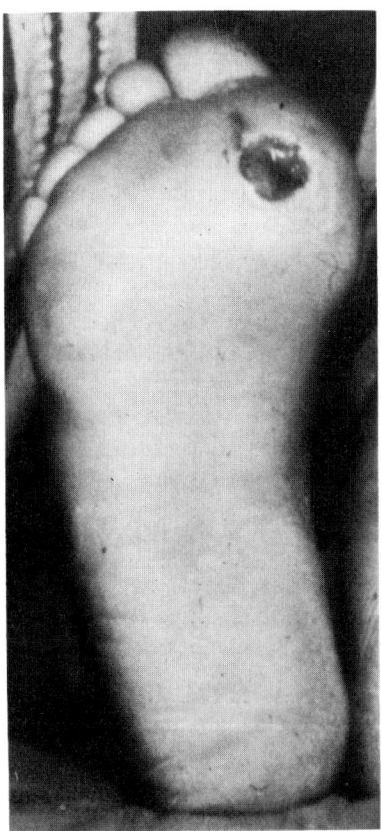

Fig. 11.12 Neuropathic ulcer over head of first metatarsal.

Doppler ultrasound can be useful in confirming arterial signs detected on examination and radiology of the foot is necessary to detect osteomyelitis.

Treatment

Careful examination of the peripheral pulses should be undertaken and, if arterial surgery is contemplated, the findings should be confirmed by arteriography. Once gangrene has developed it is unlikely that arterial surgery will be successful. In the majority of instances gangrene is of a dry type, but occasionally a 'wet' gangrene is seen demanding immediate action. Rarely, gas may be detected in tissues on radiography, but does not necessarily imply clostridial infection. If gangrene is present (Fig. 11.11) the majority of patients will require surgical amputation. In a foot where the lesion is confined to a single digit and is dry and uninfected, autoamputation may be allowed. Piecemeal surgery is not justified in the ischaemic limb and below-knee or above-knee amputation is customary. The former is preferable and may allow easier adaptation to an artificial limb. The fitting of a prosthesis, mobilisation and rehabilitation, and future quality of life depend upon good surgery.

In view of the radical nature of treatment of the ischaemic foot, prevention is a major aim. The patient should be aware of simple rules for foot hygiene and care, and toenails should be cut by a chiropodist in all but the most agile and careful patients. Prevention is of similar importance in the neuropathic foot and anyone with evidence of sensory loss should be considered at risk. Regular inspection is important.

Complications of diabetes in other systems

The occurrence of haemochromatosis and acanthosis nigricans is associated with specific aetiological types of diabetes, while xanthomata and xanthelasmata may reflect associated lipid disturbances. Necrobiosis lipoidica diabeticorum manifests as indurated plaques usually on the front of the lower legs (Fig. 11.13), but it may occur at other sites. The lesions are reddish with a pale centre which may ulcerate. It is possible that necrobiosis is due to microangiopathy, although this seems unlikely since its presence may precede the development of insulin-dependent diabetes.

Cataract is thought to occur more commonly in diabetic patients than in the non-diabetic population, but documentation of this is poor. There are good theoretical reasons for expecting the development of cataracts, since sorbitol accumulation takes place in lens as does glycosylation of lens protein. The cataract which develops is identical to senile cataract, with the rare exception of cataract occurring in young people.

DIABETIC EMERGENCIES

Hyperglycaemic coma

Three types of hyperglycaemic coma occur in diabetic patients (although mixed pictures may be encountered):

1. Ketoacidosis
2. Hyperosmolar non-ketotic
3. Lactic acidosis.

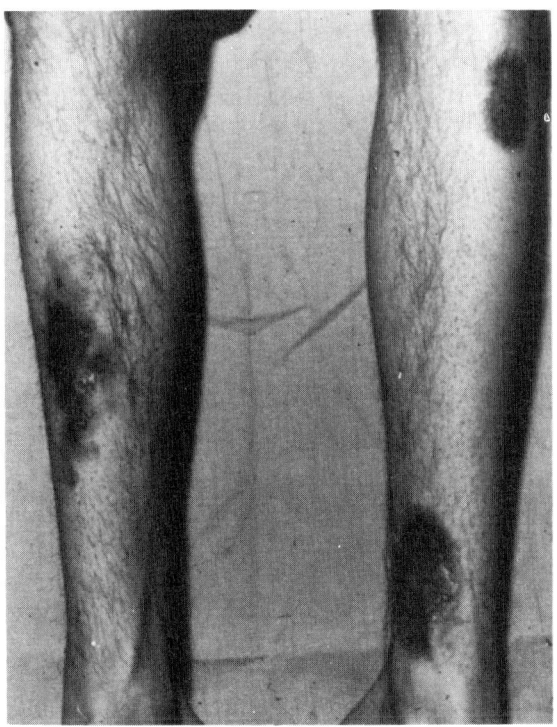

Fig. 11.13 Necrobiosis lipoidica diabeticorum.

Diabetic ketoacidosis is the commonest, exceeding hyperosmolar non-ketotic coma by about 10:1. Lactic acidosis may occur in diabetic patients although whether diabetes per se can lead to lactic acidosis is unclear.

Diabetic ketoacidosis

A working definition of diabetic ketoacidosis is severe uncontrolled diabetes requiring urgent treatment with intravenous fluids and insulin. In more precise terms, the circulating concentration of total ketone bodies (measured as 3-hydroxybutyrate and acetoacetate) should exceed 5 mmol/l and a metabolic acidosis must be present. A semiquantitative estimation may be obtained by plasma ketostix, although the severity may be underestimated by the inability of ketostix to detect 3-hydroxybutyrate.

Pathogenesis. Absolute insulin deficiency is rarely the sole pathogenic mechanism for precipitating ketoacidosis. In newly diagnosed patients with ketoacidosis concentrations of insulin range from 2–16 mu/l, which is similar to a normal man after an overnight fast but clearly inappropriately low for the prevailing blood glucose concentration. An additional precipitating factor is necessary and this is usually a rise in circulating concentrations of catabolic hormones (Table 11.9). Insulin deficiency results in increased hepatic glucose production and decreased peripheral utilisation, while lipolysis is increased. Catecholamines inhibit insulin secretion in addition to accelerating glucose production and antagonising peripheral glucose uptake and metabolism. Glucagon does not act upon lipolysis, but may alter the intrahepatic fate of fatty acids, directing them away from triglyceride synthesis and into beta-oxidation and ketone body formation. Hepatic glucose production is also enhanced. Cortisol increases glucose production and decreases

Table 11.9 Biochemical effects of catabolic hormones (+ increased, − decreased, 0 no action)

	Glucose production	Glucose utilisation	Lipolysis
Glucagon	+++	0	0
Catecholamines	+++	−	+++
Cortisol	+	−	+
Growth hormone	+	−	+

utilisation by impairing insulin receptor binding. Supply of fatty acids to the liver is enhanced. Growth hormone increases glucose production, decreases utilisation, and is lipolytic. The net result is to increase circulating blood glucose concentration and increase supply of non-esterified fatty acids to the liver. Oxidation of long-chain fatty acids in the liver occurs in the mitochondrion and the end product, acetoacetyl CoA is metabolised to acetoacetate, which is in equilibrium with 3-hydroxybutyrate. Decarboxylation of acetoacetate produces acetone.

Similar hepatic ketone body production rates can be produced in long-term fasting, but total ketone body concentrations are less than in diabetic ketoacidosis, implying a further defect in ketone body utilisation.

Clinical effects. Hyperglycaemia induces an osmotic diuresis with loss of water and electrolytes. Polyuria is considerable and, despite polydipsia, exceeds intake. Dehydration and electrolyte loss (Table 11.10) ensue and, if severe, produce hypotension. Acetoacetate and 3-hydroxybutyrate are markers of the metabolic acidosis which is accompanied by nausea, vomiting, abdominal pain and Kussmaul respiration.

Treatment. Rehydration is undertaken with normal-saline (154 mmol/l) although hypernatraemia at presentation or during treatment may necessitate use of half normal-saline (77 mmol/l). Hypotonic saline should be infused with care in view of the danger of haemolysis. The serum sodium concentration at presentation may be artefactually low due to the replacement of sample volume by large quantities of lipid.

Potassium is infused with saline. At presentation serum potassium may be low, normal, or high and rehydration and insulin can result in a rapid fall in serum potassium. Potassium is usually infused as potassium chloride but phosphate salts

Table 11.10 Fluid and electrolyte deficits in diabetic ketoacidosis

Water	5–12 l
Sodium	500 mmol
Potassium	100 mmol
Chloride	500 mmol
Phosphate	50–100 mmol

have also been advocated. Normokalaemia should be maintained by adjusting the potassium given; up to 80 mmol/l may be necessary.

Short-acting insulin is given either intravenously or intramuscularly. Insulin resistance occurs rarely and suitable regimens are 6 u/h intravenously or 20 u initially followed by 6 u hourly by the intramuscular route. Blood glucose should be monitored hourly and if there is no fall within 2 hours the dose should be doubled or the route changed from intramuscular to intravenous. If using a syringe pump for insulin delivery intravenously, a careful check of the pump should be made in apparent non-responders.

The use of bicarbonate to correct the metabolic acidosis is controversial. Acidosis can have a negative inotropic effect on the heart and cause peripheral vasodilatation thus exacerbating hypotension. Severe acidosis may cause respiratory depression. In severe acidosis (pH < 7.1) 150 mmol/l bicarbonate may be used to partially correct the pH.

When blood glucose concentration falls to 14 mmol/l, intravenous glucose (5% dextrose) is infused and insulin continued either 2-hourly intramuscularly or 4-hourly subcutaneously. Small amounts of insulin should be continued at regular intervals to avoid relapse.

Accurate monitoring of fluid balance is essential. A central venous pressure record is invaluable in elderly patients, those with cardiac disease, and in oliguric or anuric patients. Monitoring of the electrocardiogram enables early warning of dysrhythmias and is a useful guide to potassium status reflected in the height of the T waves. Rarely plasma may be needed for treatment of hypotension, mechanical ventilation may be required, and dialysis may be necessary. A precipitating cause should always be sought.

Problems during treatment. Careful monitoring of blood glucose (hourly) and electrolytes (4-hourly) should avoid metabolic problems. Hypokalaemia must be avoided because of the threat of dysrhythmias. Thrombotic episodes may occur. Vomiting is a hazard in patients with disturbed consciousness.

Mortality. In centres experienced in treating the condition the mortality is about 6%, but it is higher in certain groups such as the elderly.

Approximately half the mortality results from the precipitating illness, the major causes being overwhelming sepsis and myocardial infarction. The remaining mortality arises during treatment due to dysrhythmias, aspiration pneumonia and cerebral oedema.

Hyperosmolar non-ketotic diabetic coma

Hyperosmolar non-ketotic diabetic coma occurs when consciousness is altered in the absence of significant ketosis. Blood glucose concentration is markedly elevated (greater than 50 mmol/l) and the patient is dehydrated. Although definitive figures are not available, the elderly and West Indian patients appear to have a high incidence.

Pathogenesis. The precise pathogenesis is unknown although a common feature seems to be an attempt to alleviate the thirst of diabetes by the use of glucose-containing drinks. Precipitating factors may be identified including therapy with thiazides, which exacerbate dehydration and impair insulin secretion, and occasionally the syndrome may be produced by peritoneal dialysis against high concentration glucose dialysate. The absence of ketosis is an intriguing finding and has led to the suggestion that while insufficient insulin is secreted to promote tissue uptake of glucose, concentrations are sufficient to inhibit lipolysis.

Clinical presentation. The signs of metabolic acidosis are absent. When a history is available, thirst and polyuria are accompanied by changes in the mental state of the patient. Disturbed consciousness and coma are more usual and patients may present with neurological signs of stroke, focal fits, or generalised seizures. These changes are related to hyperosmolality. When greater than 340 mOsm/l coma usually results. Since serum sodium and potassium as well as urea are usually raised a typical calculated osmolality might be:

$$2 \times (Na + K) + urea + glucose = mOsm/l$$
$$(2 \times 165) + 30 + 60 = 420$$

Treatment. Treatment of non-ketotic coma with low dose insulin regimens is similar to that of ketoacidosis. Bicarbonate is never used and rehydration may demand the use of hypotonic saline (either 77 mmol/l or 30 mmol/l). Monitoring is similar to that in ketoacidosis, but, despite this, the mortality rate is considerably higher. Most centres report a mortality of around 50%.

Lactic acidosis

Lactic acidosis is defined as a metabolic acidosis, with bicarbonate < 10 mmol/l, accompanied by circulating lactate levels >5 mmol/l. This definition is inadequate when considering lactic acidosis in diabetes since it is well documented that lactate concentration may be raised above normal (approximately 1 mmol/l), and at times greater than 5 mmol/l, in predominantly ketoacidosis.

Lactic acidosis in diabetic patients may be classified in three ways (Table 11.11). Firstly, as in non-diabetic patients, type A lactic acidosis may occur. By definition, this is associated with hypoxia and occurs in patients following myocardial infarction, hypovolaemic shock, or septicaemic shock. Type B2 lactic acidosis is due to drugs; biguanide-induced lactic acidosis in diabetic patients is well reported. In the main, this has been due to phenformin and has led to restricted use of this drug.

Table 11.11 Classification of lactic acidosis

Type	A	Hypoxia associated
	B_1	Disease associated, e.g. diabetes, liver disease
	B_2	Drug associated, e.g. biguanides, alcohol, sorbitol, fructose
	B_3	Associated with inborn errors of metabolism

Treatment. Mortality rates in lactic acidosis exceed 50% although this can only be an approximation since the condition is often undiagnosed. Treatment is empirical and the best way to treat is unknown. In treating the metabolic acidosis two main approaches have been used. Bicarbonate may be infused in massive quantities (greater than 2000 mmol), but two problems ensue. Firstly, bicarbonate may exacerbate tissue hypoxia and lower intracellular pH; in turn this can lead to enhanced lactate production. Secondly, the ion given with bicarbonate may cause problems. This is usually sodium and infusion of large quantities may necessitate dialysis for its removal. A second approach, to lower lactate levels by dialysis, is even less successful.

Hypoglycaemia

The clinical effects of hypoglycaemia may be subdivided into those produced by the hormonal response, and those due to cerebral glucose starvation – neuroglycopenia (Table 11.12). The catecholamine response to hypoglycaemia results in anxiety feelings, sweating and a rapid bounding pulse and it is the loss of this response in diabetic patients with autonomic neuropathy which leads to hypoglycaemic unawareness. Neuroglycopenia produces alterations in mental state such as aggressiveness, paraesthesiae and ultimately fits and coma.

Table 11.12 Manifestations of hypoglycaemia.

Due to neuroglycopenia:
  Paraesthesiae
  Aggressiveness
  Altered mental state
  Fits
  Coma

Due to counterregulatory response:
  Anxiety
  Sweating
  Tachycardia
  Pallor

It is customary to define hypoglycaemia as a blood glucose concentration of < 2.2 mmol/l but this is arbitrary. Many normal people can tolerate blood glucose levels below this without hypoglycaemic symptoms and it is not uncommon to find normal pregnant women with blood glucose < 2.0 mmol/l during the night. In addition, some diabetic patients develop hypoglycaemic symptoms with a blood glucose concentration > 2.2 mmol/l; symptoms of hypoglycaemia can result from a rapid lowering of blood glucose concentrations from values above the normal range.

Treatment

Blood glucose concentration should be raised. If the patient is sufficiently conscious to swallow, oral carbohydrate should be given. It is customary to use monosaccharides such as glucose in proprietrary preparations, or disaccharides such as lactose or sucrose. If swallowing cannot be guaranteed with safety, intravenous glucose is given. Glucagon given intramuscularly or subcutaneously is an alternative which can often be given by a patient's relative. The effect of glucagon is to raise blood glucose by 1–2 mmol/l and this may be sufficient to improve consciousness and allow oral intake. The majority of patients recover immediately or within four hours, but, in some, full recovery may be delayed for several days.

Sulphonylurea-induced hypoglycaemia

This is an important condition which deserves separate consideration. It is particularly likely to occur with use of long-acting sulphonylureas, such as glibenclamide and chlorpropamide, especially if these are used inappropriately. Renal impairment may decrease excretion and accumulation may produce hypoglycaemia. Elderly patients are at special risk with long-acting sulphonylureas particularly if immobility, dependence upon social services, or occasional confusion leads to meals being omitted. A common presentation of sulphonylurea-induced hypoglycaemia is a stroke and this possibility should not be overlooked.

Treatment is similar to that of insulin-induced hypoglycaemia, using glucose orally or intravenously. Glucagon use is inappropriate since glucagon stimulates insulin secretion. Intravenous and oral glucose also stimulate insulin secretion and increase already elevated levels. For this reason, and the fact that the half-life of the activity of sulphonylureas may be long (more than 24 hours), relapse into hypoglycaemia after initial recovery is common. Patients presenting with sulphonylurea-induced hypoglycaemia as an emergency need hospital admission and infusion of glucose until the drug effect wears off.

Further reading

Becker D V 1984 Choice of therapy for Graves' hyperthyroidism. New England Journal of Medicine 311: 464–466

Besser G M, Rees L H (eds) 1985 The pituitary-adrenocortical axis. Clinics in endocrinology and metabolism, vol 14, no 3. W B Saunders, London

Bewley B R 1984 Analogues of gonadotrophin releasing hormone. British Medical Journal 288: 426–427

Bie P 1980 Osmoreceptors, vasopressin and control of renal water excretion, Physiological Reviews 60: 962–1048

Bloom S R, Polak J M 1981 Gut hormones (2nd edn). Churchill Livingstone, Edinburgh

Bloom S R, Polak J M 1987 Somatostatin. British Medical Journal 295: 288–290

British Medical Journal leading article 1981 Insulinomas 282: 927–928

Cavalieri R R, Pitt-Rivers R 1981 The effects of drugs on the distribution and metabolism of thyroid hormones. Pharmacological Reviews 33: 55–79

Clayton R N 1987 Gonadotrophin releasing hormone: from physiology to pharmacology. Clinical Endocrinology 26: 361–384

Eisenbarth G S 1986 Type 1 diabetes mellitus: a chronic autoimmune disease. New England Journal of medicine 314: 1360–1368

Graham G D, Burman K D 1986 Radioiodine treatment of Graves' disease: an assessment of its potential risks. Annals of Internal Medicine 105: 900-905

Grossman A, Besser G M 1985 Prolactinomas. British Medical Journal 290: 182–184

Heath D A 1987 Treating Paget's disease. British Medical Journal 294: 1048–1050

Hitman G A 1986 Progress with the genetics of insulin-dependent diabetes mellitus. Clinical Endocrinology 25: 463–472

Lawton N F Prolactinomas: Medical or surgical treatment? Quarterly Journal of Medicine 64:557–564

Long R G 1983 Recent advances in pancreatic hormone research. Postgraduate Medical Journal 59: 277–282

Nabarro J D N 1987 Acromegaly. Clinical Endocrinology 26: 481–512

Piccini L A, Roman S H, Davies T F 1987 Autoimmune thyroid disease and thyroid cell class II major histocompatibility complex antigens. Clinical Endocrinology 26: 253–272

Rittmaster R S 1987 Hirsutism. Annals of Internal Medicine 106: 95–107

Rojeski M T, Gharib H 1985 Nodular thyroid disease. Evaluation and management. New England Journal of Medicine 313: 428–436

Savage M O, Randall R A (eds) 1986 Growth disorders. Clinics in Endocrinology and Metabolism, vol 14, no 3. W B Saunders, London

Semple C G 1986 Hormonal changes in non-endocrine disease. British Medical Journal 293: 1049–1062

Smith R 1987 Osteoporosis: cause and management. British Medical Journal 294: 329–332

Taylor R 1986 Insulin receptors and the clinician. British Medical Journal 292: 919–922

Thomas J P 1983 Treatment of acromegaly. British Medical Journal 286: 330–332

Toft A D (ed) 1985 Hyperthyroidism. Clinics in Endocrinology and Metabolism, vol 14, no 2. W B Saunders, London

Watkins P J (ed) 1986 Long-term complications of diabetes. Clinics in Endocrinology and Metabolism, vol 15, no 4. W B Saunders, London

White P C, New M I, Dupont B 1987 Congenital adrenal hyperplasia. New England Journal of Medicine 316: 1519–1524, 1580–1586

Zerbe R, Stropes L, Robertson G H 1980 Vasopressin function in the syndrome of inappropriate antidiuresis. Annual Review of Medicine 31: 315–327

Index